The Frontier of
Brief Psychotherapy

An Example of the Convergence
of Research and Clinical Practice

Topics in General Psychiatry

Series editor:

John C. Nemiah, M.D.
Psychiatrist-in-Chief, Beth Israel Hospital
and Professor of Psychiatry, Harvard Medical School

1976:

HYPNOSIS
Fred H. Frankel, M.B.Ch.B., D.P.M.

THE FRONTIER OF BRIEF PSYCHOTHERAPY
David H. Malan, D.M., F.R.C. Psych.

In preparation:

THE PRACTITIONER'S GUIDE TO PSYCHOACTIVE DRUGS
Ellen L. Bassuk, M.D., and Stephen Schoonover, M.D.

The Frontier of Brief Psychotherapy

An Example of the Convergence of Research and Clinical Practice

David H. Malan, D.M., F.R.C. Psych.

Tavistock Clinic

PLENUM MEDICAL BOOK COMPANY · New York and London

Library of Congress Cataloging in Publication Data

Malan, David Huntingford.
  The frontier of brief psychotherapy.

  (Topics in general psychiatry)
  Bibliography: p.
  Includes index.
  1. Psychotherapy. I. Title. [DNLM: 1. Psychotherapy, Brief. WM420 M237f]
RC480.5.M318   616.8'914   76-9646
ISBN 0-306-30895-9

© 1976 Plenum Publishing Corporation
227 West 17th Street, New York, N. Y. 10011

Plenum Medical Book Company is an imprint of Plenum Publishing Corporation

Printed in the United States of America

This second book is dedicated, like the first,
to Michael Balint
and all the therapists of the Workshop

Enid Balint
J.L. Boreham
R.H. Gosling
J.J.M. Jacobs
Agnes Main
T.F. Main
M. Pines
E.H. Rayner
J.L. Rowley

on whose work I have built.

Foreword

When I was a psychiatric resident not long after the end of World War II, any patient with the wits to get himself to a psychiatric clinic was taken into long-term dynamically oriented psychotherapy. Regardless of his diagnosis or clinical need, he was seen once, twice, sometimes even more frequently a week in fifty-minute sessions. Face-to-face with the therapist, he was urged to free associate and to express his dreams, fantasies, and emotions to a usually passive listener in what often appeared to be a caricature of psychoanalysis. It was *not* psychoanalysis, of course (although the differences were sometimes hard to define), but the aims were the same—to resolve psychic conflicts through insight and to bring about an internal psychological change that would allow the individual to work more effectively and to make healthier and happier relationships.

Enough patients improved with these techniques to reinforce our penchant for using them. We were somehow able to ignore the fact that because of the limitations of time many patients withered on the waiting list. And we were able to blame our frequent therapeutic failures, not to mention the damaging regressions our narrowly restricted techniques often induced, on the patient's unwillingness to cooperate. Procrustes's couch was as inflexible as his bed.

Old customs die hard, and the mindless application of long-term therapy is still found in clinical situations where it is inappropriate or contraindicated. But change is in the air. The past decade has seen an increase in the variety of therapeutic approaches to psychological disorders, a recognition of the need to tailor the treatment to the requirements of the patient's illness, and an emphasis on making psychotherapy shorter and more effective. This has resulted no doubt in part from social demands and the dictates of health insurance payments, but of equal importance is the fact that a handful of psychiatrists have had the vision, the interest, and the patience to carry out a systematic study of the nature of psychotherapy.

One of the pioneers in this work is the author of this book. Among his virtues, three stand out: (1) He has moulded the concepts and procedures of psychoanalysis into a therapeutic technique that brings about significant psychological change in his patients in far less time than is required by classical analytic methods. (2) He has defined his treatment procedures so that they can be readily learned by others and has established a reliable set of criteria for the selection of patients for brief psychotherapy. (3) He has established a study of the outcome of treatment which provides scientific evidence that psychotherapy is effective—and effective because of the specific techniques employed.

All this and more will be found in the pages that follow. Through arresting and detailed case examples, and with the clear prose of his exposition, Dr. Malan educates while he delights his readers. This is a work of importance for the science of psychiatry and for the patients who need the skill of its practitioners.

JOHN C. NEMIAH, M.D.

Psychiatrist-in-Chief, Beth Israel Hospital
Professor of Psychiatry, Harvard Medical School

Boston, Massachusetts

Acknowledgments

My grateful thanks are due to the David Matthew Fund of the London Institute of Psycho-analysis, and to the Mental Health Research Fund, for generously supporting the work on which this book is based; and to the Sigmund Sternberg Trust for supporting the final preparation of the manuscript.

I should also like to thank Dr. Austin Case, Dr. Terry Kupers, and Miss Ellen Noonan, for permission to use their case material; and finally, Mrs. Kathleen Sargent, who as both secretary and research assistant has carried this work through from the beginning.

Contents

Part III
THE PRESENT WORK

Part IV
THE PRINCIPLES OF BRIEF PSYCHOTHERAPY

Chapter 9
SELECTION   247

Chapter 10
THE GENERAL AIMS OF PSYCHOANALYTIC THERAPY   259

Chapter 11
PLANNING AND TECHNIQUE   263

Chapter 12
CLINICAL EXAMPLES   267

Part V
EXTENDING THE LIMITS OF BRIEF PSYCHOTHERAPY

Chapter 13
THE USE OF MORE THAN ONE FOCUS   293

Chapter 14
PARTIAL FOCI IN MORE DISTURBED PATIENTS   297

Part VI
CONCLUSION

PART I

The Place of Brief Psychotherapy in Psychotherapeutic Services

CHAPTER 1

What Should Psychotherapists Be Doing?

When psychotherapists look back over the past eighty years and compare their branch of knowledge with other sciences, they can point to discoveries as fundamental—and from the point of view of problems of human existence—at least as important. These can be summed up in the ability to give meaning to a whole range of hitherto unexplained and apparently unrelated mental phenomena; and include the discovery of the unconscious, the interpretation of dreams, the part played by emotional conflict in mental illness, the effects of early experience, the phenomenon of transference, and the fine art of the psychoanalytic technique. Yet, all of these discoveries had already been made by Freud in the first decade of this century, and there remain highly practical questions that, in the excitement of our daily work, we too often overlook: How can all this knowledge best be used in the service of humanity? Or, to come down to earth, can we justify spending our time in psychotherapy? Can we ever hope to make any appreciable contribution to mental health?

When we consider that according to every estimate ever made the number of people needing help with emotional problems runs into hundreds of thousands or millions in every country in the civilized world, the answer to this last question can only be negative. The only conceivable solution to a problem of such magnitude must come from *primary prevention* through such measures as education and social reorganization; and, given the state of the world today, the solution can hardly be described as likely to be found just round the corner.

3

Should we therefore be spending the whole of our time in educating the educators and influencing those in power toward reorganizing society? Perhaps the coldly logical answer is yes; but then what should we do with the casualties? Should we leave them to the only methods of treatment that can be used on a large scale, which are purely palliative, such as tranquilizers and antidepressants? Again, perhaps the coldly logical answer is yes; but the truth is that we cannot do this. We cannot either systematically withhold, or refuse to investigate, methods of treatment based on an understanding of the causes of mental illness, which offer the only hope of radical and permanent relief. But these methods must be used with discrimination, and it is therefore our duty to see if their efficiency can be improved, their application broadened, and their impact maximized. Obviously, one possibility is the exploration of methods of brief psychotherapy.

Here we find an extraordinary state of affairs—one of the unfortunate consequences of the psychoanalytic tradition, according to which the only type of therapy worth considering must involve the long-term working through of the deep anxieties. The results of such an approach are predictable and inevitable, but until recently do not appear to have overtaxed our powers of denial. They are described very clearly by Sifneos (1965), Straker (1968), Campbell (1968), Barten (1971), and Levene, Breger, and Patterson (1972), and come under the following headings:

• Only one method of treatment is available, regardless of the social class or intelligence of the patient, and the nature of the problem.

The method is not applicable to large numbers, nor to the less intelligent, less educated, underprivileged, less introspective, or less motivated types of patients.

Therefore, patients are chosen to suit the therapy, not the therapy to suit the patient.

• All methods of treatment that are not the pure gold of analysis are depreciated.

Therefore, the briefer and more "superficial" methods are not explored, because they are assumed *a priori* to be ineffective in the long run.

• Since these methods are not explored, the fact that they can sometimes be remarkably effective is never discovered.

• Since all treatment is long-term, all vacancies are rapidly blocked, and waiting lists grow to the point at which the length of wait for therapy is quite unrealistic.

This results in a high dropout rate before the therapy starts, which is accepted as inevitable.

There is thus an inability to treat the patient in his acute state, both when the need that he feels is most pressing and when presumably the likelihood of effective help is also at a maximum.

Thus, probably, chronic maladaptive patterns are left to form and become established.

The opening pages* of Barten's book, *Brief Therapies*, describe with the utmost clarity the changing attitudes that have started the process of correcting this situation:

> (1) A growing professional commitment to provide immediate treatment, relevant and practical, to all segments of the community. The Community Mental Health Movement embodies this philosophy and has particularly stimulated its implementation. (2) An increasing shift within the mental health profession from psychoanalytic techniques to ego-oriented psychotherapy. (3) A new emphasis upon preventive and emergency therapeutic measures in addition to corrective ones. (4) A changing philosophy of treatment that often accepts limited therapeutic goals as a sufficient answer to the patient's needs and sometimes as the treatment of choice. (5) A broadening and redefining of professional roles which has enlisted as therapeutic agents a diversity of medical professionals, allied professionals in other helping disciplines, para-professionals and non-professionals, increasing the need for uncumbersome, practical but specific counseling techniques. (6) Long overdue recognition of the special needs of the poor and lower socio-cultural groups, for whom traditional techniques often have been unsuitable and ineffective. (7) Increasing consumer demand for economically feasible services. The growth of prepaid, limited outpatient psychiatric insurance coverage has been a reflection of this. (p. 3)

Barten continues:

> Short-term therapies were inevitably rediscovered as psychiatrists embraced a growing eclecticism . . . . Traditional techniques have by no means been discarded, but they have come to be used more judiciously. In some cases, they have worked better. Brief techniques themselves have expanded to include brief group and family therapies, behavior therapies, drug therapies, suggestive therapies such as hypnosis, re-educative therapies, and role-induction therapies.
>
> The traditional psychotherapist may view this as a regrettable compromise, an ignoble surrender to the pressures of circumstances which produces transient, superficial, or token results. To the eclectic, brief therapies are innovative, pragmatic developing approaches which may change our conception of the nature, objectives, possibilities and limita-

tions of psychotherapy. We should neither exaggerate the results of short-term therapy nor deprecate the rationale and objectives of long-term therapy.

At this point it is worth postponing Barten's next two sentences in order to reiterate, with him, that none of the foregoing is intended to depreciate the long-term therapies in their proper place. Without the long-term therapies, the knowledge on which the briefer therapies are based would not exist; without the insight gained in long-term therapy, and the experience in handling the phenomena that appear, no one can become an adequate psychotherapist of any kind; without continuing experience in the long-term therapies ourselves, we could not properly carry out any form of psychotherapy, nor could we supervise students, nor could we act as consultants to allied professions concerned with mental health. From the patient's point of view, there is every reason why certain privileged individuals should be treated in depth, and from the therapist's point of view, every reason why certain specialists should concentrate on doing this kind of work. I do not believe in compulsive egalitarianism, which tends to lead to situations as unrealistic or as harmful as compulsiveness in other areas.

Here Barten's words may finally be introduced:

> The brief therapies are a distillation based upon the understanding of personality dynamics and patterns of illness which traditional techniques delineated, and the latter of course are sometimes indispensable. It is their indiscriminate application which is at issue.

CHAPTER 2

The Practical Application of Brief Therapeutic Methods

One possible approach to the application of brief therapeutic methods is the attempt to concentrate on treating the patient in crisis, the point at which it is thought that the minimum intervention is likely to have the maximum effect. A second, quite different approach is not to treat the patient specifically in crisis but to try and extend the application of brief methods to as many as possible of the patients referred routinely for psychotherapy. A discussion of both approaches follows.

THE PATIENT IN CRISIS

When considering the attempt to treat the patient in crisis, we may quote Caplan (1961, p. 251):

> *The economy of crisis work.* A community programme organized along the lines suggested here will conserve professional time because patients will be treated during the disequilibrium of crisis periods. During such periods of disequilibrium it has been found that if minimal intervention is delayed until the crisis has been spontaneously resolved by the patient and his family, a great deal of professional effort has to be expended in order to get them to re-open the problems and to give up methods of solution which they have already worked out for themselves, but which the mental health specialists feel are not in their best interests.

A further quotation, from a later book by Caplan, emphasizes that crises may have highly positive effects in that they act not merely as a cause of mental breakdown but, if handled properly, as an opportunity for growth (1964, pp. 36–7):

> . . . personality . . . may suddenly change in unexpected ways during periods of crisis. The changes may be towards increased health and maturity, in which case the crisis was a period of opportunity. The changes may be toward reduced capacity to deal effectively with life's problems, and in that case the crisis was a harmful episode.

Here it needs to be said—as Caplan (1964, see pp. 105–6) recognizes—there is no *scientific* evidence that these views are correct, and we can only accept them as plausible. In our own previous work on brief psychotherapy (see Malan, 1963, pp. 183–5), *recent onset* did not correlate with favorable outcome, which seems in direct contradiction to Caplan's views, and was in direct contradiction to our own preconceptions. On the other hand, only one of our patients (the Student Thief) was seen within three weeks of onset, the maximum period during which crisis work is thought to be effective. Our results and Caplan's views are therefore still quite compatible, since our therapy did not involve crisis work in the strict sense at all.

The chance of dealing with patients in crisis is maximized by providing "early access" services, either (1) in the form of a center where patients can actually walk in and be seen at once; or (2) where they must make an appointment, but where there is a guarantee that they will be seen within a short time and, if suitable, will be given a strictly time-limited intervention. Most of the work on this type of service has been done in the United States. The following is an outline of its history:

One of the earliest programs of psychiatric emergency service was that developed at the Massachusetts General Hospital as a part of the first general hospital psychiatric department created in the United States. Initiated in 1934 under the leadership of Stanley Cobb, the department enabled members of the staff to provide help for patients with emotional crises either on the medical or surgical wards or within the setting of the general hospital emergency ward. In particular, Erich Lindemann, one of Cobb's early recruits to general hospital psychiatry, crystallized his ideas on crisis intervention in the early 1940s through his clinical involvement in the Coconut Grove fire, in which a large number of people lost their lives, and which resulted in a flood of emotional casualties (see Lindemann, 1944). When Lindemann later founded the Wellesley Human Relations Service, a pioneering community mental health center located in a Boston suburb, he included emergency facilities as an important part of its organization. And later, when he succeeded Cobb in the 1950s as chief of psychiatry at the Massachusetts General Hospital, Lindemann formalized and expanded the provision of psychiatric emergency services by organizing the Acute Psychiatric Service as one of the major segments of his clinical department.

This was followed considerably later by the establishment of similar services in other American cities. The first seems to have been the Trouble-Shooting Clinic described by Bellak and Small (1965) at the City Hospital, Elmhurst, New York, which was established in 1958. The authors emphasize that this clinic was specifically designed to attract patients of the right kind, as a contribution toward both what Caplan calls secondary prevention, i.e. reducing the duration of acute mental illness in crisis situations; and tertiary prevention, reducing the chronic impairment resulting from the maladaptive reaction to the crisis (see Caplan, 1964, pp. 16–17). Later examples of such services (see Morley, 1965) were the Emergency Psychotherapy approach introduced by Coleman and Zwerling (1959) at the Bronx Municipal Hospital, New York; Precipitating Stress Therapy introduced by Kalis and Harris at the Langley Porter Clinic, San Francisco (Kalis et al., 1961; Harris, Kalis, and Freeman, 1963); and the Benjamin Rush Center founded by Jacobson in Los Angeles in 1962 (Jacobson, 1965; Jacobson, Wilner, Morley, Schneider, Strickler, and Summer, 1965; Morley, 1965).

Moreover, in the 1960s there was a vigorous movement in the United States toward community mental health. A large amount of money was provided by the government to establish mental health centers, which were specifically required to include a provision for early access in their services. The result of all these trends has been that such services are now available at most large universities and at most of the larger general hospitals throughout the country.

The detailed questions that come to mind are concerned with whether such services are really practicable and useful: Do they get overwhelmed by demand? Are many of the patients unsuitable? Can patients be helped in any useful way? Does the help have any permanent effect?

Strictly speaking, the last two questions cannot be answered without a control sample. However, the Benjamin Rush Center has issued a report on their operating statistics for the first nineteen months, from which some tentative or partial answers to all these questions can be obtained (Jacobson et al., 1965).

When the center first opened, the staff arranged for a high level of local publicity, and during the first month one hundred patients applied; that is, an annual rate of about twelve hundred. If this had continued, the center would clearly have defeated its own aim of being able to offer immediate service, and publicity was therefore cut down. The result was a manageable intake. During the first nineteen months, patients were seen at the rate of about five hundred a year (about twice the rate at a similarly staffed clinic operating in the traditional way), and were virtually always seen within a week of application. The diagnostic impression was as follows: transient situational disorders, 16 percent; personality disorders, 28 percent; neurotic disorders, 32 percent (these three categories together making up 76 percent); psychotic disorders, 19 percent; others (e.g., organic, mental retardation), 5 percent. A precipitating stress could be identified in 73 percent; 85 percent were treated (1–6 sessions); of those treated, 74 percent were regarded by their therapists as improved at termination; at follow-up (duration not stated) 55 percent had not sought further help; and 79 percent expressed satisfaction with the service they had received.

In short, the center was able to operate effectively and seems to have provided an important service to the community. On the other hand, what does not come out of the figures is the proportion of patients who were changed in such a way as to be able to handle later stressful situations more adaptively (as in Sifneos's crisis intervention, see chap. 4), as opposed to merely being returned to the position they held before their breakdown.

The establishment of such services in Britain has very greatly lagged behind, but a comparable organization run under the National Health Service is the Young People's Counselling Service, which is attached to the Adolescent Department of the Tavistock Clinic. This is for adolescents and young adults up to the age of twenty-four. Because people of this age group are felt to be often reluctant to go to a doctor with their difficulties, there is no insistence on a medical referral. Clients may refer themselves, or may be referred by their parents or by other agencies. They will be given a first appointment within a week and will be offered a maximum of four interviews in all. The aim is similar to that of Sifneos's crisis intervention, in the sense that an attempt is made to clarify the client's current conflicts, in the hope of removing obstacles to growth and enabling him to cope better with similar situations in the future. The therapists are all nonmedical, all part-time, and all dynamically trained. Between one hundred and fifty and two hundred clients are seen in a year. However, there has been no systematic follow-up, and nothing can be said about the long-term effects to which such a service can lead.

THE EXTENSION OF BRIEF METHODS TO PATIENTS NOT IN CRISIS

When considering the treatment of the patient not in crisis, the fundamental question is a quantitative one: What proportion of such patients can be helped in any useful way? There are a number of studies that suggest that the proportion is unexpectedly high.

A very interesting development is an experiment sponsored by a New York insurance company, under which the company was prepared to meet part of the cost of psychotherapy in units of three sessions up to a maximum of fifteen (see Avnet, in Wolberg, 1965a; and Tompkins, in Usdin, 1966). Over 1200 psychiatrists agreed to participate and 1115 patients were treated. Many of the psychiatrists, initially extremely skeptical about the value of brief psychotherapy, were surprised at their own results. At the completion of the experiment, Avnet carried out a survey of therapists' and patients' opinions on improvement at termination, obtaining a 77 percent response. Fifty-three percent of the patients rated themselves as recovered or greatly improved. This sounds impressive, though of course without a control sample it cannot be properly evaluated.

The pioneer of the large-scale use of brief psychotherapeutic methods in a hospital outpatient department has of course been Sifneos, first at the Massachusetts General Hospital and more recently at the Beth Israel Hospital, in Boston. In his 1965 paper he describes the impossible situation into which all psychotherapeutic clinics inevitably lead themselves when they try to provide long-term psychotherapy for all patients who come to them:

> In some clinics one must wait for a whole year before receiving treatment. It has been argued, somewhat facetiously, that for patients with relatively mild neurotic problems, the waiting list offers the best cure. Having not been convinced by this argument, however, we decided to look into this group of fairly well-adjusted patients who, having been unable to overcome emotional crises, had developed circumscribed neurotic difficulties and symptoms. The question was: Can we offer such patients immediate, short-term psychotherapy and achieve meaningful results?

He goes on to describe how in the previous four years 450 patients have been treated by short-term methods.

He gives a further quantitative study in his paper of 1973. Here he describes how all staff members at the Beth Israel Hospital who assessed patients for psychotherapy were asked to fill out a questionnaire concerned with the suitability of each patient for brief therapy. The result was that, of 182 patients seen in the second half of 1970, 57 (32 percent) were considered suitable, not for *any* form of brief intervention, but specifically for the most radical—namely, brief anxiety-provoking psychotherapy.

A single-handed attempt to extend the application of brief therapy in a hospital outpatient setting in Britain is described by Stewart (1972) from University College Hospital, London. Here the pressure on the psychotherapeutic services was such that as many as fifteen patients had to be assessed for psychotherapy in a case conference lasting one and a half hours. Stewart undertook to offer individual psychotherapy, strictly limited to six months at once a week, to any patients thought suitable after the necessarily cursory presentation, up to the maximum that his own timetable would allow. Criteria for acceptance were similar to those used in the present work, essentially a willingness on the patient's part to work in interpretative therapy, and an ability on the therapist's part to formulate what seemed to be a feasible therapeutic plan. Therapy was thoroughly radical in its approach, being based on all forms of psychoanalytic interpretation, including extensive use of the transference and working through feelings about termination. Stewart's paper describes the first twenty patients in detail with a follow-up of nine months to three and a half years. Just as in our work, the obvious potential dangers of such an approach, such as intense dependence leading to unrealistic and traumatic attempts at termination, did not materialize; and a number of the patients seem to have received considerable help. When Stewart presented these results at a meeting of the British Psycho-analytic Society, he said that perhaps one third to one half of the patients referred for psychotherapy would be considered suitable for his approach.

All these results suggest that patients suitable for brief intervention can represent a substantial proportion of those referred routinely to psychotherapeutic clinics.

Finally, two studies—with diametrically opposed attitudes to the twin questions of *selection* and *planning*—describe the introduction to psychotherapeutic clinics of brief therapy on a large scale, and its effects both on the service provided and on the staff members. The first is by Levene *et al.* (1972), who describe the previously existing situation at the Langley Porter Neuropsychiatric Institute, San Francisco, as follows:

> . . . we believed that an excessive amount of time was being spent on screening and selection procedures of unknown validity; it seemed possible that much of the actual selection was determined by a variety of social biasing factors . . . Further, we questioned the teaching value of such a carefully screened and restricted case-load. The selection procedure served to develop a value hierarchy, at least in the mind of trainees, suggesting that long-term psychoanalytically oriented therapy was the ideal treatment, to be offered to the most qualified patients; other treatments, less valued, were for patients lower in the hierarchy. Finally, the traditional screening process isolated the trainees from the realities of the increasing community need for rapid, easily available access to psychiatric service.
>
> From these concerns we attempted to develop a research and teaching program built upon the principle that the treatment opportunities of the department should be equally open to any applicant from the community. In order to maintain our availability to a large number of unselected, unscreened patients, a brief therapy format was adopted.

After a catchment area had been defined, any patient who contacted the department was offered an appointment within four days. During the first interview the patient was offered the possibility of a maximum of ten further sessions. Patients were then randomly assigned to one of five different methods of brief therapy: two different methods based on a psychoanalytic approach, one based on behavior therapy, one on Jungian principles, and an eclectic form of group therapy.

At termination, outcome was significantly better in the *unselected* patients treated by the new methods than in the *selected* patients treated by the old methods. As far as a comparison of the five brief methods was concerned, the more active methods (behavior therapy and group therapy) tended to be most effective both at termination and at six- to twelve-month follow-up, and psychoanalytic methods to be least effective, though in fact few differences were significant. The authors say that trainees had most difficulty in learning psychoanalytic methods, which is hardly surprising and suggests that these methods are probably not suitable for use under these conditions.

At follow-up, about a third of the patients reported that they had had further therapy; while two thirds regarded their therapy at the Langley Porter as having been too brief. It is thus questionable how satisfactory the new methods of treatment were for the *patients*. On the other hand, the *staff* were clearly stimulated and satisfied by the program—"which was almost universally rated by the trainees as a highlight in their training experience at the Institute. The generally positive feelings seem to stem from the consistency between practice and philosophy."

The second article describing the introduction of brief methods on a large scale is by Straker (1968) at the Montreal General Hospital. This paper was first read at a meeting of the American Psychiatric Association, and Robert J. Campbell, one of the discussants, described similar experiences at St. Vincent's Hospital in New York City (see Straker, 1968, pp. 1225–6).

Both authors describe the effects of the previously existing traditional approach, the totally unrealistic attempt to offer long-term reconstructive therapy to all who apply. Campbell writes of the resident in such a situation, who "is in the position of having to treat every ill he encounters with the same medicine. . . The lot of the patient who enters treatment under that system is not an enticing one." Straker writes of the same situation: ". . . waiting lists produced a difficult situation for patients who were experiencing an acute emotional crisis and were not able to get psychiatric help when they most needed it . . . often the delay fostered the development of chronic maladaptive reactions. Thus continued the vicious cycle of appointment delays, clinic congestion, hurried therapy attempts, poor patient response, more clinic congestion, etc." Not only this, but the consequences were "poor diagnostic evaluations, a high patient drop-out rate, poorly planned or random therapeutic efforts, poor staff morale, long waiting lists, and frustration for both patient and physician."

This situation was dealt with at Montreal by an extensive reorganization. They established "an intake evaluation of high quality," leading to a diagnosis in depth. This was followed by an attempt to make a realistic plan for treatment of each patient in terms of what the clinic had to offer. Suitable patients were selected on this basis for *planned brief psychotherapy,* to consist of a maximum of eleven further half-hour sessions. The selection criteria were described as follows: ". . . those suffering from transient decompensations, psychotic or otherwise, from grief, mourning, or depressive reactions, or from anxiety reactions. Additional considerations include the capacity of the patients to develop useful transference feelings and sufficient motivation to involve themselves in a therapeutic relationship with the physician." Thus once more a worker who examines this problem empirically comes to emphasize motivation as an important selection criterion.

In accordance with this emphasis on motivation, while 20 percent of the *total* population were selected for brief psychotherapy, the corresponding figure for *self-referred* patients was 58 percent.

The form of brief psychotherapy offered was "perceived as an intensive interaction process, which proposes a united patient–physician effort to formulate the diagnostic dilemmas, clarify presenting problems, and search for available solutions. Treatment is related to practical and attainable goals, and adaptation is aided by giving ego support. Once equilibrium is established, the treatment relationship ends and the patient is encouraged to go unaided." This passage makes clear that the aim was to restore the patient to his previous position, as in Sifneos's crisis support, rather than to bring about deeper changes.

Straker tried to follow up a consecutive series of 220 patients two years later. He reached 107 (48 percent). Of these, 66 percent had had no further therapy (this is the same proportion as in the Langley Porter study); and 47 percent were "well, expressed satisfaction with their health, and praised the clinic services that had been provided. . . The remission rate on patients treated with brief psychotherapy reached 84 percent."

Two further important consequences were that the overall dropout rate at the clinic fell dramatically; and that there was a marked increase in the morale of the therapists, who now felt that they were participating in a realistic and effective method of treatment.

As mentioned above, Campbell reported essentially similar results in New York, with a clinic population differing considerably from that at Montreal and in particular containing a far higher proportion of schizophrenics.

In the Adult Department of the Tavistock Clinic we face exactly the same problems as have been described by all these authors. For many years our tradition has also been long-term reconstructive therapy, and we have tried to solve the problem of overwhelming demand by the use of groups. However, this too has led into exactly the same situation of long waiting lists, a high dropout rate, poor staff morale, and as suggested by our recent survey (see Malan, Balfour, Hood, and Shooter, 1976), poor therapeutic results. It has also led to another phenomenon not mentioned by these authors, namely a vicious circle concerned with referrals. Since there is a long waiting list not only for treatment but also for initial consultation, patients in crisis—and also many patients with apparently "mild" disorders—never reach us, and the patients referred to us tend to be largely those with severe chronic problems who are either downright unsuitable for interpretative psychotherapy, or only suitable for exactly what we provide: therapy of a long-term reconstructive kind. So the cycle begins again. This is reflected in our quantitative data: The proportion of patients assigned to brief therapy in our clinic is far smaller than the proportions mentioned by Sifneos (1973), Stewart (1972), and Straker (1968) and discussed above.

It is clear that any psychotherapeutic clinic that wishes to make the best use of its resources must explore to the limit the use of methods of brief intervention, and must define the characteristics of patients for which each type of intervention is suitable. It is with these problems that the present work is concerned.

PART II

Previous Work

CHAPTER 3

Brief Therapy Since 1960: I

The Work of Sifneos

By way of recapitulation, let me begin by noting that in my previous book, *A Study of Brief Psychotherapy* (1963), referred to in future mention as *SBP*, I reviewed the factors that had consistently tended to increase the length of psychoanalysis, as well as attempts by analysts to counteract this trend. Chief among the more recent efforts were those made by the Chicago school, culminating in the important book *Psychoanalytic Therapy* by Alexander and French (1946). Unfortunately, these authors presented their work as a modification of the technique of orthodox psychoanalysis, rather than as a method of brief psychotherapy based on psychoanalytic principles. They thus brought a storm of hostility upon themselves; their work—and psychoanalytic brief psychotherapy in general—fell into serious disrepute.

Any evaluation of brief psychotherapy must concern itself with three related questions—*selection criteria, technique,* and *outcome*: What kinds of technique produce what kinds of change in what kinds of patient? During the ten years after publication of Alexander and French's book, there appeared a large number of papers on brief psychotherapy, without exception based on clinical impression. A study of these works revealed an extraordinary state of confusion, which could be reduced to the polarity between the totally opposed "conservative" and "radical" views on each of the three main questions listed above. According to the conservative view, brief psychotherapy was suitable only for mild illnesses of recent onset, the techniques used should be superficial and in particular should avoid transference interpretation, and the results could only be palliative; at the extreme, this form of therapy was not worth doing. According to the radical view, far-reaching changes could be brought about in relatively severe and chronic illnesses by a technique of active interpretation containing all the essential elements of full-scale analysis. A complete spectrum of views between these two poles could be found in the literature, with no attempt to provide systematic evidence that would decide between them.

It was within this situation that in 1954 Dr. Michael Balint got together a small team of highly qualified psychotherapists to study the whole question at first hand. By 1958 the team had completed the therapy of twenty-one patients and I undertook to publish a report on our work. This appeared in 1963 as *SBP*.

The result of this study was unequivocal support for every aspect of the radical view of brief psychotherapy. Of *selection criteria,* the only factor that appeared to correlate with favorable outcome was high *motivation for insight*; and it seemed that in certain cases this was able to override such unfavorable factors as extreme chronicity and apparent all-pervasiveness of the illness. In contradiction of the conservative view, *recent onset* correlated slightly negatively with outcome. As far as *outcome* itself was concerned, long-standing neurotic patterns of behavior could apparently be reversed; and finally, the most important factor in *technique* seemed to be interpretation of the *transference* throughout the whole of therapy, with special reference to linking the transference with childhood and to working through anger and grief about the loss of the therapist at termination.

Although each separate statistical finding could only be regarded as a hypothesis needing further confirmation, the *clinical* evidence that in certain cases a radical technique could produce radical changes was sufficiently strong to be almost overwhelming. In the following pages, this clinical evidence will be a central reference point for comments on developments in brief psychotherapy that have occurred since *SBP* was published.

Here two main features are noticeable. First, the whole subject of brief therapy has aroused a steadily increasing interest, resulting in a great deal of work spread over many centers throughout the world, especially the United States, but also the European Continent and South America. In the latter two areas, Balint's work has had a direct and wide influence. On the other hand, a number of the North American centers seem to have developed their own ideas in isolation, little influenced by events elsewhere, and hardly influenced at all by our own research. The result has been many important developments on the one hand, and the needless perpetuation of certain fallacies on the other.

Of all these later developments, the most important is probably the work of Sifneos, which will therefore be considered first.

SIFNEOS: CONTRIBUTIONS TO THE PRACTICE OF BRIEF PSYCHOTHERAPY

One of the most interesting facts to emerge has been that while our work on brief psychotherapy was being carried on at the Tavistock Clinic, Sifneos was studying the same subject at the Massachusetts General Hospital in Boston; and, in a series of publications beginning in 1958, was reaching almost exactly the same conclusions. Neither he nor I knew of each other's existence until we met at the Sixth International Congress of Psychotherapy in London in 1964.

There has been a tendency in many psychiatric centers in the United States toward the development of brief psychotherapy, but the emphasis has often been largely on treating the patient in a crisis and restoring him to his previous level of functioning (see chap. 4). Sifneos, while aware that in many types of severely disturbed people this was the only method of treatment possible, also began to recognize that there was a type of patient who could be helped in a more radical way by brief psychotherapy of a different kind. He referred to this as brief anxiety-provoking dynamic psychotherapy (as opposed to anxiety-suppressive therapy, which is largely supportive). It employs all the essential types of interpretation found in psychoanalysis and is in many ways indistinguishable from the type of therapy developed by us. This was, of course—just as in our own work—a *rediscovery* of the more radical end of the spectrum of techniques used by Alexander and French. (Barten, in his important book *Brief Therapies* (1971), also emphasizes the word "rediscovery"; see p. 7.) It seems, however, that each of us has had to make this rediscovery for himself.

SIFNEOS ON SELECTION CRITERIA

From very wide clinical experience, Sifneos has developed a systematic method of selection based quite independently on many of the same principles as I suggested after studying our own cases (see pp. 277–9 of *SBP*); and in which, as suggested in *SBP*, the most important criterion is the patient's *motivation*.

Sifneos (1968a) writes that anxiety-provoking therapy ". . . focuses on the resolution of neurotic conflicts that underlie the patient's symptoms. It is offered to patients with well-circumscribed neurotic symptoms. . . ." Here we may note the words "focus" and "circumscribed," which are identical to those used by us.

The implication made by Sifneos is that the ability to see a circumscribed neurotic problem or focus is a necessary condition for selection for brief psychotherapy. This should emerge in the first interview. Additional criteria, at least three of which should be fulfilled if the patient is to be considered further, are listed below (these are taken from Sifneos, 1965; see also Sifneos, 1972, pp. 78 ff.):

1. Above-average intelligence.

2. At least one meaningful relation with another person during the patient's lifetime.

3. An emotional crisis.

4. Ability to interact well with the evaluating psychiatrist and to express feeling.

5. Motivation to work hard during psychotherapy.

6. A specific chief complaint.

If the patient fulfills three of these six criteria he is offered a second interview. This has two main purposes that are exactly consonant with our own. The first is that therapist and patient should agree on an aim for therapy: "Psychotherapy is always presented to the patient as a joint venture for the therapist and himself. . . If an area of conflict can be agreed upon, treatment will be undertaken" (Sifneos 1968b). This corresponds to one of Balint's criteria: "The patient's and therapist's aims must be the same."

The other purpose of this second interview is to assess the patient's motivation. Sifneos's procedure is much more systematic than that used by us, but works with the same concepts. For instance, we have emphasized the importance not merely of motivation for *treatment*, but motivation for *insight*; in Sifneos's statement, "There should be motivation for *change*, not motivation for *symptom relief*" (1968b), the words are different but the meaning is essentially the same.

The criteria relevant to motivation to which Sifneos directs his attention are as follows (these are taken from Sifneos, 1968a; see also Sifneos, 1972, pp. 85 ff):

1. An ability to recognize that the symptoms are psychological in nature.

2. A tendency to be introspective and to give an honest and truthful account of emotional difficulties.

3. Willingness to participate actively in the treatment situation.

4. Curiosity and willingness to understand oneself.

5. Willingness to change, explore, experiment.

6. Realistic expectations of the results of psychotherapy.

7. Willingness to make reasonable sacrifices in terms of time and fees.

To these criteria, McGuire (1968) has added two that are probably implied by Sifneos, namely:

8. That the patient should not demand that particular symptoms should be relieved.

9. That he should not regard the problem as being purely concerned with the present situation, or as being purely external.

It is important to note the conspicuous absence of severe psychopathology as a contraindication. This also accords with our own evidence.

SIFNEOS ON TECHNIQUE

Sifneos's technique is radical (Sifneos, 1966, 1967, 1972). He emphasizes the importance of early and repeated interpretation of resistance, ambivalence, and negative transference in order to maintain the therapeutic alliance; deliberately raising the patient's anxiety by concentrating on interpreting defenses; repeatedly using examples from the transference; and making the patient aware of repetitions of past patterns in the transference relationship. The technique differs from that of psychoanalysis in the following: active avoidance of deepseated characterological problems; taking advantage of the time lag in the development of the transference neurosis (also emphasized by McGuire, 1968); and early termination. All these aspects of technique are identical to those developed by us. They may be contrasted with the views of conservative authors, who state that in brief psychotherapy there is not time enough to interpret defenses or resistance, the transference should not be touched on, no reference should be made to the past, etc., etc.

However, Sifneos's technique differs—if not in kind, at least markedly in degree—from ours and that of almost all other authors in one particular emphasis, which may be introduced as follows: All psychoanalytic therapy is, of course, a *learning experience* for the patient. Not only does he learn about himself, he learns new ways of solving emotional problems, which, it is hoped, he will be able to make use of in the future. Sifneos has expanded this aspect into a basic principle of technique, making it an aim of therapy that is made explicit to the patient at the beginning: "Psychotherapy is always presented to the patient as a joint venture for the patient and himself [the therapist], in which the patient is to learn problem-solving techniques" (1968b). Correspondingly, the achievement of this aim is one of the criteria (also emphasized by McGuire, 1968) of successful outcome.

SIFNEOS ON OUTCOME

In accordance with this emphasis on learning, Sifneos regards the ability to solve new emotional problems long after treatment has terminated as a specific effect of anxiety-provoking dynamic psycho-therapy. He gives the following example (1968b): The patient was a nineteen-year-old girl who was able, after termination, to *go beyond* what she had learned in therapy. She was not only able to reapply insight gained during therapy to a new situation—one in which her original anger against her father was being redirected against her fiancé—but to reach a new piece of insight by her own efforts: that she had always used her anger as a way of avoiding sadness. She was then able to resolve the situation. Sifneos has repeatedly found that patients describe their therapy as "a new learning experience," "unique," "rare," or "unusual."

In some other statements about outcome, however, he is unex-pectedly modest. He says that patients point to only moderate sympto-matic relief; and he also says (1967) that usually "a limited dynamic change has occurred with the substitution of a new defense for an old one"; and (1966) "although no basic characterological changes seem to occur, there is some evidence that dynamic changes have taken place." I can only say that, in certain cases, our experience with an essentially similar technique seems to yield more radical improvement than this.

CONCLUSION

Although there are certain differences, the basic similarity of Sifneos's statements to the views put forward in *SBP* is obvious. This extraordinary degree of convergence of quite independent work— when taken together with the experience of Alexander and French— suggests that if well-trained analysts approach this problem with an open mind, they are likely to make the same basic clinical observations: that there is an essentially psychoanalytic technique of brief psychotherapy that, when applied to patients carefully selected according to known principles, can produce quite far-reaching dynamic improvements. This is an empirical observation that still awaits general acceptance.

CHAPTER 4

Brief Therapy Since 1960: II

THE DIFFERENT FORMS OF BRIEF PSYCHOTHERAPY

In a number of early writings, there may be found the statement or implication that brief psychotherapy is only suitable for (a) the least ill and (b) the most ill patients. One of Sifneos's major contributions has been to make sense of this utterly confusing statement, by showing that there are different forms of brief therapy that at the extreme are entirely distinct from one another. In his 1967 paper he writes: "Misunderstandings and confusion have marked the use of the terms 'brief' and 'short-term' psychotherapy. A variety of therapeutic techniques which have little or nothing in common with each other except the short time interval, have been treated as identical without an attempt having been made to define and describe the specialized features of each type." He goes on to give a classification that is summarized in Table 1.

According to this classification, there may be three quite different elements in the various forms of brief psychotherapy, which can be described as follows, beginning with the most conservative and ending with the most radical: (1) supportive measures such as environmental manipulation, reassurance, and drugs; (2) the teaching of new ways of dealing with emotional conflict; and (3) interpretation of unconscious forces.

In *crisis support* the main emphasis is on (1); in *brief anxiety-suppressive* therapy and *crisis intervention* it is on (2); and in *brief anxiety-provoking* therapy it is on (3). In practice, of course, there will be mixtures of these elements in different proportions, so that the

TABLE 1. Forms of Brief Psychotherapy

Type of treatment	Type of patient selected	Technique	Aim	Duration	Outcome
1. Anxiety-provoking (a) Short-term anxiety-provoking	As described in previous section.	Radical, essentially psychoanalytic, transference-oriented.	Circumscribed dynamic resolution. New general ways of emotional problem-solving.	Under 20 sessions.	Moderate symptomatic relief. Some dynamic change. New ways of problem-solving.
(b) Crisis intervention	Previously healthy patient in crisis.	Understanding of maladaptive reactions, learning of adaptive reactions. Essentially crisis-oriented and aimed at preventing the establishment of symptoms.	Resolution of the crisis, with ability to cope better with similar situations in future.	Not more than 2 months.	Overcoming of crisis. Able to anticipate dangers. Able to solve problems better.
2. Anxiety-suppressive. (a) Brief anxiety-suppressive	Severely disturbed patient with a history showing character defects and precarious functioning; but able to work and to recognize psychological nature of illness.	Help to understand ways of handling feelings; prepare him to avoid similar situations in the future. Drugs, if necessary.	Restoration of *status quo* with some future preventive effect.	2 months to 1 year.	Marked symptomatic relief. Ability to avoid similar situations in the future. No dynamic change.
(b) Crisis support	Severely disturbed patients showing acute decompensation.	Eliminate factors responsible for present decompensation. Drugs.	Restoration of *status quo*.	Up to 2 months. Frequent visits according to need.	Marked symptomatic relief. No dynamic change.

Note: Adapted from Sifneos, 1967; see also Sifneos, 1972.

classification really becomes a continuum. This is one of the ways in which methods of brief therapy may be classified on the conservative–radical dimension; another is discussed later in connection with the whole problem of the choice of "focus."

This continuum may be further illustrated by a discussion of *crisis theory*, by which Sifneos has been much influenced, and which itself represents an important development in the approach to brief psychotherapy (see Lindemann, 1944; Caplan, 1961; Parad, 1965).

CRISIS THEORY

According to this view, a patient in crisis has been faced with an emotional situation that is too much for him, and has developed maladaptive ways of coping with it. In the treatment of such a patient, where possible and appropriate, steps may be taken to alter the situation in such a way that the stress is reduced. However, the main aim of crisis treatment is not this, but to show him that his reactions are maladaptive and to lead him toward dealing with the current crisis in a more realistic way. The means of doing this may involve various degrees of teaching or interpretation of unconscious forces; and crisis treatment should therefore have as an additional outcome a *permanent alteration in the patient* that enables him to cope realistically, and without breaking down, with similar situations in the future. As expressed by Morley (1965), ". . . equilibrium following a crisis may be re-established at a lower *or a higher* point on the mental health continuum. Enduring positive changes can be achieved following a crisis, and crisis may have widespread results in the adjustment and coping capacity of the individual in future crises and in his overall adjustment to life." This scheme covers the main elements of three of Sifneos's types of brief psychotherapy, namely crisis support, brief anxiety-suppressive therapy, and crisis intervention; and once *interpretation* is introduced, it begins to cover brief anxiety-provoking therapy as well.

In fact, once the idea of *permanent change* is introduced, and if the word *crisis* is replaced by *current conflict*, the above scheme could equally well apply to most forms of dynamic psychotherapy. Here, as in crisis therapy, an important focus usually consists of interpretations about a current conflict; and here also the aim is to bring about a permanent change in the patient so that he can deal with such a conflict in the future. In practice this may only be possible if the *current conflict* is related to *past conflict,* and here we are led toward the childhood origins of neurosis, and through successive stages of radical dynamic psychotherapy, brief or long, toward psychoanalysis itself.

CONVERGENCE OF CRISIS THERAPY AND BRIEF PSYCHOTHERAPY

Conservative–Radical Spectra in Terms of Selection Criteria, Outcome

In the last fifteen years an interesting shift of emphasis has occurred in the literature on brief psychotherapy. Highly conservative preconceptions such as those of both Lewis and Rado (quoted by Gutheil, 1945) and also Eissler (quoted by Murphy, 1958)—see pp. 22–3 of *SBP*—that the results of brief psychotherapy are merely palliative and temporary seem to have largely disappeared. This has happened as a consequence of empirical observation that has increased to the point of being overwhelming. The main emphasis now lies in the middle of the conservative–radical spectrum and closely resembles that of crisis intervention. Again and again the opinion is expressed that brief psychotherapy is suitable for patients with *acute current conflicts,* and that the removal of such a conflict may lead to *permanent change* in which *growth and maturation* are allowed to proceed unimpeded. These opinions thus include a relatively conservative view on *selection criteria* and a more radical view on *outcome.* Sifneos's terminology may be extended by describing this form of psychotherapy as "current conflict intervention," which includes both crisis intervention and a part of brief anxiety-provoking psychotherapy.

Thus, Speers, describing brief psychotherapy with women students, (1962) writes:

> If the conflict is the result of a current situation, or the result of normal active adjustment reaction, brief psychotherapy can be effective. Students then seem to be able to resume growth toward their ultimate potential.

Hoch (in Wolberg 1965a) writes:

> Generally speaking, short-term therapy is useful in the resolution of acute conflictual problems . . . [and in many such patients] a much deeper change has been brought about than symptom control.

Bellak and Small (1965) write:

> The goal of brief psychotherapy is limited to the removal or amelioration of specific symptoms; it does not attempt the reconstitution of personality except that any dynamic intervention may secondarily, and to a certain

extent, autonomously lead to some restructuration . . . but at the same time we would stress that for many people limited psychotherapy may in itself be sufficient to help them achieve a point from which they continue autonomous improvement.

Gillman (1965) writes:

Most of the caution over the benefit of symptomatic improvement in brief therapy is due to the psychoanalytic knowledge that unconscious conflicts have remained untouched. There are now enough cases of lasting improvement in brief therapy to suggest that the reduction in anxiety that occurs in treatment can, in certain cases, permit growth and mastery to take place so that the unresolved conflicts are decreased in relative force.

Binstock, Semrad, and Bloom (1967) make the distinction between brief and definitive therapy:

Definitive therapy seeks a widening of potentialities; brief psychotherapy *may* accomplish the same, but it aims at freeing the patient from a [current] predicament which has narrowed them.

Straker (1968) writes:

Brief psychotherapy is recommended as the primary choice for patients who present a particular constellation of assets and liabilities in a setting of life crises such as are frequently seen in the outpatient clinic.
The long-range effect of such brief interventions need not be minimized. Among others Kaufman [1967] recently pointed out that the shift in ego function resulting from brief psychotherapy can secondarily mobilize an ecological reorientation of the total intrapsychic organizations and functions.

Yet, even this shift toward the radical end of the spectrum does not go far enough. None of these authors has grasped the full radical evidence that is there for those who seek it. This is that the presence of an acute current conflict is not a necessary requirement for brief therapy; that working through the long-term conflict may be made into the therapeutic plan; and that extensive dynamic change is not a sort of unexpected by-product, but something that may be aimed at from the beginning. The only author other than Sifneos who seems to have approached this realization is Wolberg, who writes as follows (1965a):

It is essential here to qualify the finding that acute problems are best suited for short-term approaches . . . I have personally treated chronic cases with short-term methods, including obsessive–compulsive neurosis and borderline schizophrenia and I have observed many gratifying results. Indeed, had I permitted these patients to continue in therapy, I am certain that some would have marooned themselves in permanent treatment waters which would have swamped their tiny surviving islands of independence.

The best strategy, in my opinion, is to assume that every patient, irrespective of diagnosis, will respond to short-term treatment unless he proves himself refractory to it. If the therapist approaches each patient with the idea of doing as much as he can for him, within the space of, say, up to twenty treatment sessions, he will give the patient an opportunity to take advantage of short-term treatment to the limit of his potential. If this fails, he can always then resort to prolonged therapy.

In a subsequent publication (Wolberg 1965b), he mentions our work and writes that he also is convinced that in patients treated by him ". . . not only have symptoms been controlled, but in a considerable number of patients reconstructive personality changes have been brought about."

TECHNIQUE: PLANNING AND FOCUSING

In *SBP* (pp. 27 ff.) I noted that perhaps the most important lengthening factor in the history of psychoanalysis was *passivity in the therapist*; and correspondingly, that the area of greatest agreement in the whole literature on brief therapy was that passivity must be replaced by *activity* in various forms. This starts with the strategic *planning* of a *limited aim* from the beginning. Earlier authors who emphasized this aspect were Alexander and French (1946), Finesinger ("goal-directed planning and management," 1948), and Deutsch ("goal-limited adjustment," "sector therapy," 1949). The limited aim can be formulated in terms of a desired *therapeutic effect*, but because therapeutic effects are difficult to predict, it is probably better to formulate the aim in terms of a particular area that needs to be worked through, and hence a particular *theme for interpretations*. Since these depend on the material that the patient brings, there arises the necessity for a more tactical form of "activity," namely *guiding* the patient during the actual sessions by means of *selective interpretation, selective attention*, and *selective neglect*. For this it is very natural to use the metaphorical verb "focus"; the therapist "focuses" attention, and tries to cause the patient to focus attention, on the chosen area. This area itself then becomes known by the metaphorical noun, the "focus" of therapy. Finally, the adjective "focal" is introduced, the technique by which the patient is guided becomes known as the "focal technique" and the method of therapy as "focal therapy."

During the course of our work Balint was responsible for introducing these words, which he did quite independently of their use by other authors. This culminated in his last book, entitled *Focal Psy-*

chotherapy, which was completed posthumously by his wife Enid and his pupil and colleague Paul Ornstein (Balint, Ornstein, and Balint, 1972). It is natural, therefore, that we should find these words used throughout the world where Balint has had a direct influence; and, apart from the writings of Ornstein (e.g., "Focal psychotherapy: its potential impact on psychotherapeutic practice in medicine," Ornstein and Ornstein, 1972), we find two German papers by Klüwer from Frankfurt with the words *Fokus* and *Fokaltherapie* in the titles respectively (1970, 1971); another German paper by Beck and Lambelet from Lausanne in which the word *Fokus* plays a central part (1972); and similarly, we find the word *foco* in Spanish in a book by Kesselman from Buenos Aires (1970, p. 93).

Nevertheless there are many centers of psychotherapy that have apparently remained unaware of Balint's work. Despite this, a most interesting observation is that in the literature on brief therapy the word "focus" now occurs almost universally. Of course, terminology is in itself unimportant, but this universality is worth emphasizing because it has deeper implications. Many centers have clearly developed these words independently; and the reason is that almost every author who studies brief therapy comes to realize the need for *planning* and *activity*, and many of them come to use the word *focus* and its derivatives to describe these elements in their technique.

The word can in fact be traced back as far as Finesinger (1948), who writes of the "focusing of material." The phrase "focal conflict" occurs in French's book, *The Integration of Behavior* (1958). Here it is used to refer to the conflict in the patient's current life (whether in the transference or outside) that is nearest to the surface in any given session; and it is contrasted with the "nuclear conflict" originating in childhood. French's term lacks the element of *planning* and has little in common with the use described here (see also Balint, Ornstein, and Balint, 1972, p. 10–11 for a discussion of this issue).

On the other hand, the word "focus" is now used in an exactly similar sense to that of Balint by a number of recent authors. As an example, in the book *Brief Therapies* containing articles by different authors and edited by Barten (1971), it occurs as follows:

Barten (p. 10): "The process of delimiting the problem area which is to be the major focus of treatment is one of the most critical operations of brief therapy."

Barten (p. 11): ". . . the therapist must be careful to maintain a realistic focus so that he and the patient are not inundated by material."

Swartz (pp. 108–9): "Once the focus is established every effort is

made to stay within the chosen area . . . The most common focus that
is chosen revolves around the precipitating stress."

Other examples are to be found in:

Harris, Kalis, and Freeman (1963): "The most important difference
between this type of brief treatment and more traditional forms of
psychotherapy is in the systematic focusing on the current situation."

Gottschalk, Mayerson, and Gottlieb (1967): "This is a report
of a . . . study examining the effectiveness of short-term focal
psychotherapy."

Fox (1972): ". . . most of these post-combat adaptational problems
could be resolved using a focal psychotherapeutic approach."

The following delightful quotation is from Wolberg (1965a):
"Anathema to short-term therapy is passivity in the therapist. Where
time is no object, the therapist can settle back and let the patient pick
his way through the lush jungles of his psyche . . . Treatment failures
are often the product of lack of proper activity . . . Focused interviewing in the sitting-up position is almost mandatory."

McGuire (1965) describes a similar approach in different terminology, writing of the "dissection" of a "treatable emotional conflict from
its deeper and more expansive connections."

Finally, the clearest statement of all on these issues comes from
Mann (1973). He emphasizes that "a central problem or focus" must be
defined at the beginning, and like Sifneos, he discusses and agrees on
this directly with the patient. He goes on to say that in the early stages
of therapy the patient is "inclined to pour out much important
anamnestic data and secret feelings and fantasies. The therapist will
be tempted to explore one or other fascinating avenues of data, and it
is in this setting that any variety of psychotherapy may become
excessively diffused and the goals of treatment increasingly blurred.
The therapist must remain insistent in confining attention to the
central issue, and use only those data that relate to it." In his 1969
paper he writes: "If the therapist resists every effort to divert him from
the agreed area of investigation, the area of regression in the transference will remain limited."

Thus this aspect of general agreement reported in *SBP* has
continued and developed further in the later literature.

THE CONSERVATIVE–RADICAL SPECTRUM IN TERMS OF FOCUS

As I pointed out in *SBP*, selection criteria, technique, and outcome are inextricably intertwined, and it is impossible to consider one

without reference to the others. The choice of focus, which concerns *technique*, will depend both on *selection*—the type of patient or problem thought suitable—and the type of *outcome* desired or thought possible; and there now arises another conservative–radical spectrum in terms of focus. Here French's term, the "nuclear conflict" becomes useful. Therapies can then be classified in terms of the "depth" of the focus, which will in turn depend on both the depth of the nuclear conflict, and the extent to which the focus can be taken as the nuclear conflict itself, or only parts or derivatives of it.

This is once more an area in which very few authors have seen to the heart of the matter. With the exception of Sifneos, Mann, and Wolberg, almost every author implies that the focus is always something more superficial than the nuclear conflict. It needs to be said again and again that the work reported in *SBP* demonstrated that this is not necessarily so, and that a complete spectrum can be found between what may be called partial or derivative foci on the one hand, and nuclear foci on the other, and that even the partial foci can be at a very considerable depth.

I think it is probably true that Michael Balint himself, and certainly some of his close associates, never fully realized this. Balint was so anxious to emphasize the active nature of the focal technique, which implied formulating a circumscribed area for interpretation, that he did not see that the patient's nuclear conflict might itself be a circumscribed area and thus might automatically provide a circumscribed focus.

Of course, one does not want to get too involved in splitting hairs over the meaning of the term "nuclear conflict." There may be those who believe that every patient's nuclear conflict must be concerned with primitive mother–child relationships. But if one takes a middle-of-the-road view that some patients have nuclear conflicts that are (for instance) essentially Oedipal, then it needs to be said that such a conflict has repeatedly been taken as focus, and at depth, in our work. It is worth studying the following edited quotation from the thirteenth session of the highly successful fourteen-session therapy of the Neurasthenic's Husband (see *SBP*, pp. 99–103):

> He went on with a story about his father coming back from the war, with gifts for the family. It was a tragi-comedy, for all these gifts were no good—a watch which fell to pieces for the daughter, some silver thing that almost broke in your hand for the son, etc. I interpreted this in the transference, how he appreciated my goodwill but thought little of what I had given him, and I pointed out how his father, impotent and unable to be anything but laughable, was his view of all men including himself and me. He went on to say that of course he hadn't known his father much—

when he was near puberty his father had gone away to the war. The hint here was that his father had not helped him with his sexual problems as I had not, and I took this up. He repeated that he had been independent from an early age. I pointed out that he was now being "independent," and that on three occasions when the prospect of ending the treatment had occurred he had become independent and threatened to leave—rather than be deserted he was doing the deserting, to avoid having feelings of disappointment, longing, and dependency on a man. I pointed out his loneliness all his life, his need for men, and this really shook him. He paused, sat back in his chair and thought, and said, "I have always felt my independence to be virtuous and never allowed myself to be owned by anybody." I pointed out that his ancestors included men as well as women, and contrasted his view of women as being people who had sexual tensions that "needed relief" with his view of men who brought home broken toys and gifts. I pointed out how he castrated his father regularly and denounced his potency in order to have his mother for himself. He again took this soberly and said, "Like Moses, like the Virgin Birth," and went on with a dawning realization that he had never allowed himself to have a father.

It is difficult to see how much more "deeply" an Oedipal problem could be interpreted even in a full-scale analysis; and it is certainly arguable that this was the patient's nuclear conflict.

It also needs to be said again and again that this is not a new discovery, but a *re*discovery of principles made clear by Alexander and French. Here I only need to quote once more their Case P, a young man of nineteen whose severe depression was resolved in thirty-five sessions by uncovering his feelings about the death of his mother when he was three. This therapy culminated in an intensely moving transference experience in which he put the woman therapist in the position of his mother and symbolically reincorporated her into himself.

Again, it needs to be said that the most successful therapies reported in *SBP* were those in which the focal conflict was linked with childhood (see pp. 246–60), and thus in which not merely derivatives of the nuclear conflict were interpreted, but at least aspects of the nuclear conflict itself.

There is an intermediate type of therapy in which the nuclear conflict is left severely alone, and the therapist makes as his focus what may perhaps be termed a subsidiary conflict, though even this may occupy a considerable portion of the patient's make-up and itself possess very considerable depth. The clearest example is when the patient is psychotic but the therapist carefully confines his interpretations to an Oedipal focus. An example was the Paranoid Engineer reported in *SBP*. The recently published book, *Focal Psychotherapy* (Balint, Ornstein, and Balint, 1972), is entirely concerned with a similar but much more striking therapy (taken from the present series), that of the Stationary Manufacturer, in which the therapist was Michael Balint. The patient, a man of forty-three, suffered from a severe "jealousy paranoia," the history of which went back at least six years. His Rorschach contained a preoccupation with women as phallic, sinister, and dangerous, together with sadistic attacks on them; and we may suppose that his "nuclear" conflict was at a very primitive level indeed. Balint chose to confine his interpretations to the patient's much less primitive relations with men in a triangular situation, taking as his focus the patient's homosexually tinged inability to accept that he had won his wife from a rival, because this would mean that the rival was an enemy. This theme was consistently interpreted throughout therapy, and was linked with the transference and the patient's relation with his father. This amazingly successful therapy is discussed in detail later (see chap. 14).

At the conservative end of the scale, there are many case histories reported in the literature in which some current conflict is taken as focus, and in which this is interpreted only so deeply as is necessary to help the patient. An excellent example is given by Ornstein and Ornstein (1972), in which the basic interpretation given to a thirty-year-old man was that he was unable to assert himself with his wife because of his fear of losing her, this in turn being based on the feeling that because his penis was too small he would not be acceptable to any other woman. No transference interpretations were made in this therapy, and no direct reference to Oedipal conflicts. The therapeutic consequences of this six-session therapy spread throughout the patient's whole life. Case histories of this kind demonstrate beyond doubt that deliberately keeping to a relatively superficial focus is a perfectly legitimate operation. The error is to assume that deeper foci are not possible.

SELECTION CRITERIA

The implication of much of the literature mentioned in preceding sections seems to be that almost all acute current problems are suitable for one or other of the techniques included in "current conflict intervention," and few authors seem to consider explicitly the obvious point that this kind of therapy requires certain special characteristics in the patient over and above the passive willingness to accept what he is offered. Thus, Mann (1969) writes:

> The selection of patients for this kind of time-restricted psychotherapy
> remains to be satisfactorily defined . . . My present experience indicates
> that it can be useful to any patient in whom a fairly clear central present
> issue can be defined.

Where other factors in the patient are mentioned, *motivation* and
related dynamic criteria such as *ability to work in interpretative therapy*
and *congruence of aims between patient and therapist* occur most often
and will be the only ones considered here. Thus, Hollender (1964)
emphasizes that these criteria are more important than severity of
pathology, and adds correspondingly that ". . . if the prospective
patient demands that the therapist take over, treat him as though he
were helpless and do whatever seems to be required, it is glaringly
evident that most forms of uncovering therapy and a relationship
based on mutuality are out of the question." Similarly, Wright,
Gabriel, and Haimowitz (1961) refuse all patients who come for any
reason other than wanting help for themselves; and, as a further test of
motivation, insist that patients pay a limited fee out of their own
earnings. Straker (1968) made the important related observation that
self-referral was highly correlated with both termination by mutual
consent and favorable outcome.

Here it should be mentioned that there is one study of motivation
that did not confirm the above views, namely that by Schoenberg and
Carr (1963). These authors repeated Seitz's experiment (1953) on
treating neuro-dermatitis by encouraging the overt expression of
hostility. An inspection of their figures, however, suggests to me that
among their twenty-six patients the distribution of degrees of motivation—with eighteen patients showing "moderate" motivation, and
only eight showing the extremes of "marked" and "slight"—was such
that a significant result could hardly be expected.

VIEWS ON TECHNIQUE, WITH SPECIAL REFERENCE TO TRANSFERENCE

These also can be dismissed relatively briefly. There is exactly the
same spectrum of conservative and radical views as was found in the
earlier literature. At the conservative end, Straker (1968) writes:

> In essence, the aims of brief psychotherapy are to provide ego support and
> some gratification of oral needs while there is concurrent exploration of
> current external interpersonal, family, and intrapsychic conflicts. The main
> problems are clarified, together with the patient's characteristic defenses

and methods of problem solving. Transference interpretation is avoided where possible.

Bellak and Small (1965) write:

> . . . in brief psychotherapy positive transference is sought and maintained from the beginning to the end. . . The emergence of negative transference is avoided as much as possible and referred to only on rare occasions when it can, in a helpful way, be related to other manifestations or when it stands in the way of therapeutic progress.

At an intermediate stage, transference may be an important factor without being explicitly interpreted (Wright *et al.*, 1961):

> . . . as in all psychotherapy, the relationship with the therapist is the focus of the treatment through which other goals are realized. In time-limited psychotherapy, however, these are often not analyzed with the patient, nor understood by him, but utilized to achieve the underlying goals established at intake.

Further toward the radical end, transference may be regarded as central to treatment, but it is not explicitly linked with the past (Binstock, Semrad, and Bloom, 1967):

> *Transference* and its interpretation are a crucial element in a treatment relationship. Transference interpretations are not withheld because a "transference neurosis" has not had a chance to develop. Rarely does the therapist encounter a panorama of the patient's past relationships beyond an unconscious revival of what is most relevant to the current dilemma . . .

In contrast, Mann (1969) regards the link with the past as an essential part of therapy, and makes a clear reference to Menninger's (1958) concept of the "triangle of insight"—the link between the transference relationship, current external relationships, and past relationships—though with some reservations about the depth of interpretation that is appropriate:

> Transference is interpreted within the framework of the focused central conflict . . . The interpretation includes the past, the present, and the therapist but is not couched in libidinal developmental terms even though these may be expressed unknowingly but very clearly by the patient.

Finally Whittington (1962) explicitly mentions the triangle of insight and makes one of the clearest statements of the radical view:

> In summary, then, it is suggested that the process of brief psychotherapy be viewed within the framework of psychoanalytic theory as a technique involving the effective utilization of the transference manifestations to complete the "triangle of insight." Further, it is suggested that attempts to understand the transference pattern and to respond—either interpretatively

or by attitudes—in a therapeutic manner, are important to the outcome of psychotherapy, no matter how brief the course of such treatment.

Thus, whereas the need for planning and focusing remains as before an area of striking convergence, the role of transference remains an area of total disagreement—where, more than anywhere else in the whole field, there is a need for definitive empirical evidence to clear up the confusion.

NUMBER OF SESSIONS, TIME LIMITS, TERMINATION, AND THE WORK OF MANN

The various forms of long-term therapy may last for hundreds of sessions spread over many years, and "brief" therapy is a relative term. As far as the definition of "brief" is concerned, I have tended to use an upper limit of forty sessions, which of course is entirely arbitrary and is probably longer than most workers in this field would accept.

Far more important is the question of whether a definite time limit should be set and agreed with the patient from the beginning. In the work reported in *SBP* we did not have the confidence to do this, both because we did not know how many sessions would be appropriate, and because we felt that it would put pressure on the patient that might well be antitherapeutic; and although we made it plain that therapy was to be relatively short, we left vague the exact number of sessions. This has considerable disadvantages: Both therapist and patient tend to become deeply involved, and the therapist may find it very difficult to interrupt work that is going well by suddenly introducing the subject of termination.

Mann (1973) also strongly criticizes this practice as I described it, and he may be glad to hear that I have for many years independently adopted his own practice of setting a time limit from the beginning, as indeed have many other workers in this field. I have also independently reached his conclusion that it is far better to set the limit in terms of a *date* calculated on the basis of a number of sessions rather than the number of sessions itself. With the latter arrangement both patient and therapist tend to lose count, and there are further difficulties concerned with whether or not to add on sessions that the patient has missed, for what may or may not be reality reasons.

It seems clear that there is no special magic in any particular number of sessions, and that patients can work within any number, provided they know what it is from the beginning. Barten (1971) says that most therapists use six to twenty sessions. As has already been described by Avnet (in Wolberg, 1965a), therapists supported by an insurance scheme used a maximum of fifteen, rising in units of three. In my own practice at the Tavistock Clinic I now use twenty sessions for an experienced therapist and thirty for a trainee. An interesting variant is described by Swartz (1971), in which a total of twelve hours may be distributed in any way that the therapist chooses, such as one hour a week, one every two weeks, or half an hour a week.

It also seems clear by now that an initial time limit is beneficial rather than harmful, and the main reason is that it highlights the termination issue from the very beginning. The importance of working through disappointment and anger at termination was much emphasized by Balint and his team, and in *SBP* I reported considerable evidence that this did in fact tend to correlate with favorable outcome (see pp. 225–31).

Mann (1973) has carried this emphasis on termination to the limit, making it the central issue in his system of brief therapy. As already described, the patient is set a limit of twelve sessions, and this is put to him in the form of an exact date for the last session. Mann believes that termination must appear to the patient to be absolute, and that no hope of any further sessions must be held out. Thus, no mention whatsoever may be made of the possibility of follow-up—which, if it occurs, must come out of the blue. Though I agree with much of what Mann says about termination, I do not think this absolute approach is necessary. In my experience, even when it is stated clearly to the patient that he may come back to discuss further problems as required, to his unconscious the last regular session is the end of the relationship.

Mann goes on to describe the typical course of a therapy that starts in this way. He says that the prospect of termination tends to bring out in the patient four basic and universal conflicts:

1. Independence versus dependence;
2. Activity versus passivity;
3. Adequate self-esteem versus loss of self-esteem; and
4. Unresolved or delayed grief.

All these conflicts will have been generated in the patient by his past experience, and Mann uses this to create a situation in which the links between the transference, the current conflict, and the past, become the central issue of therapy: "Knowing the termination date at the start increases anxiety in respect to loss as well as defenses against loss. The termination date is quickly repressed, and the intensification of the defenses against separation and/or loss serves to highlight much of the nature of the present central issue, and the means employed to master it."

Because the issue of termination has been repressed, the patient enters into therapy with enthusiasm and tends to bring interesting material on all sorts of different issues. The therapist, however, sticks to the central focus as originally defined. The result is now a loss of enthusiasm, manifestations of resistance, and, if there has been symptomatic improvement, there is often a relapse. All this tends to occur after six or seven sessions, and most of the rest of therapy must "deal insistently with the patient's reaction to termination."

The importance that Mann attaches to this phase, to the way in which it brings out past conflicts, and to the way in which it fosters a therapeutic rather than an idealized relationship with the therapist after termination, may be illustrated by the following quotations: "It is in this end phase that the definitive work of resolution will be done, and it will incorporate, of necessity, understanding of all the highly concentrated and intensely experienced dynamic events that have preceded it . . . The genetic source of these affects is relived in the disappointing termination and separation from the therapist in whom he has become heavily invested." He goes on to say that the appropriate management of termination will allow the therapist to be internalized: "This time the internalization will be more positive (never totally so), less anger-laden, and less guilt-laden, thereby making separation a genuine maturational event."

We thus end this survey of recent work with one of the most radical approaches to be found anywhere.

CONCLUSION

An overall view of these developments since 1960 thus reveals that there has been some shift toward the radical end of the spectrum, but that much of the literature still bears a considerable resemblance to that reviewed in *SBP*. The same irreconcilable views still exist side by side, and the consensus still seems to be essentially conservative.

Here it needs to be repeated that no one should disagree with a conservative approach in its proper place. The mistake is to suppose that this is the only way of working, and therefore to fail to explore the possibility that more ambitious therapeutic aims can be achieved, with more radical techniques, in patients with more severe and more long-standing disorders. That this was in fact possible was the main clinical finding that emerged from the work of Balint's team. In addition there was, however, an even more important *research* find-ing, namely that with appropriately selected patients the more radical the technique the more apparently deep-seated were the therapeutic results obtained. Yet, all this work was carried out on a very small sample; and whereas the clinical results might easily have been some kind of never-to-be-repeated therapeutic miracle—often seen after the introduction of a new technique—the research results might equally have been simply due to chance; and all the findings could therefore be regarded as nothing more than useful hypotheses. The present work is a replication, in which these hypotheses can either be contradicted, or, if confirmed, can begin to claim the right to be regarded as conclusions.

PART III

The Present Work

CHAPTER 5

Results of the Second Study of Brief Psychotherapy

While the results on the *first series* of twenty-one patients (those reported in *SBP*) were being worked up, Balint's team continued to function and treated a further thirty-nine patients in all. These patients, the *second series*, were thus available for a replication of the original study, for which we were given grants by the David Matthew Fund of the London Institute of Psychoanalysis and the Mental Health Research Fund, which we here gratefully acknowledge. The aim was to replicate the previous study with longer follow-up and more rigorous scientific safeguards.

The main *clinical* results of this previous study had been as follows:

1. That important and apparently permanent dynamic changes could follow brief psychotherapy (ten to forty sessions);

2. That these could occur in patients with relatively extensive and long-standing psychopathology;

3. That the technique used could be thoroughly radical and involve all the main types of interpretation occurring in full-scale analysis, including interpretation of dreams and fantasies, analysis of resistance, interpretation of the transference, and the link between the transference and childhood.

It must be said at once that these observations were entirely confirmed.

With a purely clinical approach, however, only the following kinds of statement can be made with any certainty: These were the patients selected, this was the technique used, and these were the therapeutic effects found at follow-up. Although it is certainly possible to form many clinical impressions about which patients are suitable and which techniques are effective, this way of reaching conclusions is extremely unreliable, as is very clearly shown by the many false ideas that have been perpetuated in the literature. The only way of reaching any valid conclusions must involve statistical evidence, in which all of the following are considered: (1) the nature of the sample; (2) the correlations between various factors on the one hand and outcome on the other; (3) the interpretation of these correlations in terms of cause and effect; and (4) possible fallacies in this interpretation. These questions are considered in detail in *Toward the Validation of Dynamic Psychotherapy* (Malan, 1976). Here, only the results will be presented, together with a discussion of their main implications.

NATURE OF THE SAMPLE

This is considered in detail in chapter 7. In a few words, patients were included in the study for whom a *prima facie* case for brief therapy could be made out. This involved (1) eliminating patients who seemed obviously unsuitable, particularly those who did not appear to have the basic strength to stand up to uncovering psychotherapy; and (2) including those (a) who were responsive to interpretation, and (b) with whom some conceivable circumscribed focus could be formulated. Within these limits, severity of pathology and chronicity of disturbances were not considered to be contraindications, so that the range of patient chosen was very wide.

CHANGE IN THE METHOD OF SCORING OUTCOME

In both series certain therapies resulted in failure to terminate within an arbitrary limit of forty sessions, and the problem arose of how outcome in these therapies should be scored. In the first series I regarded them as failures of brief psychotherapy and scored them as zero. When I came to study the second series, I soon found that to do this destroyed all the important correlations. I therefore adopted two alternative procedures and calculated the correlations for each: (1) to omit the longer therapies, giving $N = 22$; and (2) to include all therapies ($N = 30$) but to use the score for final outcome whatever the length of therapy. The first procedure results in a study of various factors in genuinely brief therapy; the second, in a study of factors in "psychotherapy," regardless of length. With either of these procedures a number of significant correlations reappeared. If I then went back to the first series and used either of these procedures, the original significant correlations were almost always preserved. An important inference from these observations is that many of the important factors in *brief* therapy and in the longer forms of dynamic psychotherapy are the same.

It thus remains possible to say that certain significant correlations have been obtained in two successive series; but it must also be freely admitted that any alteration in the method of scoring, deliberately chosen in order to preserve correlations, results in a weakening of the evidence.

SELECTION CRITERIA

First Series. We started with two basic hypotheses:

1. The less dynamic or "static," Hypothesis A: The prognosis is best in *mild illnesses* of *recent onset*.

2. The more dynamic Hypothesis B: The prognosis is best in patients who show evidence from the beginning of a willingness and ability to *work in interpretative therapy*.

Each of these two general hypotheses was broken down into subcriteria, the most important in Hypothesis A being (1) mild psychopathology and (2) recent onset; and in Hypothesis B (3) response to interpretation and (4) motivation for insight.

The results in the first series were as follows: Within the limits of the patients selected neither *severity of pathology* nor *chronicity* seemed to have any bearing on outcome. The only criterion that showed any hope of being of value was *motivation for insight*, especially if it was judged during the first few therapeutic sessions and not only in the initial interview. Finally, the other main subcriterion of Hypothesis B, namely *response to interpretation*, could not be evaluated because it constituted one of the criteria on which patients were accepted for the study in the first place.

It is important to note that this *research* finding on motivation corresponds exactly with an entirely independent *clinical* finding made by Sifneos, who devotes a special interview to assessing this factor because he regards it as of such central importance.

Selection Criteria at Initial Assessment, Second Series. Here we studied the same two basic hypotheses, but divided them into a larger

TABLE 2.   Selection Criteria Studied in the Second Series

"Static" criteria	Dynamic criteria
Mild psychopathology	Motivation for insight
Recent onset	Manner of cooperation
Propitious moment	Contact or response to interpretation
Good outside relationship	Ability to find a focus
Absence of deprivation	
Heterosexual experience	

number of subcriteria, ending with ten on which two independent judges could reach reasonable agreement. These were judged on the *initial interview and projection test,* and are shown in Table 2.

At first sight the results were disappointing. None of the ten gave a positive correlation with outcome that reached the 5 percent level of significance. However, two important considerations increase the value of these results: (1) The lack of confirmation for Hypothesis A is really a positive rather than a negative finding, because it means that some patients with relatively severe and chronic illnesses can be helped by brief therapy; and (2) of all the ten criteria, the one that gave the highest correlation with outcome was, once more, *motivation* (p > .05 but < .1). Nevertheless the correlation was too small for this criterion to have been of any practical value.

TWO VARIABLES IN THE INITIAL STAGES OF THERAPY— MOTIVATION AND FOCALITY

We went on to study fluctuations in motivation during the first eight contacts with the clinic, and their relation to outcome; together with fluctuations in another variable over the same period, namely *focality.* This latter variable can be defined for each session as the extent to which the therapist can stick to his therapeutic plan, or a single theme for his interpretations.

The results here were of extraordinary interest. Shorn of excessive detail, they were as follows:

1. Neither motivation nor focality showed a significant correlation with outcome during the first four contacts with the clinic.

2. Both motivation and focality tended to show a significant correlation with outcome during contacts 5 to 8.

3. Both variables tended to start unrelated to each other but to become *highly correlated with each other* during contacts 5 to 8.

4. During contacts 5 to 8, high-motivation/high-focality tended to

lead to short, successful therapy; low-motivation/low-focality to short, unsuccessful therapy; and high-motivation/low-focality to long, successful therapy.

All these findings can not only be seen to have clear clinical meaning but might be used for practical purposes in selection.

First, the clinical meaning can be formulated by the following argument: Careful thought suggests that these two variables are measures of what may be called *successful dynamic interaction* between patient and therapist. In the very early stages of therapy it may often happen that neither patient nor therapist has really settled down. The patient is not yet aware of the implications of the type of therapy that he is being offered; and the therapist is not yet certain of his therapeutic plan or focus. During the course of the first few sessions the therapist offers a tentative or partial focus in the form of interpretations, and the patient reacts either positively, by increased motivation; or negatively, by decreased motivation, resistance, or withdrawal. Increased motivation is likely to lead to clearer communication on his part and a clearer therapeutic plan on the part of the therapist. Conversely, decreased motivation and increased resistance are likely to lead to lack of clear communication from the patient and the therapist's inability to see the correct interpretation. Moreover, it can be seen at once that there will be a tendency for each of these situations to result in a self-perpetuating cycle: Therefore, therapies will tend to polarize into those that are high-motivation/high-focality on the one hand, and low-motivation/low-focality on the other; and statistically, this will reflect itself in the development of a positive correlation between the two. Finally, it can also be seen (1) that high-motivation/high-focality should tend toward the rapid working through of the focal problem, and hence to short, successful therapy; (2) that low-motivation/low-focality should tend toward failure to work the problem through and premature termination, and hence to short, unsuccessful therapy; and (3) that high-motivation/low-focality may result in a long search for what may eventually transpire to be a complex focus, leading therefore to longer therapy; but since high motivation may carry patient and therapist through all the difficulties, therapy may tend to be ultimately successful.

Second, as far as practical considerations are concerned, these results suggest that the study of motivation and focality during an extended diagnostic period may resolve uncertainties about whether a patient is suitable or not. The way in which these statistical findings have converged with my own clinical practice will be discussed more fully in chapter 9.

CHARACTERISTICS OF SUCCESSFUL TECHNIQUE

In the First Series.   The aspects of technique studied in the first series consisted essentially of the relation between outcome on the one hand and various aspects of *transference interpretation* on the other. Here it emerged that those therapies tended to be successful in which:

1. Transference arose *early;*
2. The *negative* transference was thoroughly interpreted;
3. The link was made between the transference and the relation to *parents* (the transference/parent or T/P link); and
4. The patient was able to work through grief and anger about *termination.*

The most striking of these correlations was with the transference/ parent link. I studied this not only by clinical judgment but also by a semiobjective and purely quantitative method involving a content analysis of the accounts of therapy (which, it must be remembered, were dictated by the therapists from memory). Here I marked off each *interpretation* and made a judgment of whether or not it made the T/P link. As a measure of the emphasis laid on the T/P link in each therapy I took the *number of interpretations making the T/P link,* divided by the *total number of interpretations recorded* for that therapy. The resulting figure was called the "transference/parent ratio." When these figures were compared with the scores for outcome over the whole series, the resulting correlation was positive and significant.

There thus seemed overwhelming evidence from the first series against the conservative view that in brief therapy transference interpretations are harmful, and strongly suggestive evidence that on the contrary they may constitute a major factor leading to therapeutic effects.

In the Second Series.   Again shorn of excessive detail, the results in the second series were as follows:

The finding on the *negative transference* was not confirmed; those on *early* transference and *termination* were also probably not confirmed; while that on the *transference/parent link* was confirmed in a most striking manner: In a very detailed content analysis, the correlations between outcome and a large number of different kinds of interpretation were studied, and the transference/parent link not only headed the rank order by a large margin but gave the only correlation that was significant.

TWO FURTHER CORRELATIONS IN THE FIRST SERIES THAT WERE NOT CONFIRMED IN THE SECOND

In the first series a very striking correlation was found between *emphasis on transference* on the one hand and *behavior over follow-up* on the other. Briefly, those patients with whom the transference had been thoroughly interpreted tended to accept termination and to come back for follow-up without acting out, whereas those with whom less emphasis had been laid on the transference tended to show either (1) failure to terminate, (2) acting out over follow-up, or (3) refusal of follow-up altogether. However, this was not confirmed for the second series. I am still inclined to believe that the original observation was genuine, and I think the discrepancy may be due to the fact that follow-up was much longer in the second series, so that unresolved transference feelings had been softened by the passage of time.

The second observation was that each therapist tended to be successful with his *first case* when presumably his enthusiasm was highest. When the final results on both series became available, however, a most strange observation emerged, which needs to be introduced by some preliminary explanation of the constitution of Balint's research team: The meetings were held at the Tavistock Clinic but included not only Tavistock therapists, but also therapists from the Cassel Hospital in Richmond. When the full results from both series became available, it now appeared that there was no overall tendency for "first cases" to be successful, but on the other hand, whereas the Cassel therapists *all* did well on their first case, the Tavistock therapists *all* did badly. (The distribution was significant at the 1 percent level, two-tailed test). There are various ways of explaining this observation, but it is probably best regarded as simply due to chance.

The results on the *first series* could be summed up in the following words adapted from *SBP* (p. 274):

The prognosis seems to be most favorable when the patient has a high motivation; the therapist has a high enthusiasm; transference arises early and becomes a major feature of therapy; and grief and anger at termination are important issues.

These conditions seem to contain a single unifying factor of extraordinary simplicity:

That the prognosis is best when there is a willingness on the part of both patient and therapist to become *deeply involved,* and to bear the tension that inevitably ensues.

However, now that the full results on first cases from both series have become available, the evidence for therapeutic *enthusiasm* and hence involvement on the part of the *therapist* is much more doubtful, and this part of the original hypothesis has to be abandoned. On the other hand, evidence about involvement on the part of the *patient* still stands. Clearly, the result that is most strikingly confirmed is that patients do best who *involve themselves by repeating a relation to parents in the transference.*

Nevertheless, the part played by the therapist now returns in the form of a new variable, focality, which is concerned with his ability to keep interpretations on a basic theme. We now can see a rather different unifying factor, which may be introduced as follows:

Every therapist who bases his work with patients on psychoanalytic principles can recognize clinically the characteristics of a therapy that seems to be going well: a patient who has a strong wish to understand himself, who makes clear communications leading to clear understanding and hence to a clear theme for interpretations, who responds to these interpretations with increased communication rather than withdrawal, and finally whose transference feelings are such that they can be clearly interpreted as repeating a relationship from the past.

These features can be summed up in the phrase already used, "successful dynamic interaction." It now appears from the present work that *successful dynamic interaction tends to be associated with favorable outcome.*

SIGNIFICANCE OF THE STUDY AS A WHOLE

The consequences of these observations seem to be as follows:

1. The previous finding is conclusively confirmed that with carefully selected patients the radical rather than the conservative view is correct on all the three main aspects of brief psychotherapy: selection, technique, and outcome; that is, that relatively disturbed patients can be helped toward permanent major changes by a technique that contains all the essential elements of full-scale analysis. Moreover, with these patients, the more radical the technique the more favorable the outcome.

2. Thus, as I have written before (1975), the conservative view of brief psychotherapy—according to which only patients with the most mild and recent illnesses can be helped, the technique should be superficial and should not involve transference interpretations, and

the results are only palliative—has been disproved, and should disappear from the literature, together with the view that the *only* patients suitable for brief psychotherapy are those in crisis.

3. Research support is given to two of the criteria that I have used for many years to select patients for brief psychotherapy, namely (a) that it is possible to formulate a circumscribed focus; and (b) that the patient appears to have the motivation to work with this focus within therapy based on interpretations.

4. Since the central therapeutic mechanism in psychoanalytic therapy, emphasized by so many writers, is the working through of the transference relationship in terms of the relation to people in the patient's past, the fact that the transference/parent link has been shown to have an important relevance to outcome in both series constitutes a *scientific validation in a clinical setting of a fundamental psychoanalytic principle.* To my knowledge this has never happened before.

5. Therefore, these results also offer an indirect validation of the effectiveness of psychoanalytic psychotherapy.

It should be stated here that there are a number of possible fallacies in drawing this kind of conclusion, particularly those arising from problems of interpreting correlations in terms of cause and effect. This whole question is discussed fully in *Toward the Validation of Dynamic Psychotherapy* (Malan, 1976). Nevertheless, the final conclusion is that the validity of psychoanalytic principles and therapy is the *most probable* of the various possible interpretations of the evidence.

6. Finally, an important characteristic of this work has been the use of *clinically meaningful variables* based on *judgments made by experienced clinicians,* which has led in turn to research findings immediately applicable to clinical practice. This should serve to counter some of the despairing opinions about the clinical irrelevance of research expressed by so many leading researchers to Bergin and Strupp (1972). Moreover, the convergence between research and clinical practice will be illustrated clearly in Part IV of the present book, which deals with the clinical principles of brief psychotherapy.

CHAPTER 6

The Psychodynamic Assessment of Outcome

Written in Collaboration with E. H. Rayner, E. S. Heath, H. A. Bacal, and F. H. G. Balfour

---

Before the clinical material is presented it is necessary to give an account of our method of assessing outcome.

Until recently two outstanding features of psychotherapy research have been, first, the lack of impact of research on clinical practice; and, second, the despair about research expressed by many leading workers in the field. My own belief is that both these features are largely due to the failure to devise outcome criteria that do justice to the complexity of the human personality. Obviously, without valid outcome criteria, much of psychotherapy research is meaningless.

I have written extensively in other publications about the problem of assessing outcome on psychodynamic criteria (Malan, 1959, 1963; Malan, Bacal, Heath, and Balfour, 1968, 1975; Malan, 1975) to which the reader is referred for further discussion. Here I shall summarize the principles of the method and go on to discuss its conversion into a rating scale.

In each patient we take the whole evidence provided by the initial assessment material (in the present work, this consisted of the psychiatric interview, projection test, and first therapeutic session), and first try to define a *basic neurotic conflict* that lies at the heart of the patient's difficulties. This is referred to as the *psychodynamic hypothesis*.

These hypotheses are kept relatively simple and are always carefully based on the available evidence. They avoid technical terms as far as possible, and employ only the simplest and most widely accepted aspects of psychodynamic theory. They serve several important and related functions, namely, to define by implication for each patient: (1) a *specific kind of stress* to which he is vulnerable; (2) the main criterion of recovery, which must obviously consist of his ability to overcome his central difficulty, or to face his specific stress and to cope with it in a new way without developing symptoms; and (3) various ways in which he may *appear* to be recovered without actually being so, which mostly consist of *avoiding* his central difficulty or specific stress rather than facing it and overcoming it.

On the basis of this psychodynamic hypothesis, we then define *criteria of maximum improvement*, tailored for each patient, and—like the hypothesis—formulated before the patient is seen for follow-up. Theoretically, of course, a patient's improvement should be formulated in terms of "resolution" of his conflicts, which is the aim of all forms of psychoanalytic therapy. However, this is a concept that is difficult to define, let alone to measure, and it is therefore necessary to fall back on an operational definition based on behavior or feelings that can be observed or described. According to this definition, resolution is assumed to have taken place when "inappropriate" responses, which include especially the inappropriate reaction to specific stresses, do not merely disappear, but are replaced by the corresponding "appropriate" responses.

The final step consists of a comparison of the actual findings at follow-up with the criteria already laid down, and the giving of a global score.

DISCUSSION OF DYNAMIC HYPOTHESES AND CRITERIA OF IMPROVEMENT

The following passage is adapted from our second paper on untreated patients (Malan *et al.*, 1975):

There are two main possible types of objection to our procedure, which come from opposite ends of the theoretical spectrum. The first, from the more strictly scientific and less dynamic approach, may suggest that the hypotheses are too subjective and contain too much unvalidated theory, and that the criteria are based on a series of value judgments that are not made explicit and can only be a matter of opinion. The second, from a more psychoanalytic approach, may suggest that the hypotheses are too superficial, often say nothing about certain causal factors, may ignore overdetermination, and may leave the inner mechanisms of some manifestations of the illness quite unexplained. Both objections are best answered by a description of how our procedure developed.

When we started we tried to make our hypotheses "deeper" and more psychoanalytic in an attempt to answer the second type of criticism. The result was absolutely clear, fully justifying the first type of criticism: The independent judges imposed their own theoretical bias on the material, often producing hypotheses that had little in common with one another. The policy that we then needed to adopt in reaching a consensus became equally clear: The amount of theory had to be reduced to the point at which agreement could be reached, and the final result was the *highest common factor* among all the hypotheses that had been made independently. In fact this process coincided exactly with the universal scientific principle of keeping the hypotheses as close as possible to the available evidence.

As far as the criteria are concerned, we accept unashamedly that they contain value judgments, which we believe cannot be avoided. This was discussed at some length in *SBP* (see pp. 49–50). We can only say in the end that since the evidence is published in detail any reader is free to formulate his own hypotheses and criteria, and with these as a basis, to make his own judgments of improvement.

A Note on the Dynamic Hypotheses in the Present Series. An important question is whether two teams working independently— which was the situation in the present work—can reach similar hypotheses. Unfortunately this cannot be fairly tested. The reason is that the accounts of interviews were written on special forms in which the interviewer was asked to put forward his own views about the patient's psychopathology. Thus, any judge was immediately able to base his hypothesis on that of the interviewer, and it is not surprising that on the whole the hypotheses made by the two teams should have borne a strong resemblance to one another.

It also needs to be said that the hypotheses given in the clinical material as presented here are those made by Team 1, Malan and Rayner. Being members of the workshop, we were often contaminated by knowledge of subsequent events. I do not believe this matters. We were very careful to base our hypotheses on the evidence available from the initial assessment material only. Moreover, we have demonstrated on two other and larger series (forty-five untreated patients, fifty-five group patients) that relevant hypotheses that make the assessment of follow-up meaningful can be made by judges who are entirely blind to subsequent events.

THE OUTCOME SCALE

In *SBP* the scale used (see p. 50) consisted of the four points 0, 1, 2, and 3. In the present work this scale has been extended and refined to include (a) a score of 4, (b) half-points, and (c) negative scores where the patient was judged to be "worse." As described in chapter 9, the final score was taken as the mean of four independent judgments. Since the minimum interval in the scale used by each judge was half a point, the minimum interval on the final scale was one half divided by four, or one eighth of a point (0.125).

It needs to be emphasized that patients are so diverse and so complicated that the scale has to be used in an essentially intuitive manner, in which the changes are fed into the computer of clinical judgment, are weighted and integrated, and finally emerge as a global judgment of "improvement" in the form of a single score. For this reason, requests for schedules of the scoring system, which we fairly often receive, can only be met by a series of clinical examples. Nevertheless, our experience has been that psychoanalytically trained research workers have little difficulty in grasping the principles, and can achieve reasonable agreement after practice on no more than three or four cases.

Clinical Example.   The system is best illustrated by a type of case that occurs quite frequently, namely, a patient suffering from:

1. Symptoms;
2. Problems concerned with rivalry, hostility, or self-assertion, in relation to people of the same sex; and
3. Problems of full closeness and sexual satisfaction in relation to the opposite sex.

The best example in the brief therapy series is the Pesticide Chemist, who suffered from:

1. Obsessional anxiety about work;
2. Inability to assert himself at work in such a way as to get his legitimate needs met; and
3. Emotional withdrawal from his wife, together with lack of sexual satisfaction on both sides.

The hypothesis made on the basis of the initial assessment material was approximately correct, but was expressed less clearly than what emerged during therapy, namely that (1) he felt resentful about having responsibility put on him; (2) he felt guilty about this resentment and afraid of expressing it; and therefore (3) defended himself by an exaggerated preoccupation with meeting the demands of others, a position that he could not maintain. The criteria for full "resolution" follow more or less automatically if the three main disturbances are replaced by the corresponding appropriate feelings and behavior.

We may now examine various hypothetical situations that might be found at follow-up, and the scores for them:

1. The only change observed is *loss of obsessional preoccupation*, but this has clearly been bought at the price of emotional disengagement from his work, and is accompanied by some loss of efficiency. This is a clear-cut false solution and scores 0.

2. The only change is *loss of obsessional preoccupation*, but there is apparently no disengagement or loss of efficiency. The mechanism of such a change would be obscure, but the result would definitely be something of value. This is a standard situation: loss of symptoms without other detectable changes. The score is 1.0 and no more, no matter what the severity of the original symptoms had been.

3. The patient is now found to be able to *demand his rights at work in a constructive and effective way, and his obsessional preoccupations have disappeared. There is no change in the relation with his wife.* This also is a standard situation: apparently genuine "resolution" of the problem with the same sex, accompanied by loss of symptoms, but no change in the problem with the opposite sex. Because of our emphasis on the importance of close relations with the opposite sex, this scores 2.0 and no more, leaving two whole points for further improvement in this latter problem.

4. This is the situation actually found at follow-up: *All the changes described in 3 had occurred, but in addition there was some limited improvement in the relation with his wife* (see Assessment and Therapy Form for details). All four judges scored 2.5.

5. A score of 3.0 would be given for "substantial resolution" in the problem with his wife as well, but with some important reservations: 3.5 if there were few reservations; and 4.0 if there were hardly any.

Once more it must be emphasized that although many of the types of change described above represent standard situations found in practice, the changes do not necessarily occur in any clear-cut sequence; and the scale cannot under any circumstances be regarded as one in which half a point is awarded for such and such a change, one point for another, etc., and these points are summed to give a final score. The scale is intuitive and global and represents simply the number of points out of a maximum of 4 that a judge awards to the changes found, when these are weighted and compared with the criteria laid down beforehand.

As already stated, when the final score is the mean of four judgments, it rises in intervals of one eighth of a point, or 0.125. Comparison with verbal judgments of improvement suggests the following rough correspondences:

0–0.5	essentially unchanged
0.625–1.875	slightly to moderately improved
2.0–2.75	improved
2.875–3.375	much improved
3.5–4.0	recovered

A study of our actual cases suggests that any score below 2.0 is not really satisfactory, and thus therapies can be arbitrarily divided into "successful" (≥ 2.0) and "unsuccessful" (< 2.0).

Clinical Meaning of the Scale. The scale has *grown* out of the necessity for treating the outcome of psychotherapy statistically, and some of its properties need to be examined, together with the mental processes involved in arriving at a score.

Introspection suggests that a judge naturally makes his measurement from the end that is nearest, i.e.; (1) toward the lower end of the scale he mainly bases his score on *degree of improvement*; while (2) as he approaches the upper end he is to a greater and greater extent influenced (in the opposite direction) by *residual disturbance*. This subtle alteration is reflected in the frequently used qualitative scale by a transition in the phrasing, from "much improved" to "recovered." Toward the lower end, therefore, the scale measures "improvement," whereas toward the upper end it tends to measure "mental health." Nevertheless, it is not a true mental health scale like the Health–Sickness Rating Scale used by the Menninger workers, in which there is room for differences in *initial* as well as final scores (Luborsky, 1962; Kernberg, Burstein, Coyne, Appelbaum, Horwitz, and Voth, 1972). In our scale, as in the Menninger Absolute Global Change Scale, all patients start from zero, and the extent of possible change is encompassed by the same number of points no matter what the severity of the initial pathology. This means, for instance, that possible improvements in the severe pathology of such patients as the Stationery Manufacturer and Dress Designer have to be compressed into the same range as those in the relatively mild pathology of the Almoner and Gibson Girl (see Assessment and Therapy Forms). This disadvantage has to be accepted.*

Although, therefore, scales of this kind contain less information than mental health scales, they have one important advantage. This is that they avoid a statistical artifact that otherwise has to be eliminated by various sophisticated mathematical techniques: namely, that where there is room for more change because of the more severe initial disturbances, an inevitable statistical result is that the more severely ill patients tend to show greater improvement, and hence, apparently, a better prognosis—which contradicts clinical common sense. For a discussion of these issues in the Menninger study, see Kernberg *et al.* (1972, pp. 20–39, 35, and 249–50).

RELIABILITY

Although this is a subject that is not likely to arouse any great passions and may well be passed over by the reader who wishes to commence with more interesting matters, it in fact contains a result of almost incalculable importance. This is that the inter-rater reliability for our judgments of outcome has always been satisfactory and most of the time has been strikingly high. In a sense this could be said to be the most important result presented in this book, because it points forward to the proper scientific study of all kinds of psychotherapy, whereas the present work is concerned only with a particular type of patient and a particular type of therapy. Since the opinion has always been widely accepted that such judgments are so subjective and unreliable as not to be worth attempting, this would be publishable in its own right even if the result of our whole study had been entirely null.

The two teams worked in slightly different ways. The contaminated Team 1 (DM and ER) never modified their independent scores after discussion; the blind Team 2 (HB and EH or FB) sometimes did so. Inter-rater reliability between the two members of Team 2 therefore has little meaning. Also whereas Dr. Bacal, the first member of Team 2, remained throughout the study and scored all thirty patients, Dr. Heath left for Canada after scoring nine patients, and was then replaced by Mr. Balfour.

---

* An attempt, probably misguided, to compensate for this was made for the Stationery Manufacturer by one of the judges (DHM), by extending the scale to include a score of 5. In fact this probably just resulted in an overvaluation of outcome in this particular patient.

Counting the composite judge EH/FB as a single judge, this gives five meaningful inter-rater reliabilities. These varied from $r = +0.67$ to $r = +0.82$ with a mean of $r = +0.76$. Perhaps more important, the reliability between the mean of the contaminated Team 1 and that of the blind Team 2 was $r = +0.83$. Comparison of the actual scores on the individual patients (Mean Team 1/Mean Team 2) showed the following:

1. For twenty-one patients (70 percent) the difference was half a point or less.

2. For two patients the difference was more than half a point and less than one point.

3. For five patients the difference was one point.

4. For two patients the difference was more than one point (1.125 and 1.5, respectively).

We can now add to these reliabilities those obtained in our long-term follow-up study of patients who had had group treatment at the Tavistock Clinic (Malan, Balfour, Hood, and Shooter, 1976). In this study, also with four independent judges, two of whom were the same as in the present study, inter-rater reliability varied from $r = +0.73$ to $r = +0.83$ with a mean of $r = +0.80$; and the blind/contaminated reliability (usually based on the mean of two judgments in each case) was $+0.89$ ($N = 51$). Thus, the satisfactory agreement obtained in the present study has been not merely repeated but increased.

The generally high values for the inter-rater reliability go some way toward justifying the statistical studies described in *SBP*. These were based on my own single-handed judgments, which now have been shown in two other series to agree to a considerable extent with those of five independent judges. (My own inter-rater reliabilities with these judges have varied from $r = +0.70$ to $r = +0.82$, mean $r = +0.78$.).

Here I should add the following important notes:

1. For eight of the thirty patients one or other member of Team 1 (DM or ER) was the therapist. One might suppose that these judges would have an unconscious interest in scoring their own patients more highly. In fact in only two cases was the score given by the therapist higher than the mean given by the other three judges, in one it was equal, and in the other five it was lower. Whatever this means it is at least good public relations!

2. It needs to be asked whether the scores are in accord with clinical judgment. My short answer to this question is yes; and moreover, where clinical judgment suggests the possibility of reconsi-

dering a score in a particular situation, the result is usually a strengthening of the important correlations.

3. In some cases we have follow-ups later than those on which the scores are based. Again, in almost all cases, the result is to strengthen the correlations. The most important example of this is the Contralto (not included in the present book). At the time of assessing her follow-up, she was still continuing her analysis, and improvements seemed to be minimal. Because the initial stages of her therapy were highly dynamic, she stands out as a glaring exception in several of the important correlations, making a considerable negative contribution. However, she has since completed her analysis with apparently major benefit, and if her probable new score of 3.0 to 3.5 were introduced, this would strengthen the correlations and eliminate her anomalous position altogether. The same applies—though to a much smaller extent—to the most anomalous patient of all, the Dress Designer, who has shown certain improvements since the follow-up on which her score is based.

These considerations can only strengthen one's belief in the clinical meaning of the conclusions reached.

Finally, it is worth comparing our reliabilities with those obtained in the Menninger study. Their outcome measure most relevant to ours is the scale of Global Change (see Kernberg et al., 1972, p. 219), which was rated by two judges using the method of paired comparisons in overlapping batches of twelve patients, and which contained a maximum of twenty-two points that could be awarded by each judge to each patient. They obtained an average rank order reliability of $\rho = +0.93$ at termination and $\rho = +0.74$ at follow-up. Thus, our reliabilities and theirs appear to be of much the same order of magnitude.

When I met Dr. Kernberg at the meeting of the Society for Psychotherapy Research in Philadelphia in 1973, he said that he regarded the problem of measuring outcome on psychodynamic criteria as essentially solved, and I could only agree with him.

CHAPTER 7

Criteria for Rejection

This is an important chapter for two main reasons. First, it gives a detailed account of the criteria that we used for judging that patients were *unsuitable* for our kind of brief psychotherapy, which, from a clinical point of view, is as important a subject as the criteria used for judging them to be suitable. Here it needs to be said that since in general we did not take such patients on, our rejection criteria have not been properly tested out and are based essentially on clinical common sense. Second, this chapter defines the characteristics of the sample of patients whom we did take on, a preliminary step that is essential to creating a situation in which statistical analysis can become meaningful.

Although much of our own selection procedure was not fully thought out at the time, the following retrospective analysis shows that it was in fact based on clear-cut principles.

Patients were brought for discussion to the workshop at two main stages. The first was the *referral stage*, before the patient was seen, when the information available would consist of an application form and/or a report from a referring agency. At this stage certain types of patient were never considered. The following list of "excluding factors" is taken from the work of H. P. Hildebrand (unpublished), who has introduced it into the screening process for patients applying to the London Clinic of Psycho-analysis:

> Serious suicidal attempts
> Drug addiction
> Convinced homosexuality
> Long-term hospitalization

More than one course of E.C.T.
Chronic alcoholism
Incapacitating chronic obsessional symptoms
Incapacitating chronic phobic symptoms
Gross destructive or self-destructive acting out

On the other hand, certain positive criteria were used at this stage, which were thought to constitute a *prima facie* case for brief therapy. The underlying principle here was the search for a *discernible simplicity* that, it was hoped, would lead to the possibility of discovering a "focus." By a focus is meant, as always, a unifying theme that can be made the basis of interpretations.

This simplicity might mean (1) simplicity of complaints (though we were quite aware that it was naïve to suppose this necessarily implied simplicity of pathology); (2) apparent simplicity of current issues in the patient's life; or (3) the appearance of symptoms in relation to some definite precipitating event. These three often came together in the form of a *current or recent crisis*, which in fact was present in a high proportion both of patients finally accepted and of those accepted for interview and then rejected. This might or might not imply *recent onset*, and it does not introduce as much bias into the sample as might be supposed, since there must always be some reason why a patient seeks treatment at one particular point in time rather than any other.

The second stage at which the patient might be brought for discussion was the *interview stage*. This happened when a member of the workshop, on the lookout for suitable patients, felt that he had found a *prima facie* case in a patient already seen in routine consultation. Here the *prima facie* case might include the factors mentioned above, but in addition it could now be based more firmly on knowledge of the pathology, the degree of contact and response to interpretation, and the interviewer's ability to think of a possible focus. If accepted at this stage the patient would go on to *projection test*.

Once the full initial assessment, consisting of interview and projection test, had been completed, the members of the workshop were in a position to project themselves into the future and to undertake an imaginary therapy. It must be emphasized (1) that this can only be done with extensive experience of what actually happens in analytically oriented psychotherapy; and (2) that since our experience was mainly with long-term methods, it was much easier to forecast what would happen in those patients who would need long-

TABLE 3. Types of Event Forecast in Rejected Patients

Event forecast	Specific danger
1. Inability to make contact.	
2. Necessity for prolonged work in order to generate motivation for treatment.	Inability to start effective therapeutic work within a short
3. Necessity for prolonged work in order to penetrate rigid defenses.	time.
4. Inevitable involvement in complex or deep-seated issues that there seems no hope of working through in a short time.	Inability to terminate.
5. Severe dependence or other forms of unfavorable intense transference.	
6. Intensification of depressive or psychotic disturbance.	Depressive or psychotic breakdown.

term therapy, i.e., easier in those whom we rejected than those whom we accepted.

An analysis of patients interviewed, brought up for discussion, and rejected, shows that the negative criteria that we used can be formulated quite specifically. They consist essentially of various aspects of *inability to find a feasible focus*, which may mean either (1) inability to see any focus or unifying theme for interpretations at all; or (2), with emphasis on the word "feasible," that a unifying theme can be seen but will involve certain specific dangers if an attempt is made to use it in brief therapy. These dangers are summarized in Table 3.

It is so important to convey the basis on which this kind of prediction was made that it seems worthwhile to describe our rejected patients in some detail. I have succeeded in collecting nineteen on whom full information is available, and details are shown in Table 4. The "implied predictions" have been formulated retrospectively by myself from transcripts of summaries of workshop discussions recorded at the time. These predictions are summarized in Table 5.

It must be emphasized once more that our predictions of failure of brief therapy in these rejected patients were never directly tested. Yet, a partial test by implication can come from a study of what happened in those patients whom we accepted and treated. In none of these did nothing of importance happen; in none was contact never made or only made after months of apparently fruitless work; only one patient was worse at follow-up, while all of the others were at least slightly

TABLE 4. Details of Patients Rejected for Brief Psychotherapy

Patient	Referral	Complaint (duration)	Prima facie case for brief psychotherapy	Details	Implied prediction	Summary of reasons for rejection
Miss Ca. 39 Art teacher	Request for urgent appointment by G.P.	Recently caught stealing.	Current crisis. Deeply felt tears at interview when she spoke of her adoptive mother's death.	1. She only discovered at 21 that she had been adopted at the age of 14 months. 2. The inference was that she had been severely deprived, which included a period in the hospital, in the first 14/12 of her life. 3. Inadequacy of supporting background; apparently she had no real current relationships. 4. Workshop couldn't find a focus.	Any attempt at dealing with the presenting symptoms would become involved in problems of early deprivation. Dependence on the therapist would be marked, with no person in the patient's outside life to deflect it onto.	No focus. Deep-seated problem (severe childhood deprivation). Inadequate current support. Likelihood of intense dependent transference.
Mr. Cr.	By Tavistock-trained (woman) G.P.	The G.P. was in difficulties over treating the wife for frigidity. The patient has no complaints of his own.	None; referral only.	1. An extremely well-defended patient with no complaints of his own. 2. The projection test suggested latent homosexuality.	It would be a difficult task to get him to want therapy for himself at all. If this was successful it seemed likely that deep-seated homosexuality would be exposed.	No motivation. Deep-seated problem (latent homosexuality).
Mr. D. 41 Salesman	By G.P. currently in Tavistock seminar.	Leg fetishism (as long as he can remember).	Good basic personality. High motivation. Marked response to interpretation.	1. His parents quarrelled constantly and were eventually divorced. His own sexual upbringing, at the hands of his father, was extremely strict.	Although a possible focus could be seen in the patient's homosexuality and his confusion about his mother's sex, the fetishism is well recognized to be complex and to be in-	Chronic, deep-seated problem. Although a focus can be seen, analysis, which was possible in practice, was the treatment of choice.

70

tractable even in analysis, and it seemed a long shot to expect brief therapy to help.

2. His mother was very proud of her legs and used to stroke them.

3. Besides his fetish, he is excited by watching courting couples and by exhibiting his penis.

4. The interviewer felt there was a strong homosexual component, and that a focus could be found in the patient's bisexuality. (There were factors that might have led him to be confused about the sex of his mother).

Miss Da. 39 Secretary	By Tavistock-trained G.P. with a view to brief therapy.	Attacks of nausea, vomiting, dizziness, for 2 years, since the first anniversary of the death of her father.	Referral for brief therapy. Recent onset in relation to a specific event.	That it would be extremely difficult to get her to accept treatment at all; and that if any progress was made it would lead to very complex and deep-seated issues, and probably severe disturbances that could probably only be dealt with in analysis, if at all.

1. The whole interview was characterized by denial of there being anything wrong, of her own badness, of her need for help, of having any sexual or other human feelings. The interviewer commented on her "tiresome saintliness."

2. She had been extremely close to her father, whom she had nursed through 5 years of illness.

3. She had the almost delusional feeling that her mother knew everything she was doing.

4. Severe Oedipal problems would provide a clear focus,

Severe psychopathology. Poor contact. Poor motivation.

Continued

TABLE 4. (Continued)

Patient	Referral	Complaint (duration)	Prima facie case for brief psychotherapy	Details	Implied prediction	Summary of reasons for rejection
				but she showed no wish to give up her denial and little response to interpretation. 5. The Rorschach showed a split between (a) a world inside herself in which everything is beautiful, feminine, and idealized and (b) a world felt to be outside herself, masculine, violent, unpleasant. Responses were almost bizarre in the use of fantasy. Borderline paranoid condition diagnosed. Any stress situation that threatened this split might lead to a breakdown. 6. She was relieved when told psychotherapy was not the right treatment for her.		
Mrs. Du. 21 Housewife	By G.P.	Vaginismus after 2 years marriage; marriage in effect unconsummated although she	Current crisis. She is full of intense feeling that she cannot speak of but can express in	1. There was a deprived background—neither parent seemed to be interested in children. Her brother is delinquent. Her husband is the only good relationship she has ever had.	It is not impossible that this patient could have been helped by brief therapy, using the focus of trying to help her to express her feelings verbally: but with such a patient a direct physical ap-	No real focus.

	has had a baby. Recently returned to U.K.	writing	2. She was unable to tell stories to the O.R.T. 3. The only possible focus seemed to be to help her to express feelings directly to another human being, which was felt to be too ill-defined.	proach would seem much more appropriate. In fact she was referred to a Balint-trained gynecologist who examined her physically, prescribed some lubricant, and advised her about the best positions for intercourse. Soon after this the patient wrote that she had had successful intercourse and did not consider she needed further treatment.	No focus.
Mrs. Go. ? age	By woman G.P. who had been treating her.	Travel phobia (2/12).	Recent onset. Marked response to interpretation of her need for self-control.	1. Marked dependence (probably homosexual) on G.P. 2. Patient went into resistance when treatment was discussed (probably because she was afraid of losing the G.P.). 3. Her phobia makes it difficult for her to attend as an outpatient. 4. It was not clear what impulses she needed to control, and the interviewer could not think of a focus. "I hoped the projection test would suggest one" (but it didn't).	There would be difficulty over both the transfer from her G.P. and getting her to attend. If this was successfully achieved therapy would probably become involved in intense and complicated feelings, including problems of dependence.	
Mr. Gr.	By Tavistock-	Being upset by criticism, leading-	None. Referral only. Re-	1. The interpretation that he responded to was that he felt	Since there was no discernible focus, therapy could only	No focus. Severe psychopathology (?schizophrenia).

Continued

73

TABLE 4. (Continued)

Patient	Referral	Complaint (duration)	Prima facie case for brief psychotherapy	Details	Implied prediction	Summary of reasons for rejection
	trained G.P. with a view to brief psychotherapy.	ing to depression and migraine.	sponded well to interpretation.	like an adolescent, neither a schoolboy nor an adult. 2. The interviewer was quite unable to get an idea of the psychopathology. 3. Test: Highly resistant, concrete thinking, unable to tell stories to O.R.T., sorted Rorschach cards according to their "obscurity"—suspicion of schizophrenia.	aim at exposing his deeper feelings, which would almost certainly result in intensification of his psychosis.	
Miss L. 34 Public relations officer to an industrial firm	By Tavistocktrained G.P.	She consulted her G.P. for frequent menstruation. It then emerged that she was unable to form deep and lasting relations with men.	No real positive criteria.	1. An outstandingly beautiful girl who had had 14 offers of marriage. 2. She had great difficulty in communicating—she was apparently unaware of deeper feelings. 3. Factors seemed to be (a) a longing for her mother's interest, (b) an inability to mourn her bad-tempered father. 4. There was clearly no definite focus. 5. She had little therapeutic drive or understanding of what treatment is about.	That it would take a long time, against considerable resistance, to enable this girl to face any deeper feelings at all; and it would need a long working through of a transference relationship to help her over her main problem. In fact what happened was that she was taken into group treatment, where she showed very little capacity to talk about anything beneath the surface, and broke off treatment within a few months.	No focus. Poor contact. Poor motivation.

Mrs. M.₁ 28 Teacher	By Tavistock-trained G.P.	G.P. had seen the husband, who had asked in passing if anything could be done about his wife's unwillingness to have children.	None in particular, except clear-cut problem seriously affecting her marital life.	1. She married 6 years ago and told her husband then that she did not want to have children, which he accepted. He has now changed his mind, and is pressing her to have children. 2. At interview this seemed to be a very chronic, depressive problem. The patient said she felt like an empty shell; and that if she didn't have treatment, life would hold nothing for her.	Therapy would rapidly become involved in deep-seated depressive problems that only a long analysis would be likely to help.	Severe depressive psychopathology. Severe dependence.
Miss M.₂ 28 Secretary	By G.P.	Tunes in her head (4/12).	Recent onset.	1. Her mother, who died 4 years ago, was given a terrible life by her father, who was dirty and financially irresponsible. 2. She said at interview that she couldn't stand men who were sloppy, and suddenly realized then the connection with her father. 3. She shares music in common with her father. 4. She financed her sister's wedding because her father wouldn't do so, but now resents doing so. 5. She shows a pattern of allowing other women to steal men who are interested in her. The interviewer sus-	That her vindictiveness was deep-seated and would probably lead to a malignant clinging to the therapist, which would require prolonged working through; and that if this was penetrated, severe depressive problems would emerge.	Severe psychopathology (depressive and obsessional). Poor motivation.

Continued

TABLE 4. (Continued)

Patient	Referral	Complaint (duration)	Prima facie case for brief psychotherapy	Details	Implied prediction	Summary of reasons for rejection
				pected a homosexual element in this. 6. There was thus an obvious focus in terms of the relation with her father, but she seemed to be a lifelong depressive and obsessional character, full of vindictiveness, and was openly skeptical of anyone trying to help her.		
Mr. Na.	By psychiatrist.	Anxiety attacks and feeling that he is about to lose consciousness; 10 years, especially bad in last 3 years.	Onset of symptoms in relation to specific event.	1. His symptoms started at about the time he returned from the war and found that his wife had left him, presumably for another man, though he never verified this. 2. He remarried 8 years ago but he and his wife have not been able to have any children. 3. Sexual relations with the second wife are much less satisfactory than with the first. 4. He remembered practically nothing before the age of 13 and could give little informa-	That it would take a long time to penetrate his defenses of denial and obsessional rumination.	Severe psychopathology (weak ego, strong defenses, danger of depression).

			tion about relations in his family. 5. He was very unsophisticated psychologically, but showed the beginnings of being able to relate symptoms to feelings. 6. Projection test (ORT): Ego weak; well-defended ruminatory obsessional, focal problem of potency difficulties felt to be optimistic; real danger of depression. 7. The actual disposal was to group treatment, in which he stayed for 3 years. There was gradual lessening of both his defensiveness and his symptoms.	? No focus. Intense sexual transference.
Miss Ni. 26 Secretary	By G.P.	Two attacks of abdominal pain and diarrhea 6-7/52 ago.	Acute and recent symptoms clearly reactive to her relation with a married man. Clear focus. 1. She had a very bad relation with her father, who has never shown any affection. She was close to her mother. 2. She showed a pattern of forming relations with men who ill-treat her. 3. She has only had orgasm once, when a man was trying to rape her. 4. There was a highly seductive transference at interview, but this was thought quite likely to be a "false sexuality" masking sexual anxieties.	A possible focus might be violent feelings against men, but it was felt that (1) it would be a long task to penetrate her false sexuality, and (2) the result would be to become involved in very complex issues. This was later confirmed by information obtained at follow-up.

TABLE 4. (Continued)

Patient	Referral	Complaint (duration)	Primia facie case for brief psychotherapy	Details	Implied prediction	Summary of reasons for rejection
				5. Test (ORT): There was a continual shift in stories from men to women and back again, the two rarely being brought together. Though she did not appear to be very ill, her pathology seemed to be complex, and no focal issue emerged. 6. She was finally rejected on the grounds that the sadomasochistic transference that would develop would need a long working through. 7. Follow-up (7 years 11/12): She was still in relation with same married man. She still has sadomasochistic relations with men. She now has a symptom of preoccupation with her bowels for which she sought treatment 1 year ago. What had precipitated her coming here originally had been the fear that a Tampax had got lost in her vagina.		

Miss R. 23	By psychiatrist.	A few months ago she was told she had an "innocent" heart murmur, and since then she had not been able to get out of her mind that there is something wrong with her heart.	Recent onset.	1. Other complaints: (a) the feeling that she cannot face life, especially when she first wakes up. (b) Refusal of food; vomiting. 2. She was full of self-reproaches at interview. 3. She showed a long-standing pattern of overcompensating for strong dependent feelings. She feels her parents have not allowed her to live her own life. 4. A clear focus might be guilt about anger with her parents, but there was little response to interpretations about this. 5. Diagnosis: fairly severe depression. 6. Action: admitted to hospital.	That the only possible focus, guilt about anger with her parents, would lead into deeply depressive feelings, quite possibly accompanied by a depressive breakdown.	Poor contact. Severe psychopathology (depression). Dependence.
Miss Se.₁ 24 Student nurse	By psychologically minded G.P. with a view to possible brief psychotherapy.	Two attacks of physical symptoms (shivering, pain, numbness) in last 3/12.	Acute and recent onset.	1. Her upbringing, on the Continent of Europe, was much disturbed by the war and her father's infidelity. Her parents divorced when she was 8. She is engaged to be married but her fiancé asks repeatedly for postponement. The patient has recently been frigid. 2. She showed *belle indifference* at interview with no response to interpretation.	That it would take a very long time to penetrate the *belle indifference* and that if this was successfully done, primitive dependent transference would emerge, with no effective support in the patient's outside life.	No focus. Primitive dependence.

Continued

TABLE 4. (Continued)

Patient	Referral	Complaint (duration)	Prima facie case for brief psychotherapy	Details	Implied prediction	Summary of reasons for rejection
				3. There were indications of primitive dependent transference. 4. Our judgment was of a diffuse illness, with no focus definable.		
Miss Se.₂ 23 Teacher	By G.P. to a psychiatrist at another hospital who referred her for psychotherapy to the Tavistock Clinic.	Longstanding homosexual feelings. When her fiancé recently returned from overseas, she confessed these to him and he insisted on her seeing a doctor.	Current crisis.	1. Her mother died when she was 12 and her father remarried when she was 14. She had a poor relation with her stepmother. 2. She has tried to like men and last year became engaged. She had intercourse but was disgusted afterward. When her fiancé returned she found she couldn't stand him. 3. A recurrent dream of sexual assault by her father provides a possible focus. 4. But at test she appeared to be defending herself against deep feelings, with fear of complete breakdown (story of a house in danger of falling off a cliff). 5. Both at consultation, and	That it would be very difficult to penetrate to deep feelings, and that if this were successful, there would be a danger of breakdown. The homosexuality was probably more than just Oedipal in origin. (In fact the patient was taken into a group, in which she made little progress and eventually went abroad. She wrote twice from abroad asking to be referred to psychiatrists there.)	Poor contact. Deep-seated problem (female homosexuality).

Miss Si. 35 Hospital sister	A friend persuaded the G.P. to refer her to a workshop member, and the patient spontaneously rang up asking for treatment.	Patient had recently broken off a 6-year affair with a man.	Recent crisis.	in test, contact decreased as the interview went on. 6. Marked dissociation between fantasy and real life. 1. Choice of work thought to be an overcompensation for destructive impulses. 2. No actual internal crisis discernible. 3. Disturbed Rorschach with two paranoid responses.	It would be necessary (1) to interpret her defense of overcompensation, and then (2) to deal with primitive destructive feelings in the transference over a long period.	No focus. Severe psychopathology.
Mr. T. 27 (Pakistani)	By Tavistock-trained G.P. "clearly a long-term case."	Premature ejaculation (married 11/12).	Current crisis. Good contact at interview. Problem seemed clearly concerned with his conflict with his father.	1. Failed to attend for test first time. 2. Test (second appointment) showed marked impoverishment of relationships. Patient not interested in sex for his own sake; women demand it. 3. Doubts about sincerity of motivation.	The implication here was that the premature ejaculation was part of a general impoverishment of relationships to women, which it would be very difficult to deal with in long-term, let alone in brief psychotherapy.	Deep-seated problem. Poor motivation.
Mrs. W. 28 Solicitor's wife	? By G.P.	Kleptomania (3 years).	Current crisis.	1. Her husband is mean with money and the marital relation has deteriorated; stealing is most marked from her husband. The patient herself won't spend money.	Any attempt to deal with the presenting symptom would quickly become involved in problems of early deprivation.	No focus. Deep-seated problem.

Continued

TABLE 4. (Continued)

Patient	Referral	Complaint (duration)	Prima facie case for brief psychotherapy	Details	Implied prediction	Summary of reasons for rejection
Miss Y. 24 Secretary	By physician who noticed on several occasions that she had been drinking.	Depressed 18/12 since abortion. Nervous 7/12 since breaking off engagement.	Acute and recent onset in response to life events.	2. Insecure childhood, parents eventually divorced; mother alcoholic. 1. There was a background of conflict with her father and little contact with her mother. 2. She had been engaged to a man who got her pregnant but then wouldn't marry her. 3. The patient has recently been drinking heavily. 4. Motivation seemed to come from others. 5. The patient was very guarded and there was no contact at interview. 6. The patient was ½ hour late for test; there was little content in her stories; a deep feeling of unworthiness; probably pregenital problems; impoverished ego.	That contact would be very difficult to make and it would be difficult to hold the patient in treatment; and that even if both these were successful the therapist would eventually become involved in deep-seated depressive problems.	Poor contact. Severe, probably depressive, psychopathology. Poor motivation.

82

TABLE 5. Summary of Implied Predictions in Rejected Patients

Patient	Inability to make contact	Prolonged work to generate motivation	Prolonged work to penetrate rigid defenses	Inevitable involvement in complex or deep-seated issues	Severe dependence or other unfavorable transference
Miss Ca.				+	+
Mr. Cr.		+		+	
Mr. D.				+	
Miss Da.		+		+	
Mrs. Du.					
Mrs. Go.		+		+	+
Mr. Gr.					
Miss L.			+		
Mrs. $M_{.1}$				+	
Miss $M_{.2}$				+	+
Mr. Na.			+		
Miss Ni.			+	+	
Miss R.					
Miss $Se_{.1}$		+			+
Miss $Se_{.2}$			+		
Miss Si.			+		+
Mr. T.			+		
Mrs. W.				+	+
Miss Y.	+	+		+	

improved; in only one of those followed up had there been a suicidal attempt or evidence for hitherto undetected borderline disturbance (both of these events occurred in a single patient, Mr. Upton); only two patients (Mr. Upton and the Dress Designer) were admitted to the hospital; and although eight therapies could not be terminated within forty sessions, all but two were terminated within one hundred sessions; and of these two, one was eventually strikingly successful. Indeed, no patient at follow-up showed total relapse from the position achieved at termination, and many showed marked further improvement. It therefore seems reasonable to suppose that many of the specific dangers included in our implied predictions were in fact eliminated in our selection procedure.

Nevertheless, the differences between accepted and rejected patients were subtle and amounted to no more than a matter of degree. They are best presented as the following negative statements: No patient was accepted with whom practically *no* contact could be made;

who had *hardly any* motivation for treatment; with whom the workshop could see no *conceivable* focus, however dimly; or with whom
nobody—especially not even the therapist—believed there was the
slightest chance of success.

When these statements have been made, however, there were
several patients accepted who were generally believed to be unsuitable, and who were taken on to test our predictions that therapy would
fail. Probably the least suitable according to our criteria was the
Playwright (not included in the present book), of whom the psychologist wrote, "This is most definitely not a focal problem but a chronic
character problem." Here, nevertheless, it was felt worthwhile to use
the current crisis to see if something could be achieved; but the
patient was thought basically unsuitable and the statement was
specifically made that the long-term aim was analysis.

A situation that sometimes developed was that the workshop
member who had seen the patient thought that he could see a possible
focus, against the overwhelming skepticism of the rest of the workshop; and he was then encouraged to go ahead in order to test the
overall prediction of failure. This happened most clearly (1) in the
Stationery Manufacturer, where the summary of the discussion states,
"The general feeling was that this was outside the framework of the
workshop," and where the therapist's optimism was spectacularly
vindicated; and (2) in the Receptionist, where the summary states,
"We all have the impression that this is not a focal therapy case," and
where the improvement achieved was much more limited.

In two other severely disturbed patients who were accepted, the
possibility of breakdown was clearly envisaged; but it was felt that
this could be avoided either by keeping the focus superficial (Mrs.
Morley) or by exploring very carefully and gradually (the Military
Policeman). In both cases the implied prediction was fulfilled.

Thus, the characteristics of our sample of accepted patients can be
relatively simply defined, as follows:

Some contact had been made and there was some response to
interpretation.

Some conceivable focus could be seen.

The dangers (see Table 3) of attempting brief therapy did not
seem inevitable.

CHAPTER 8

The Clinical Material

I have chosen eighteen case histories to illustrate the types of patient selected, the techniques used, the changes found at follow-up, and the method of assessing outcome. These have been chosen as follows:

1. Six successful brief therapies with relatively healthy patients: In three, the Buyer, the Gibson Girl, and the Indian Scientist, the focus was Oedipal; in the Almoner and the Pesticide Chemist, the main problem seemed to be concerned with self-assertion, the first clearly in an Oedipal setting, while the second received a number of interpretations about anal impulses; and finally, the Zoologist suffered from a pattern of self-destructive anger when he was let down by people he loved (his therapy is considered in detail in chap. 12). All these examples show one or more of the following features: high motivation, high focality, and a high emphasis on transference/parent interpretations, thus illustrating the patterns that tend to be found in successful brief therapies.

2. Two successful brief therapies with more disturbed patients, in which the focus was deliberately kept superficial: In the Stationery Manufacturer, who suffered from severe paranoid jealousy, the focus was confined to a carefully circumscribed area of the Oedipus complex. This is the best example of the focal technique and is considered in detail in chap. 14. The other example was Mrs. Morley, who was thought to be in danger of a severe depressive breakdown. Therapy consisted basically of no more than pointing out her possessive relation with her grown-up daughter.

3. Three therapies in which early termination became impossible, but where the ultimate outcome after medium-term therapy (forty to one hundred sessions) was favorable. I think it is true to say that in

none of these cases could the necessity for longer therapy have been foreseen. Hindsight suggests the following reasons: With the Personnel Manager the Oedipal focus quickly gave way to a working through of deeply depressive problems; with Mrs. Craig the factors included both the presence of deep-seated depression and the lack of true support from her husband; with the Oil Director the lifelong neurotic patterns needed a great deal of working through, and even then began to reassert themselves during the follow-up period. Finally, if anyone wishes to see what a good result of psychotherapy is really like, I would urge him to read the account of the Personnel Manager.

4. One therapy, the Dress Designer, in which early termination became impossible and the ultimate result of very long therapy (over two hundred sessions) was thoroughly unsatisfactory. This patient was wrongly assessed at the beginning and turned out to be suffering from a far more deep-seated disturbance than had been foreseen.

5. Six basically unsuccessful brief therapies: The Bird Lady, the Cellist, the Receptionist, and the Sociologist show an essential pattern of limited or poor motivation and a confused focus; the Military Policeman is an example of a patient in danger of breakdown with whom a very limited intervention (five sessions) gave a useful but very limited result; and Mr. Upton is another example of a patient who was wrongly assessed and turned out at follow-up to be much more disturbed than anyone had suspected (he is the only patient in the whole series who was judged to be "worse.") The overall emphasis on transference/parent interpretations in these examples was low, thus illustrating one of the important characteristics of the less successful therapies.

Apart from these *research* findings already mentioned, the therapies presented illustrate all the essential *clinical* features of brief psychotherapy in the present work. Above all it will become clear that the technique used contains most of the elements of full-scale analysis and little else, and that—when appropriate—deep and disturbing interpretations were given in full and were in no way watered down. Examples of all these features are as follows (for the Zoologist, see chap. 12; for the Stationery Manufacturer, see chap. 14):

> Interpretation of resistance: Zoologist, session 4.
> Sociologist, repeated examples.
> Pesticide Chemist, session 3.
> Interpretation of dreams: Zoologist, session 16.
> Stationery Manufacturer, session 9.
> Buyer, session 14.

Primal scene material: Gibson Girl, session 10.
Highly disturbing material: Buyer, session 14.
                          Indian Scientist, session 4.
                          Zoologist, sessions 31, 32.
                          Stationery Manufacturer, session 5.
Anal impulses: Pesticide Chemist, session 3.
Interpretation of primitive self-destructive mechanisms and their
    resolution: Zoologist, sessions 9, 16, 17.
Strong dependence on the therapist: Zoologist, throughout.

It should also be clear that the *therapeutic results* often go deep and
survive very long follow-up. The chief general characteristics of many
of the favorable changes consist of the *removal of a pathological defense,*
the *disappearance of a symptom,* and the *release of the underlying
instinctual impulse,* which can then be *used constructively in the patient's
outside life.* Thus, the Indian Scientist appears to have resolved his
Oedipal anxieties to the point at which he lost his symptom of
premature ejaculation and became able to function as a man in all
spheres of his life; the Almoner lost her defense of having to keep
everything "nice" and used her aggressive feelings to improve the
relation with her parents; the Zoologist partly (but only partly)
overcame a deep-seated pattern of self-destructive anger; and the
Pesticide Chemist lost his obsessional ruminations and became able to
assert himself constructively at work. For examples of therapeutic
effects that actually appeared during therapy, apparently in response
to a particular piece of interpretative work, see the Indian Scientist,
sessions 4 and 5; the Almoner, session 9, the Pesticide Chemist,
session 11; the Zoologist, sessions 16 and 17; the Stationery Manufacturer, session 8; and the Gibson Girl, sessions 13 and 14, and 23 and
24.
    The following notes may be helpful:

    1. The material is set out in Assessment and Therapy Forms as in
SBP, arranged in alphabetical order of pseudonyms. Each form begins
with a brief summary so that the reader can choose those of most
interest.
    2. In this summary I have included an indication of the contribu-
tion of each therapy, whether positive or negative, to the main
significant correlations with outcome, i.e., those given by motivation,
focality, and the transference/parent link.
    3. The case histories are, of course, disguised. The names are
fictitious.

TABLE 6. List of Patients

Patient	Sex	Age	Marital status	Complaints	Time of onset	Psychiatric diagnosis	Number of sessions	Outcome
Patients followed up								
1 Almoner*	F	22	Single	Difficulty in deciding and remembering	A few months	Mild depression[2]	11	3.25
2 Au Pair Girl	F	21	Married	Fatigue; irritability; headaches	6 months	Depression	9	2.5
3 Bird Lady*	F	35	Divorced and remarried	Phobia of birds	Life-long	Phobic anxiety	9	1.375
4 Buyer*	M	27	Single	A single blackout	2 days	Hysteria	18	2.75
5 Car Dealer	M	48	Married	Pains in feet and legs.	5 years	Hysteria, reactive depression	54	2.25
6 Cellist*	M	32	Married	Stiffness in his bowing arm.	Several years	Phobic anxiety	9	1.875
7 Contralto	F	34	Single	Wanted cosmetic surgery	?	Character disorder	>400	0.9375
8 Company Secretary	M	43	Married	Indigestion, impotence	6 years	Character disorder	12	1.0
9 Mrs. Clifford	F	23	Living with a man	Temper tantrums	Some years	Marital problems	90	2.75
10 Mrs. Craig*	F	37	Married	Frigidity	Many years	Depression, frigidity	76	2.875
11 Dress Designer*	F	26	Married	Crippling panic attacks	3 months	Acute anxiety state	>200	1.25
12 Factory Inspector	M	41	Married	Impotence	11 months	Impotence	19	0.83
13 Gibson Girl*	F	18	Single	Agoraphobia	5 months	Phobic anxiety-hysteria	28	2.875
14 Gunner's Wife	F	23	Married	Nausea and vomiting	5 years	Hysteria, depression	6	2.125
15 Mrs. Hopkins	F	36	Married	Frigidity	Many years	Anxiety-hysteria	33	0.875
16 Indian Scientist*	M	29	Single	Premature ejaculation	6 years	Anxiety state	12	3.5
17 Mrs. Lewis	F	23	Married	Nonconsummation of marriage	5 years	Anxiety-hysteria, depression	20	2.83

88

	Sex	Age	Marital status	Complaint	Duration	Diagnosis		
18 Maintenance Man	M	39	Married	Panic attacks	5 weeks	Acute anxiety state	30	3.0
19 Military Policeman*	M	38	Married	Acute anxiety attack	Few weeks	Acute on chronic anxiety state	5	1.375
20 Mrs. Morley*	F	60	Widowed	Difficulties with her grown-up daughter	Many years	Character disorder, potential severe depression	9	2.25
21 Oil Director*	M	49	Married	Anxiety	1 year	Anxiety state, depression	46	2.0
22 Personnel Manager*	F	40	Single	Phobia of driving her car	Few months	Phobic anxiety	62	3.25
23 Pesticide Chemist*	M	31	Married	Outburst of rage	4 weeks	Obsessional personality	14	2.5
24 Playwright	M	28	Single	Severe panic attacks	5 years	Anxiety attacks; severe character disorder	93	2.25
25 Receptionist*	F	21	Single	Depression, irritability	1 year	Character disorder, depression	9	1.875
26 Representative	M	21	Single	Blushing	2 years	Phobic anxiety	3	2.125
27 Sociologist*	F	25	Married	Dermatitis on neck, frigidity	5 years	Character disorder, depression	26	1.25
28 Stationery Manufacturer*	M	45	Married	Preoccupation with his wife's former relation to another man	7 months	Incipient psychosis ("jealousy paranoia")	28	3.75
29 Mr. Upton*	M	18	Single	Anxiety, depression	1 year	Anxiety state, depression	5	−0.625
30 Zoologist*	M	22	Single	Conflict over his studies	2 years	Character disorder, reactive depression	32	2.5
Failed follow-up								
31 Character Actor	M	34	Married	Panic about forgetting his lines	Some years	Phobic anxiety	15	
32 City Solicitor	M	28	Single	Headaches, hot flushes, depression	1 year	Character disorder	7	
33 Mrs. Curtis[2]	F	20	Married	Abdominal pain, depression, since miscarriage	10 months	Hysteria	5	

Continued

TABLE 6. (Continued)

Patient	Sex	Age	Marital status	Complaints	Time of onset	Psychiatric diagnosis	Number of sessions	Outcome
34 Interior Decorator	M		Married	Inability to consummate marriage	3 months	Impotence	18	
35 Manicurist	F	26	Single	Shyness and loneliness	Some years	Character disorder	11	
36 National Assistance Officer	F	40	Married	Worry about hair on her face	Some years	Character disorder	20	
37 Rhodesian	M	22	Single	Fear that he was homosexual	Few weeks	Latent homosexuality	5	
38 Trawlerman	M	22	Single	Impotence	?Some years	Character disorder	7	
39 Dr. X.	M	32	Single	Loss of drive	Few months	Character disorder, depression	?15	

[1] The word "depression" refers to depression near the "neurotic" end of the scale throughout.
[2] This patient was followed up but was clearly not telling the truth and the result was found impossible to score.
* The assessment and therapy forms of patients marked thus are included in the following pages. Those not marked (excluding those not followed up) are given in *Toward the Validation of Dynamic Psychotherapy* (Malan 1976).

4. The names of therapists have been omitted in order to make patients less easy to identify.

5. The criteria, hypotheses, and assessments of outcome are those of Team 1 (DHM and EHR). They are reproduced exactly as written except for slight editing.

6. Sessions are numbered from the first interview with a workshop member, except that the projection test is not counted. The initial consultation is therefore usually the same as session 1. Unless otherwise stated, sessions were at the rate of once a week and all patients were seen face-to-face.

7. The number of sessions is measured from session 1 to termination.

8. Length of follow-up is measured from the date of termination.

9. In order to link the clinical material more closely with the statistical evidence, I have laid emphasis on four important variables: (1) motivation, (2) focality, (3) interpretation of the transference/parent link, and (4) interpretations about termination. The projection tests used were the Rorschach and the Object Relations Test or ORT (Phillipson, 1955). The latter is similar to the TAT, consisting of a series of pictures about which the patient is asked to tell stories. It differs from the TAT in that the pictures are drawn less clearly, thus giving more room for the patient to project his own fantasies onto them, and also they are more specifically designed to evoke the kinds of feeling and anxiety commonly dealt with in psychoanalytic therapy.

10. Some details of all thirty-nine patients in the second series are shown in Table 6. Those whose Assessment and Therapy Forms are included here are marked with an asterisk. Those not included (excluding those not followed up) will be given in *Toward the Validation of Dynamic Psychotherapy* (Malan, 1976).

The Almoner

SUMMARY

Category: Short, favorable (11 sessions, outcome 3.25).

A single girl of twenty-two with a pattern of having to keep everything "nice," now complaining of mild depressive symptoms. Interpretations were made of a number of different themes, and exactly what happened is not entirely clear, but therapy culminated in a violent row between the patient and her parents, after which the patient felt much better and the parents felt on better terms with her. The patient clearly thought that enough had been accomplished and withdrew from treatment against the therapist's wishes.

CONTRIBUTION TO THE CORRELATIONS

Motivation. Positive (moderate motivation, very favorable outcome).
Focality. Disagreement between the judges.
Transference/Parent Interpretations. Strongly positive (very high score, very favorable outcome).

DETAILS OF PATIENT AND THERAPIST

1. Patient

Sex	F.
Age	22.
Marital status	Single.
Occupation	Almoner at a hospital.
Complaint	Difficulty in deciding and remembering things (a few months).
What seems to bring patient now	Her parents are worried about her and are pressing her to seek help.

2. Therapist

Code	J
Sex	M

PSYCHIATRIC DIAGNOSIS

Mild depression in an inhibited personality.

DISTURBANCES

1. Symptoms. (a) *Difficulty in remembering things* (e.g., she forgets the names of the patients under her care); and *difficulty in making decisions.*

She feels she hasn't a mind of her own. At present she has given in her notice at her job, but everyone is telling her to withdraw it, and she feels she cannot cope with taking a decision over this.

(b) *Depressive Manifestations.* She wakes early in the morning and dislikes the idea of another day. She feels people have a poor opinion of her and she has an exaggeratedly poor opinion of herself.

2. Difficulties Over Aggression. At no time in the assessment period was there any indication of aggression toward anybody. She has a general defense of keeping everything "nice." She has difficulty in asserting herself at work. In the ORT, whenever there was any possibility of aggression or resentment she changed the story.

3. General Social Difficulties. She is not outgoing. She can't make easy contact with people, and never knows what to say to them.

ADDITIONAL EVIDENCE

1. Her father is a naval officer and her home life was very unsettled because the family was constantly moving around.

2. She was very fond of her father and admired him, but never really knew him.

3. She was much closer to her mother, but the picture that she gave of her mother seemed to be idealized.

4. She was unhappy at boarding school, but has a very good academic record.

5. There has been much quarreling between her parents, who seem to be on the point of separation. One of her mother's main complaints is that because the patient's father is in the Navy, she has no proper home life.

6. The recent difficulties were precipitated by an incident in which a man at work, whom she was fond of, threw something at her, and since then seems to have turned against her.

7. At interview she mostly maintained her smiling, proper, middle-class façade; but when the interviewer pointed out that her recent disappointment with this young man had meant more to her than she was willing to admit, she became moist-eyed and said it was ridiculous but it did.

8. With the psychologist (who also became the therapist) she communicated much richer material. Important themes in her ORT were: (a) jealousy and anger when other people love each other; (b) her wish to be loved by a man but her fear of a woman's jealousy; (c) anger with a paternal figure for not loving her exclusively; and (d) the theme of betrayal, which it was thought must refer to her fear of betraying her

parents by admitting her true feelings about them. She is intensely guilty about all these feelings.

HYPOTHESIS

The evidence suggests that she feels guilty about aggressive feelings toward both her parents: toward her father for not being close to her, and toward her mother for standing between her and her father. These feelings have interfered with the development of mature sexuality. She defends against it by idealizing her parents and herself behaving in a very proper and conventional manner.

CRITERIA

1. Loss of symptoms. (a) Ability to remember things, (b) ability to make decisions and to feel that she knows where she is going, and (c) she should lose the depressive manifestations, have an improved view of herself, and feel that she can enjoy life.

2. She should shed her defense of keeping everything "nice" and be able to be aggressive and assert herself in appropriate circumstances.

3. She should be able to be socially confident and be able to make closer contact with people in general.

4. Although there is little evidence about difficulty with men, we feel this exists. She should be able to get close to a man and enjoy a satisfactory emotional and sexual relation with him.

REASON FOR ACCEPTANCE AND THERAPEUTIC PLAN

The psychologist liked her, felt he had made contact with her, and was eager to take her on. He made a formulation based on *anger* within the *Oedipal situation:* (1) that she was angry at her parents when they were close to each other but excluded her, (2) that she was afraid of her mother's anger if she had a man of her own, and (3) that she was angry with her father for not loving her exclusively. The discussion was confused and rather skeptical, and the opinion was expressed that she was very heavily defended and it would be impossible to get at her anger with her parents short of a full analysis. No definite plan was made, but the implication was that she needed to face her true feelings about her parents.

SUMMARY OF COURSE OF THERAPY

With hindsight it seems certain that the important factor in therapy was that the therapist got her to face her anger with her parents much more quickly and easily than anyone had expected. This anger does not really seem to have been Oedipal in origin, but was just about her feeling that they had not been good parents to her. It is this theme that will be picked out from a very complex brief therapy.

In sessions 2 and 3 an important pattern emerged that played a part later (see session 10). She gave in her notice at the hospital where she worked, then decided she wanted to stay and withdrew her resignation, but it was now too late. The hospital would have liked her to stay if only she hadn't resigned so many times, and everybody told her how well she did her work. The therapist suggested that she used threats of leaving as a way of proving to herself that other people wanted her, with which she agreed.

Much of the rest of session 3 was concerned with her relation with her mother. Her parents had quarreled again, and now the patient had no social life because she felt so guilty about her mother being lonely that she felt compelled to visit her on weekends. The theme of the therapist's interpretations was that when her parents quarreled (with the implication that she felt she had separated them) she became very guilty and then surrendered her life to her mother; and that independence meant expressing hostility. The patient left this session deep in thought.

An important feature of session 4 was then the emergence of a much less idealized picture of her mother. The patient spoke at great length and with considerable contempt of the way in which her mother had quite childish tantrums.

In both sessions 4 and 5 she said she was feeling much better. In session 5 she spoke of how she had never had any permanent friends because the family moved around so much when she was a child. The therapist said she must be blaming her father. She went on to say that her father could never talk about his real feelings; nor could anybody else in the family—they just talked commonplaces. She went on with further resentment against her mother, saying that she felt her mother was jealous of her youth and almost seemed pleased to see her in a mess. She added that other people thought her parents were wonderful but it was a sham. She said she didn't blame her father for preferring the Navy; it must be peaceful compared with living with her mother. The therapist pointed out how a few weeks ago everything had been confusion and self-blame. Now she was blaming her parents and felt much more peaceful.

In session 6 she reported excitedly that she had got a new, and very good, job. In session 7 the therapist told her the dates of his forthcoming holiday (to come after session 8), and she said that she felt so much better than she didn't really want to come any more. The therapist interpreted that this might be a punishment to him for going off and leaving her, like her father (transference/parent interpretation). This led to her saying that her father always seemed to be displeased by the things she did. She ended by shrugging her shoulders and saying, "Well, I know it's like that now." The therapist made further attempts at transference interpretations, which the patient could not accept.

She began session 8 by saying that everything had been going very well and she didn't think she needed to come any more. The therapist made a number of interpretations about *jealousy*, in particular that she dealt with jealous feelings about his going away on holiday by going away herself. Although she denied all these interpretations, she went on to say that during the war her father had been away most of the time; and when he came back the family situation seriously deteriorated. Her father and mother quarreled, and she became so difficult that she was sent away to boarding school. Her parents then seemed to get on all right when the children were away. She said that her father was very *jealous* of the children and resented the attention that her mother paid to her.

Session 9 was six weeks later. During this time she had gone to stay with her parents, but things got so bad between them that she had left after four days. She said that she had made a clean break and felt much better. She spent most of the rest of the time complaining about her parents, and the therapist repeatedly tried to relate this to the transference. She ended by giving the therapist a lecture, and he interpreted that she was whipping him with her tongue just as she whipped her parents (transference/parent interpretation). She agreed with this and became anxious that she might have hurt him. During this session she continued saying that she wanted to stop coming, to which the therapist said that she was just beginning to show her fire, and surely this was the time to stay.

The climax of therapy came in session 10. She said that her father always criticized her and her mother would never let her grow up. Then, referring to herself, she said she was reminded of a book about a cat by Paul Gallico, who, whenever a situation became intolerable, just went out. The therapist interpreted her pattern of leaving when she was afraid she herself would be thrown out. This had happened with her parents, with a number of jobs, and it was now happening with treatment—where, he suggested, the situation was also becoming intolerable for her. This led her to speak of a hospital that she had left, where several people had been fired, and where she had refused a plea to come back again. "Anyhow, they were too busy to help when I needed it." The therapist suggested she always left to forestall being thrown out, and that she felt he was too busy with other patients. He linked this with the fact that she had been sent away to boarding school when her father returned from the war (implied transference/ parent interpretation). It then turned out that her mother was perpetually threatening to leave, and the therapist pointed out the parallel. During the course of this, the patient told how she herself was good at many artistic things, and while her mother appreciated this, her father seemed merely contemptuous of her efforts. Yet, she and her father had sometimes gone to art galleries together, and he had even tried to do some painting himself. She said that he wanted to do this in order to express himself, because he couldn't express himself in words at all, whereas often she herself was absolutely boiling over with the wish to say what she felt. The therapist asked her what she did feel, and she burst out in fury at her parents, but particularly at her father, who, she said, really wanted to paint himself and expressed his jealousy by being comtemptuous of her. She said that her father always thought she was accusing her parents of being philistine, but really she could teach them a lot. She had mentioned previously that when she left home she had started to do some music teaching, and the therapist suggested this was a substitute for teaching her father, and said that it showed how important her relation with her father was. He added that in the last session she had given the therapist a lecture, and thus was trying to teach *him* (transference/parent interpretation).

In session 11 the main theme seemed to be the idea of being self-contained and not becoming involved. The therapist made a number of interpretations suggesting that this was a defensive maneuver, but she eventually said she didn't want to talk about it and left.

A week later she wrote, thanking him very much for all his help and saying that she didn't want to come any more. He wrote back, suggesting that they should talk about it, but in her reply she refused, and added "I really do feel a completely different person from when I first came." She sent him a box of chocolates.

There were a number of interpretations about *termination,* mainly on the theme that she was leaving to forestall being left, to which there was never a very clear response.

It is worth noting that this extremely successful therapy was highly transference/parent oriented, there being fifteen transference/ parent interpretations recorded out of a total of ninety-four (16%).

Total number of sessions   11
Total time   5 months

FOLLOW-UP

6 Months

The important thing that emerged was that since the row she had had with her parents, not only was she getting on better with them but they were getting on better with each other. They seemed to realize how they got on her nerves and how she had to be independent. They didn't seem to make such impossible demands on her. She quite looked forward to the idea of visiting them at weekends. She said that treatment had showed her how her worries about school were really connected with her worries about her parents, and this had helped a lot. She was now extremely happy in her job, and she said that she felt she had a lot of her father in her in the sense that she had a profession like him. She also now had a boyfriend, and she said she thought this might be "it." She said that her only trouble at present was that she hated being alone in the evenings, and supposed that this had to do with a fear of burglars. The therapist pointed out that although she hated being alone, nevertheless she felt that she needed to manage everything on her own, and this was why she had broken off treatment. She said it was quite true she never felt she could wholly commit herself to anybody. The therapist raised the question of whether she wanted to come back for treatment about these problems, but she said she still wanted to see how things would go.

The picture of things being so much better between her and her parents was confirmed when, four months later, the therapist received a brief letter from the patient's father, from which the following are quotations: "This is a note to thank you most sincerely for the help you have given my daughter. I returned from being at sea three months ago, and since then my wife and I have seen her most weekends. She is much more relaxed and cheerful and able to cope with her life very much better than when I first referred her."

1 Year 1 Month

There was now a marked change in her appearance, in that she was dressed in a much more attractive way. She was bubbling over with enjoyment, which the therapist felt had a slightly hypomanic quality. Things continued to go well, and the picture was much the same as in the last follow-up. Much of the session was taken up with recalling her original breakdown, and wondering about what it meant. She thought that is was due to the fact that it was her first job, and that her parents were in difficulties. She said there was an obvious parallel with the time that she first was sent away to boarding school.

She still found it difficult to be alone, and she wanted the assurance that if she had another breakdown she could come back.

5 Years 8 Months
General. Although almost everything that she had to report was favorable, it was also true that the therapist felt she was rather drawn-looking, "like a careworn young mother," and that beneath an air of calm and honest thoughtfulness, there was also something of an underlying sadness.

Four years ago she had married the man mentioned in the previous follow-up reports. They now have two children. He is housemaster in an important state school that also takes some boarders. He is very devoted to his work and she also has a lot to do as housemaster's wife. The result of this is that they have very little time for family life during term time. In order to cope with this problem, they have bought a cottage in the country where they spend the school holidays. "I think it is when you have almost stretched yourself to the limit that you can really enjoy getting away from it all and we do this during the holidays."

1. Symptoms. (a) *Difficulty in Remembering Things.* On the whole she has no trouble here. Sometimes, when very busy, she finds she has become flustered and forgotten something; but she no longer actively worries about this as she used to do. (b) *Difficulty over decisions.* The difficulty over minor decisions has disappeared. There is still a good deal of worry over major decisions. As far as knowing where she is going is concerned, she has completely accepted her role as wife to a schoolmaster and mother to her children. She plans to do part-time work at some time in the future. (c) *Depressive manifestations.* There has been no serious or lasting depression, but she gets depressed if her husband is away often. She no longer suffers from early waking. As far as feeling that people have a poor opinion of her is concerned she said, "No, I don't bother. People take us as we are. I hadn't really given it much thought." She no longer has a poor opinion of herself and recognizes her husband's appreciation of her. There is no doubt of her ability to enjoy life.

2. Need to Keep Everything "Nice." She straightforwardly explains the reality of home—overwork, untidiness, the wish to see more of her husband. She recognizes her parents' failings.

3. Ability to Assert Herself. She and her husband behave as equal partners in the marriage. The therapist made the judgment that she has not tried to assert herself enough over the problem of her husband giving more of his time to her and the children during term time. Instead, she just sadly accepts the situation. He felt that this accounted for her rather haggard and careworn appearance. He felt there might well be residual difficulty here.

4. Social Confidence. She seems fully confident socially and has much closer contact with people.

5. Relation With a Man. She has married someone whom she appreciates and who appreciates her. She shares his work with him in term time; and in the holidays they are able to relax together. The sexual relation is apparently satisfactory in the holidays, though infrequent and less satisfactory in term time when they are both so tired.

SUMMARY

Considerable resolution in the main problem. She has certainly shed her defense of trying to keep everything "nice"; and she has been able to assert herself to the extent of getting away from home and knowing where she is going. It was striking how her self-assertion with her parents improved the relation with them. There may, however, be residual difficulties in asserting herself with her husband.

Team 2 also laid emphasis on the residual difficulties over standing up for her rights for her husband's time and for sexual attention.

SCORES

Team 1	4.0	3.0
Team 2	3.0	3.0
Mean	3.25	

The Bird Lady

SUMMARY

Category: Short, unfavorable (9 sessions, outcome 1.375).

A woman of thirty-five suffering from a lifelong fear of birds. Therapy was confused, motivation steadily decreased, and though apparent progress was made in session 7, the patient then broke off.

CONTRIBUTION TO THE CORRELATIONS WITH OUTCOME

Motivation and Focality. Strongly positive. (Scores low, decreasing; unfavorable outcome)
Transference/Parent Interpretations. Strongly positive (low score, unfavorable outcome).

DETAILS OF PATIENT AND THERAPIST

1. Patient

Sex	F.
Age	35.
Marital status	Divorced and remarried.
Occupation	Secretary.
Complaint	Lifelong fear of birds.
What seems to bring patient now	Recently, while driving, she panicked at a flock of birds and lost control of the car. Her husband now won't let her drive. She has been seen by a Tavistock trained (woman) G.P. for several interviews, who has persuaded her that she needs treatment and who referred her specifically for brief therapy.

2. Therapist

Code	G
Sex	M

PSYCHIATRIC DIAGNOSIS

Lifelong phobic anxiety with depression.

DISTURBANCES

1. Symptoms. (a) *Lifelong fear of birds flapping that started with a nightmare about birds when she was very young.* It has been much worse recently and now she can't go out without great fear of meeting birds in the street. Her husband now won't let her drive because of a recent incident in which she panicked at a flock of birds and lost control of the car. She would "throw herself under a bus rather than face birds." (b) *Fear of meat* (no further details known). (c) *Alternating constipation and diarrhea.* She also presumably suffers from some menstrual disturbance as she is shortly to go into the hospital for curettage.

2. Problems Over Femininity. She is apparently frigid and her first marriage led to divorce because of this. According to the therapist, she regards herself as unattractive, a "silly, clumsy, useless woman who can't make any use of femininity . . . Women understand each other but there can be no useful contact between women and men." She is jealous of men. She doesn't like men's bodies, "nor women's either unless they are young and glamorous." She "never wanted to have children except to prove that she could do better than other women whose children she criticizes." She does not feel that she has any personality except at the office. She is afraid she is wrecking her present marriage.

3. Depression. She seems depressed and hopeless.

ADDITIONAL EVIDENCE

1. She was an only child whose parents quarreled violently. She did not like her father who died when she was thirteen.

2. She would give little information about her previous marriage, but we knew from her G.P. that after her divorce she went back to live with her mother. Her mother was planning to remarry a man who later died, and the patient married this man's son. She has been married five years and has no children.

3. The therapist commented on the initial interview that she presented herself as a challenge to show how powerfully destructive she could be to a man's potency; and that she seemed to enjoy the sexual undercurrent of this in an almost teasing way. At the projection test she said in a very seductive way how much nicer the psychologist was than the psychiatrist who had interviewed her.

4. Themes in her projection test were: (a) Identification with quarreling parents and indecision as to whose side to take; (b) stories of murder and violence; (c) later stories of reparation; (d) her final story contained the clear communication that she felt she was wrecking her marriage.

HYPOTHESIS

We do not think the evidence is clear enough for a definitive hypothesis, but the following explains much of the evidence:

The impulses against which she is defending herself are: (1) in a two-person situation with a man, vicious sexual teasing; and (2) in a three-person situation (herself and a man and a woman), playing off one against the other.

She defends against this by rejection of femininity.

CRITERIA

1. Loss of Symptoms. (a) Fear of birds; (b) fear of meat; and (c) gastrointestinal symptoms.

2. Enjoyment of sexuality with a man. Ability to value both his masculinity and her femininity.

3. Ability to be constructively self-assertive or aggressive where appropriate.

4. She should maintain her ability to get along well with women.

REASON FOR ACCEPTANCE AND THERAPEUTIC PLAN

The patient was referred specifically for brief therapy by the G.P., and although this seemed to be probably unrealistic, the therapist made some contact with her at interview and wanted to try. He formulated his aim as "to deal intensively with her struggle in the transference, leading to problems of sexual development and identity." The general consensus in the workshop was that this was a complex case and probably unsuitable for brief therapy. (It should be noted that this patient was seen at the clinic before the arrival of behavior therapy as an accepted form of treatment.)

SUMMARY OF COURSE OF THERAPY

In session 2 the therapist stuck to his plan and made a number of transference interpretations such as (1) that she wanted him to chase her and then to prove him useless, and (2) that since he had the penis, he must do all the work and have no fun. This seemed to bring out her envy of men, and her attitude to bodies and to children. The patient canceled her next appointment. In session 3 the therapist tried to make some links between current situations and her feelings about her quarreling parents, without much clear response. In session 4 the patient seemed to be controlling the session, and the therapist interpreted that she had sexual feelings for him and was trying to pretend she didn't enjoy the sessions. She seemed to enjoy this, but then said that she couldn't come next week because of pressure of work.

She then canceled two more sessions after the Christmas break. She returned defensive, and the therapist repeatedly interpreted that she needed to control the situation in order to avoid getting in contact with deep feelings. When, in session 6, she again said she couldn't come next week, the therapist put it to her that unless she took treatment seriously she would get nothing out of it. Thus, the evidence for decreasing *motivation* was overwhelming.

In session 7 there was apparent progress: The therapist interpreted that she was provoking him into being aggressive with her, and she herself then admitted that her teachers used to accuse her of "dumb insolence" as a child. She said she never understood this—she was only frightened of them—and she related this to her feelings about her parents' quarrels, in which she was quiet because she was terrified. The therapist suggested that she was afraid of her own anger and really wanted to join in, and she admitted that she had once or twice rushed downstairs as a child and screamed at them.

During the next week the patient's husband rang up to say that she always came home very upset from the sessions and was talking about giving up coming. In session 8 the therapist told her about this and said that to his face the relationship had to appear useless and empty, while when she was away from him it was obviously highly important. He suggested that this was like the relation with her father, that he mustn't know that he means anything to her and must think that her loyalties lie with her mother (this was the more important of two recorded transference/parent interpretations throughout the whole therapy). Her only response to this was to say that the male members of the family were usually to be despised.

There then developed a situation revealing most pointedly her paradoxical motivation and basic resistance to change. She canceled the next session but came up to session 9 almost dramatically different—friendly, talking freely, and obviously wanting to make use of the session. She began to speak of her fear of destructiveness in her relationships and her hopelessness about being able to control this. For the first time she admitted terrible tempers as a child. She was teased by all the women in the family and was filled with fury and hate against them all. She said that her mother used to provoke her father, who was very jealous, and she tricked him and played about with other men.

After this session of apparent major progress the patient broke off treatment. There was, obviously, no work on feelings about termination.

Total number of sessions   9
Total time   4 months

FOLLOW-UP (5 years 1 month)

Subsequent Events. She said that her husband had died suddenly two years ago, and when the therapist tried to get her to talk about him, she immediately burst into tears. She now has a gentleman friend.

1. Symptoms. (a) *Fear of birds.* This is entirely unchanged. (b) *Fear of meat.* She doesn't like cutting up meat but will do it. This symptom is unchanged but not important. (c) *Gastrointestinal symptoms.* The alternation of constipation and diarrhea has altered to constipation alone. She also used to get attacks of severe abdominal pain. These have now gone.

2. Enjoyment of Sex With a Man; Valuation of Her Femininity and His Masculinity. Here the facts as reported are (a) that she was completely frigid in both her marriages; but (b) that her second husband was impotent; and (c) that she now enjoys sex very much (though probably without orgasm) with a man resembling her first husband—with whom she has "a lot in common" but "wouldn't think of marrying because they are incompatible" (note the contradiction), and whom she almost certainly neither loves nor respects. She spoke with genuine surprise about her discovery that it was possible to enjoy sex. There also seemed to be considerable idealization of her late husband and an inability to admit any faults in him.

3. Ability to Be Constructively Aggressive. She said she was still terrified of any aggressive situation, as it reminded her of the quarrels between her parents. The evidence is that this problem is unchanged.

4. Ability to Get Along With Women. The therapist said that she retains this ability in general, but her relation to her mother is clearly an exception. She cannot stand up to her mother in any way and remains tied to her. As far as general social life is concerned, she seems to be behaving in such a way as to confirm her own fear that people do not want her for herself.

5. Depression, Hopelessness, Clumsiness. (a) *Depression and hopelessness.* She is clearly still depressed about her husband's death two years ago and has been drinking heavily. On the other hand, there does appear to be more hope in her life, as shown by her ability to enjoy sex and the fact that she said she would like to marry again. Her social difficulties make it difficult for her to meet people whom she would like to marry. (b) She still presents herself as clumsy and anxious in any new situation.

SUMMARY

Since, even after the follow-up, we still have little idea of the dynamics, this is a very difficult case to score. The improvements are (1) the ability to enjoy sex, (2) the improvement in gastro-intestinal symptoms, and (3) perhaps some increase in hope. On the other hand, the main symptom remains entirely unchanged, she is depressed, and she still has social problems and problems over aggression. The score depends on how important the sexual change is considered to be, and how much it is regarded as an inner change as opposed to the result of a change of partner. DHM and EHR differed on this.

SCORES

Team 1	1.5	0.5
Team 2	2.0	1.5
Mean	1.375	

The Buyer

SUMMARY

Category: Short, favorable (18 sessions, outcome 2.75).

This was a single man of twenty-seven in an "Oedipal" crisis involving his fiancée and her father, who started with very poor motivation, and who had to be "interpreted into" therapy. Once this had been accomplished he worked very hard, but the therapist probably paid too little attention to the transference and termination was unsatisfactory. Outcome was fairly favorable, but there was evidence for major deficiencies in his central problem in relation to women.

CONTRIBUTION TO THE CORRELATIONS

Motivation and Focality. Initially negative (both factors low), then positive (both factors high), with favorable outcome.
Transference/Parent Interpretations. Negative (low score, favorable outcome).

DETAILS OF PATIENT AND THERAPIST

1. Patient

Sex	M.
Age	27.
Marital status	Single.
Occupation	Assistant buyer.
Complaint: what seems to bring patient now	He had a blackout in his office two days ago and was referred to the Tavistock Clinic as an emergency.

2. Therapist

Code	F
Sex	M

PSYCHIATRIC HISTORY AND DIAGNOSIS

1. He described himself as having been "nervous" as a child and having suffered from frequent illnesses.

2. He had done his National Service in the R.A.F. He had been posted to a unit under a C.O. whom he disliked and who had left him with too much responsibility. While there he had had a blackout

similar to the present one. He had been transferred to another unit where he got on well with the C.O. and there had been no further trouble.

3. His present attack had come on him suddenly in the office. He had lost consciousness and been unconscious for one and a half hours. He had been examined in the casualty department of a hospital, and had been told that there was nothing physically wrong with him and that his problem was psychiatric.

4. The current stress apparently associated with his present attack was as follows: A few weeks ago he had become engaged to a girl called Pamela, whom he had known for five months. Her father had taken an instant dislike to him and had forbidden him the house. The day before his blackout, she had broken off her engagement with him, telling him a rather novelettelike story as an excuse for doing so. **Diagnosis.** Hysteria.

DISTURBANCES

1. Blackouts. (a) In the R.A.F. when given too much responsibility; and (b) in the context of the present situation with his fiancée and her family.

2. Difficulty Over Being Effective. He gave the impression of having done his best to be "reasonable" at all costs both with his fiancée and with her parents, and he had been unable to deal effectively with the situation. The theme of anxiety about "making the grade" ran through his story.

3. People Dislike Him. In the present story, this applied especially to his prospective father-in-law. Both the psychiatrist who interviewed him and the psychologist who tested him were irritated by his obviously false politeness.

4. Overdramatization. Both the present story and certain incidents in the past had a distinctly novelettelike flavor to them.

ADDITIONAL EVIDENCE

1. In the initial interview the interviewer, feeling that he was not very seriously disturbed, decided to give him a push toward being effective, pointing out how mildly he had handled the whole situation, and telling him that if he really wanted Pamela he had better go out and get her.

2. In his projection test (ORT), older men were seen as weak

people, hiding behind a façade of effectiveness, and his fear seemed to be that in order to get a woman he would have to engage in rivalry with the man, who would crumble and be destroyed. An important story was of a military exercise in which, because the fog came down, the enemy position was captured without a shot being fired. The psychologist's interpretation of this was that the patient's problem was that he was in a situation requiring aggression, and he did not know how to achieve anything without hurting someone.

The interviewer spent two sessions trying to help him over the current situation, and thus got little information about his background.

HYPOTHESIS

He is afraid that he cannot cope with the responsibilities of masculinity. To take responsibility entails being agressive, and his fear is that this will result in (1) triumphing over a father, and possibly (2) damaging the woman.

He defends against his anxiety about not being able to cope by overdramatization; and he expresses the anxiety by losing consciousness and thus withdrawing from the situation completely.

CRITERIA

1. No further blackouts or substitute symptoms.
2. Ability to be effective (a) with men without inappropriate hostility; and (b) with women, including a satisfactory emotional and sexual relationship.
3. Inner feeling of confidence in himself as a man.

REASON FOR ACCEPTANCE AND THERAPEUTIC PLAN

This was a psychiatric emergency, the immediate origins of which were obvious. The interviewer (who became the therapist) initially hoped to help him over the current crisis simply by giving him a push; and when this did not work, realized that his background problems—which were clearly Oedipal—needed to be dealt with. There was thus no difficulty in making a therapeutic plan: to deal with Oedipal problems, in the transference to the male therapist where necessary.

The only trouble with this plan was that the patient's initial motivation for looking at himself was minimal. The therapist nevertheless felt that this could be overcome.

SUMMARY OF COURSE OF THERAPY

As will be seen, the actual focus of therapy was not so much Oedipal problems as *conflict over aggressive feelings,* though these feelings were certainly expressed within Oedipal situations. It emerged that the patient's aggressive feelings were directed toward (1) Pamela's father, (2) Pamela herself, (3) the patient's father, and (4) the patient's elder brother; and moreover, that the patient's rebelliousness was not merely *directed against* his father but also expressed an *identification with* him, and in addition involved direct conflict with the patient's Christian values.

First Phase: Work on the Defenses. In response to session 1 the patient reported in session 2 that he had "taken the therapist's advice" and taken a tough line with Pamela. He had made her put on the engagement ring that she had given back to him; and he had also told her that he was going to confront her parents, and that if he heard any more slander from her father he was going to take legal action. Pamela was delighted and said how much good it had done him to see a psychiatrist. This didn't last, however. When she went home for the weekend, she got under the influence of her parents again, and was now being distant and snappy with him. He now began to feel that if he just "bulldozed in" it would only make the situation worse, and he didn't known what to do.

In session 3 he reported that Pamela had broken off the engagement once more. When he remarked that he felt Pamela's story all sounded a bit dramatic, the therapist took this as his cue to tell the patient that *his* story was all a bit dramatic, too; and that this false dramatization must be because he was really afraid of his real feelings. The patient couldn't face this and always veered away to talking about Pamela's problems rather than his own.

In session 4 the patient started by spending a long time talking about Pamela's "mother complex," etc., and after some unsuccessful attempts at bringing him to his own feelings, the therapist said to him flatly that it appeared he did not want treatment. Some further rough handling of this kind eventually induced in him some serious communication. He began to say that he had sometimes wondered if there was something not quite nice in him, and particularly if his sexual instinct might be too strong. There then emerged the true story of what had led up to one of his previous broken engagements. Instead of the novelettelike story to which he had previously attributed this, the true reason now appeared to have been that he was afraid to express his sexual feelings when clearly invited to do so. The therapist interpreted that the patient had adopted the values of the English gentleman as a way of escaping from the down-to-earth side of his nature, and the result had been that he was never quite real in the things he did and therefore never quite succeeded. The therapist then led him in the direction of Oedipal problems by adding that perhaps this was all bound up with the problem of growing up and becoming a man.

Breakthrough: the Emergence of Aggressive Feelings. In session 5 there was a complete transformation of atmosphere, which now became one of serious thought on the part of the patient. This represented a sudden *increase in motivation.* The important things that emerged were (1) that his father seemed to have a fear of the subject of sex; and (2) that up to the age of seventeen the patient had been very aggressive, and used to have terrific verbal battles with other people in a number of societies to which he belonged. Since then, however, something seems to have gone wrong, and he can't express these feelings any more. In this session the therapist for the first time felt able to discuss the plan of therapy, and set the patient a limit of a total of sixteen sessions (i.e., counting the initial interview, therapy should end at session 17).

In session 6 there emerged for the first time *aggression toward his father.* He spoke of how in his job he had to be "nicey'nicey" to people whom he'd rather *kick.* He went on to speak of his father, telling (1) of having a recent row with him, (2) of having originally tried to follow his father's choice of career for him, and then breaking away, and (3) finally speaking of him with real contempt—"he is so narrow that I could shake him."

A new theme that emerged in session 7 was the possibility of *aggression toward women.* The patient spoke of how some wives seemed to thrive on being inconsiderately treated by their husbands. The patient said he didn't understand this and it was contrary to his Christian values. The therapist said that it was no good trying to pretend one didn't feel things that one did, even if it was contrary to one's principles. The patient became deeply thoughtful and went on to say that once he had been an "Angry Young Man," but he wasn't any more. It later came out that when he had been aggressive with people at the age of seventeen, it has been his father who had encouraged him in this.

Session 8 was notable for the emergence of possible *aggression toward the therapist.* The patient said that he felt he had been wrong to doubt Pamela's story that had led to the broken engagement. The therapist said that he felt the patient was challenging him, and the patient agreed with this and then said in a much more relaxed way, "I feel much happier these days." The therapist later said that the patient could not get away from the fact that he must be angry with Pamela. To this the patient answered, "Yes, I've several times thought I'd like to spank her. It would probably do her good." The patient ended up by speaking of his *conflict between his sexual feelings and his Christian values,* a theme that he continued in the next few sessions.

In session 9 one of the things that emerged was that the patient kept having the thought that he might be homosexual; it was almost as if there was another person inside him taunting him with this suggestion, and that this tended to occur in church. The therapist interpreted that trying to live up to a standard of values was imposing authority on himself, and it sounded as if there was another part of him trying to rebel against this authority. The patient said this made sense to him.

Session 10 started with a long story about how the patient's brother had had a protracted quarrel with a superior. The patient said that the truth was that this wasn't really his brother doing the quarreling, but his father, who had always had a chip on his shoulder about authority. The therapist said that the patient must be in great difficulty over rebelliousness, since on the one hand he wanted to *rebel against his father,* but on the other hand rebelliousness was just *being like his father.* The patient went on to speak with some contempt of the "nicey-nicey" atmosphere when guests came to his home. The therapist compared this with the patient's excessive politeness when he had first come to treatment, to which the patient said in a really heartfelt way, "Yes, and how on earth am I to get rid of it?"

The Link Between the Current and the Past Triangular Situations. Session 11 was probably the most dramatic and important of the whole therapy. The patient started defensive and the therapist eventually interpreted that the patient was afraid that some hostile feelings for him, the therapist, might come out unexpectedly. This led the patient eventually to speaking of (1) lying terrified in bed as a small boy listening to his mother and father quarreling, and (2) of a time when his father had come up "white with rage" because the patient and his brother had been making a noise when they slept in the same room together. "I can see his face as plain as I can see yours—there was really murder in his eyes." The therapist pointed out the parallel between these two situations, and suggested the patient must have had murderous *impulses* against his father. The patient said that indeed he had had murderous impulses against *Pamela's* father. On one occasion when he was having a quarrel with this man, "I said to myself, 'I wish to high heaven he would strike me. I really wish that he would strike me.' And I would have killed him. I am certain of that. I would have killed him." The therapist immediately linked this with the triangular situation between the patient and his parents, suggesting that he might have felt he wanted to kill his father in order to take his mother away from him, but felt terribly guilty about this. The therapist linked this with the patient's inability to be effective in taking Pamela away from her father. The patient then spoke of how his father had always disapproved of his having girl friends.

One of the things that he said in session 12 was that when he read in the paper about a girl being raped and murdered, he couldn't help feeling that he understood what the murderer had felt. The therapist tried to make use of this in order to suggest that the patient was angry not only with his father but with his mother also, and tried to link this with the primal scene. This did not lead to any useful response.

The Therapist Mistakenly Takes Sides in the Conflict Between Impulse and Conscience. In session 13 the patient spoke of finding all sorts of unacceptable impulses in himself, and said with great intensity, "There is constant tension . . . constant tension." The therapist here invited the patient to have a fantasy about what he would like to do if he had no conscience. This merely increased resistance. The therapist therefore changed his approach, interpreting that the patient's conscience was brutally authoritarian with the other part of him and thus resembled his father. The patient immediately spoke of an incident in which, while he was driving a car, a policeman had beckoned him on despite the fact that there was a stream of pedestrians crossing the road in front of him. He had waited for them, and the policeman had spoken rudely to him, and he had been absolutely furious. The therapist interpreted that it was almost as if the policeman had been inviting him to run the pedestrians over, and that this was like him, the therapist, asking the patient to have fantasies against his conscience. This aroused in him quite violent hatred, but perhaps the real reason for this was that these clashes with people outside represented the conflict between two parts of the patient, his impulses and his conscience. The patient said he partly understood this.

The Highly Ambivalent Relation With His Elder Brother. Session 14 was another session of high intensity. The patient told of a childhood dream: In this his father was taking his elder brother, Richard, to the dentist, while the patient was left in the car outside. He had been told not to touch any of the instruments in the car. He could see a blue flame through the window of the dentist's house and was terrified by the thought of what they were doing to Richard. He took the brake off the car, which started rolling down the hill.

What emerged in the association to this dream were highly ambivalent feelings toward Richard, e.g., (1) when they were small the two brothers were always fighting; but on the other hand, (2) once, when at school, he had inadvertently got left with Richard's sandwiches in addition to his own, and he had become terribly upset. The therapist interpreted that he both loved his brother and wanted to knock him down as a rival, but felt guilty and sorry about the latter. Taking his brother's sandwiches would be like stealing his strength. In the dream Richard's teeth had been drawn, so to speak, and this might represent his strength being taken away. Perhaps Richard had represented to him the father that he would have liked to have had, but about whom he still had mixed feelings. In response to this the patient said that he did remember once wanting to kill his father as a child, and feeling very guilty about this. He went on to speak of a fight that he had had with Richard at the age of about eighteen, the cause of which was that he didn't like the way Richard treated his own wife. By this time he was strong enough to stand up to his elder brother and the fight had been a draw. The two were eventually reconciled and they have been good friends ever since. The therapist said that only when his anger with his elder brother and his rivalry had been both admitted and expressed could their relation become complete. He related this to the patient's murderous impulses toward his father, and rivalry for his mother.

Suddenly the patient said, "Do you think that there was something wrong in my relationship with Pamela because I couldn't express any anger in it?" The therapist said that Pamela had obviously put him through a lot of anguish and had ended up by rejecting him, and it must certainly be true that underneath he felt angry with her. During his associations to the dream the patient had mentioned that taking the brake off the car seemed in some way related to the blackout that had brought him to treatment; and the therapist said that all these mixed feelings must have come together in this blackout. He went on to emphasize that the patient seemed to be angry with women as well as with men, and he related this to the patient's feelings of insecurity with his mother.

Unsatisfactory Termination; the End of the Relation with Pamela. In session 15 the therapist was very conscious that, according to the original time limit, there were now only two more sessions, and termination hadn't yet been mentioned. In this session the patient mentioned two incidents involving stealing, one of which involved his brother. This eventually led to interpretations about guilt-laden wishes to steal power from either his brother, his father, or the therapist (transference/parent interpretation). At mention of the relation with the therapist the patient became slightly confused, and he made some remarks about psychiatrists in the clinic and their rather offhand behavior. This was discussed for a short time, and then the therapist reminded the patient that there were only two more sessions. The patient's reaction to this was to say, "Just where do you think treatment is getting me?"

In session 16 there was no mention of termination, and the subject of Pamela was brought up once more. He had recently been meeting her again, but when her parents had found out about this and caused trouble, she had again said that she didn't want to see him any more. The therapist emphasized the triangular situation between the patient, Pamela, and her father, and the patient spoke once more with great intensity about the wish to kill her father. The therapist emphasized how his guilt about this must have interfered with his being able to deal with the situation effectively, and reminded the patient of the story of the fog coming down in his ORT.

In session 17 the patient looked subdued and upset and his hands were shaking. The other day he had visited the house that he and Pamela were to have lived in, and there had welled up in him more anger against her than he had ever known he had. He had rung her up and more or less ordered her to see him the evening after the present session. When she had demurred, he had told her that unless she came he would go round and cause trouble with her parents.

Sometime after this there was a rather confused discussion about the patient's feelings about the therapist. This ended unsatisfactorily, and the therapist felt he had to suggest another session.

For this session the patient arrived twenty-five minutes late, and it was clear that his feelings were very mixed about coming back at all. He said that perhaps he just wanted to be free of having to come here any more.

In this session the therapist got the story about the final meeting between the patient and Pamela. What had happened was that she had brought a girlfriend along with her to their meeting, and had said that she couldn't see him because the two of them were going off to have a meal. He said he knew very well that she was lying, so he let her go and then went and waited for her at the Tube station near her home. Sure enough, she arrived. She tried to get out of this, but he said to her, "Look, I don't want any more lies." Some sharp words passed between them and they parted. He went into the garden of his house and started to do some digging and said that he had felt very much better about the whole situation since. In fact, he said, he had been setting about getting one or two other girl friends.

In his final thanks to the therapist, it seemed as if his old defensive politeness had returned.

SUMMARY

This was a therapy with the following main characteristics:

1. Initial very low motivation, increasing dramatically in session 5 after much hard work on the therapist's part.

2. Two inter-related foci, (a) anxiety-laden hostility toward Pamela's father, linked with the patient's own father, and (b) anger against women.

3. The transference and the transference/parent link were relatively little emphasized, though there were six T/P interpretations recorded out of a total of 136 interpretations (4 percent).

Total number of sessions   18
Total time   5 months

FOLLOW-UP

4 Months. There was a sequence of misunderstandings over the arrangements for this meeting, much of which was clearly due to the patient's mixed feelings about coming back. The interview was mostly taken up with trying to deal with this and his relation with men in general. He said that there was constant tension inside him, and the therapist interpreted this as being due to intense feelings of antagonism to people that the patient had to hide. The patient told a story in which he had had a rather vindictive running battle by letter with an older man, which had ended in complete friendliness after the two had had a confrontation and spoken their minds to each other.

1 Year 7 Months. There was no acting out over this follow-up. The patient had now been married for nearly a year, and his wife was now expecting their first child. He said that the meeting with her had been providential; he had been "on his knees" and badly in need of "help, comfort, and support," On questioning, he admitted freely that in the early months of their marriage their relation had not run smoothly, and there had been a good deal of bickering. An important cause of this had almost certainly been his wife at times making him feel inferior. Their sexual relation had been disappointing, largely because of his own lack of desire, and intercourse was infrequent.

As far as symptoms were concerned, the patient said that for the past few months, ever since his wife had had an illness, he had had considerable difficulty in sleeping. He suffered first from early waking, and then from difficulty in getting to sleep. The patient provided some evidence that this might have been due to unconscious guilt at taking his wife away from her father, to whom she had been very close.

The patient's relation with his own father had improved very considerably. They now no longer quarreled and his father often came to him for advice.

1 Year 10 Months, Re-test. There were considerable changes from the first test, in three main areas, but only the first of these indicated any real resolution of his problems:

1. In his original test his first story had been about a man whose car had broken down in the middle of a storm and he had lost his way. In the re-test the story to this same card consisted of thinking over unsolved problems, reaching decisions, and putting them into effect successfully.

2. As far as problems over aggression against men were concerned, the impression that he gave the psychologist was that these had been bypassed rather than solved.

3. As far as his relations with women were concerned, the psychologist wrote that whereas in the first test the problem was getting a woman at all, now he had "got his woman but didn't know what to do with her." There was poverty of imagination in his stories concerned with this area, for which the patient apologized during the test.

7 Years 3 Months

General. The patient showed considerable unwillingness to come back, but was eventually persuaded to do so. In the interview it was quickly possible to relate this to his feelings about his former superiors at work and to his father, who he felt had driven him without any regard to the pain they were causing. The interview then became honest and easy.

1. Symptoms. (a) *Blackouts or substitute symptoms.* There have been no symptoms. On the contrary, he had handled a situation of great stress at work (see below) in a highly effective, independent, and appropriate way. (b) *Overdramatization*. This has disappeared. (c) *Overpoliteness*. This was almost absent at interview. He seemed much more sincere and able to admit his own shortcomings. There was, however, a rather patronizing attitude to certain people. (d) *Compulsiveness*. Whereas it had emerged in therapy that he had a compulsive need to plan everything ahead, he now clearly took great pleasure in having to cope with unexpected things at work.

2. Ability to Be Effective in General, and With Men in Particular. At interview the therapist reminded him that his two blackouts seemed to have been on occasions when he felt he couldn't cope, and asked him whether anything like this had ever occurred since. The patient said that he recognized this feeling of being unable to cope, and that it had in fact recurred about two and a half years ago, but that on this occasion he had reacted more "positively" to it. What had happened was that there had been a series of "political" changes in his work that made the position of a number of the staff intolerable. He had felt that either he was going to fold up or else he had to get out. What he had done was to start building up a private business of his own, while still keeping on at his job, and then to resign when he felt ready. His business consisted of dealing in secondhand precision instruments, and he had built this up to a point at which it was now really very successful. He said that he got along well with people of all kinds whom he had to deal with in his business. Moreover, he told a story in which he had dealt with some rather underhand methods of competition from a rival in a quite legitimate and highly effective way. His relation with his father had remained good, as in the previous follow-up, and he also told a story of putting his father in his place most effectively when this was necessary.

3. Ability to Be Effective With Women. The evidence about his relation with his wife was very clear. Whereas, before, he had had an overdramatized and largely fantasy-based relation with his former fiancée, in which he was quite unable to act effectively; now he had a real relation with a woman whom he valued, in which he could admit considerable difficulties, and in which there seemed to be a large amount of companionship and mutual cooperation. He had also changed from getting irritable when his wife made him feel inferior, to being able to admit without apparent anxiety that she was "streets ahead of him intellectually."

On the other hand, his marked lack of sexual drive remained, and he seemed to be unaware that this might be a serious privation for his wife.

Although it was clear that he enjoyed his family life, he also gave the impression that his main energy was poured into his business. This did not, however, involve excluding his wife, since she gave him a considerable amount of help in it.

4. Inner Feeling of Confidence in Himself as a Man. This seemed to be completely fulfilled in relation to men; but very partly fulfilled in relation to women (see above).

5. There were reservations over his limited ability to express concern for certain people, though not for others.

SUMMARY

We felt that although there had clearly been many changes, his preoccupation with his business and his ability to deal with men served to disguise a basic unresolved difficulty in relation to women.

The conclusions of Team 2 were essentially the same. They noted that the attempt to manipulate his environment passively—through his blackout—had changed into the ability to be aggressive directly and effectively. On the other hand, they noted that the patient did not seem to have mentioned love and affection at all.

SCORES

Team 1	2.5	3.0
Team 2	2.5	3.0
Mean	2.75	

The Cellist

SUMMARY

Category: Short, unfavorable (9 sessions, outcome 1.875).

A married man of thirty-two, a musician, whose livelihood was threatened by a symptom that affected his playing. The psychodynamics were extremely unclear. Early sessions contained many Oedipal interpretations; but the moment of greatest communication seemed to occur in session 7, with the emergence of guilt-laden hostility toward his mother, soon after which he broke off treatment. At follow-up there were considerable improvements, but—apart from an intense moment of self-assertion with his mother—many of these could be attributed to a realistic adjustment of his life to his symptom, which was basically unchanged.

CONTRIBUTION TO THE CORRELATIONS WITH OUTCOME

Motivation. Positive (moderate motivation, intermediate outcome).
Focality. Marked disagreement between the judges.
Transference/Parent Interpretations. Strongly positive (intermediate score, intermediate outcome).

DETAILS OF PATIENT AND THERAPIST

1. Patient

Sex	M.
Age	32.
Marital status	M.
Occupation	Cello player in an orchestra.
Complaint	Attacks of stiffness in his bowing arm (some years).
What seems to bring patient now	The fear that he will lose his job because of his symptom.

2. Therapist

Code	J
Sex	M

PSYCHIATRIC DIAGNOSIS

Phobic anxiety in an inhibited personality.

DISTURBANCES

1. *Symptom.* He plays the cello and his bowing arm gets stiff during pianissimo passages, so that he draws the bow jerkily across the strings. There is no difficulty with loud passages or when playing by himself. These attacks start with a racing in his heart that he is afraid will get out of control and will lead to his having to walk off the stage, and then to the loss of his job and his security. These symptoms are relieved by his drinking a pint of beer beforehand, and he is afraid he will become a "drinking musician."

He first noticed these symptoms several years ago, but they have become much worse since he had a row with his mother a few months ago.

2. Difficulty Over Aggression. He avoids disturbances at home by saying nothing, letting others have their own way, and waiting for them to get over their moods. His attitute to troubles is a passive acceptance.

3. History of Sexual Inhibition. He was always timid over seeking girls and he had no sexual contact before marriage. Now his wife is dissatisfied with the lack of frequency of sexual intercourse.

ADDITIONAL EVIDENCE

1. His father died when he was two and he was brought up by his mother. She used to have severe rages. She is at present living with him and his wife.

2. He played the cello from puberty, determining to be a musician when an old male friend of the family used to come and play the cello at his home. He practiced for hours, especially when beset by longings for a girl friend. The psychologist who tested him (who was also his therapist) wrote, "He has gone on finding one father after another who will help him to play well."

3. The interviewer described him as a quiet-voiced, gentle man, who avoided contact extremely well. The interviewer deliberately made somewhat disturbing interpretations about aggressive sexual feelings, including the suggestion that the jerky bowing movement was a masturbatory equivalent. There was a limited response to this, the patient becoming able to speak more easily about his loneliness as a child.

4. In the projection test, it seemed that the interview had been a considerable experience for him; and the psychologist wrote that he

wanted to communicate a host of feelings, particularly anger, envy, and a wish to punish other people.

5. In session 2 the therapist (who was the psychologist who had tested him) succeeded in bringing out daydreams of racing off on his motorbike and doing something violent.

HYPOTHESIS

It seems that his cello-playing has always represented for him an expression of his inner fantasy life, and he is afraid of unacceptable impulses breaking through into open expression. The main evidence suggests that these impulses are aggressive, but they are probably sexual as well. There is a general characterological defense against aggressive impulses consisting of passivity in the face of conflict with others.

CRITERIA

1. Loss of Symptoms. There should be an increased freedom in his playing, and he should be able to enjoy it to the full without disturbance or anxiety.

2. He should become free to assert himself constructively and to be angry in appropriate situations.

3. There should be an increased freedom and enjoyment of sexual feelings, and increased involvement in his relation with his wife and family.

4. He should become freer in making contact with people in general.

REASON FOR ACCEPTANCE AND THERAPEUTIC PLAN

The psychologist felt he had made contact with him and was eager to take him on. As far as understanding the psychodynamics was concerned, it was possible to make all sorts of psychoanalytic speculations about the meaning of his symptom, and it was obviously a significant fact that his father had died when he was two, but such speculations were based on very little direct evidence. The implied plan was to try and interpret sexual, aggressive, and Oedipal feelings that were presumed to underlie his symptom.

SUMMARY OF COURSE OF THERAPY

Much of therapy seems to have consisted of a search for a focus, with a number of interpretations being made on different themes.

With hindsight, including the information given at follow-up, it really looks as if the current problem worrying the patient was his inability to express anger against his mother, an interpretation of which was reached in session 7, with a very marked response, and that even when there did appear to be a response to Oedipal interpretations earlier in therapy, this was not the main point.

One of the early themes was hostility against and rivalry with men, father-figures such as conductors in the present, and the patient's brother in the past. The therapist interpreted how important the patient wanted to feel in relation to the women in his present household—which included the patient's mother—and yet how weak and impotent he feared he really was. This was linked with the childhood situation, in which he wanted to be more important to his mother than his brother or his dead father. Work of this kind seems to have disturbed him, because he began to say that he didn't know what to say next, and would be worrying himself sick as to what he was going to say next week. A comparison between this anxiety and his anxiety about playing the cello gave the patient considerable relief. In session 6 he reported a quarrel with his wife, in which she had complained about his going out to play chamber music. He said he felt fulfilled and relieved playing chamber music, which was quite different from how he felt when playing in an orchestra.

The climax of therapy came in session 7. The patient spoke of always being in rivalry with his brother, who as a child used to get into all sorts of scrapes, quite unlike the patient. The therapist pointed out that the brother was showing his independence and his hostility to his mother, and that although the patient had never been able to do this openly, it was now coming out in relation to his wife—his wanting to go out and do something violent on his motorbike or go off with another girl, etc. The patient agreed that his feeling of duty to his wife was similar to what he felt for his mother when he was a child. The patient went on to speak about an old man who used to come round to the house and say how wonderful the patient's mother was. He said this moralizing made him sick. The therapist interpreted that the moralizing frightened him because he felt he ought to be grateful to his mother for not leaving the children and going and finding another husband. The patient smiled in great relief and said, "Yes, of course."

The aftermath of this session was two sessions in which hardly any communication took place, followed by a letter to the therapist, saying that he felt unable to continue with treatment and apologizing for wasting so much of the therapist's time.

Throughout therapy there were a number of transference/parent interpretations, with the therapist interpreted as either the patient's father or mother. They were on various themes and their significance was never clear.

Total number of sessions   9
Total time   3½ months

FOLLOW-UP (4 years 8 months)

1. Symptoms.

2. Problems Over Aggression. These are best considered in the light of the whole sequence of events since termination:

He said that in therapy he felt he had put forward the whole history of his life, and that he was waiting for the therapist to do something, which of course the therapist didn't. This was why he had stopped coming. A few weeks after termination, however, he began to realize that he must do something himself. Things had come to a head between him and his mother, who was living in his house. He said that she was a depressed person for whom nothing was ever quite right, and that he saw that she was doing to his children what she had done to him as a child. So he had a row with her and told her she must go. She went back to where she used to live, where she had a number of friends, and she now seems to be reasonably happy there. She still visits him from time to time and they seem to be on quite good terms. He spoke of his therapy with appreciation, saying that he thought it had somehow got things moving.

This change in circumstances made the situation very much easier at home, but his symptom remained unchanged, and he began to get increasingly anxious about playing in the orchestra. Eventually a G.P. put him on a drug for this (perhaps an MAO inhibitor) that very greatly helped. One day, however, he panicked while playing and collapsed, was found to have a raised blood pressure, and had to be taken off the drug. This forced him back into coping with his symptom, which finally became so bad that he asked to be seen at the Tavistock Clinic once more. Here he saw a doctor who told him that perhaps he was in the wrong job. After much conflict he then resigned from the orchestra; and after trying other work for a short time, he returned to cello-playing, but this time free-lance, both in small orchestras and in chamber music. He has been very successful.

This change was both the fulfillment of a long-held ambition and an avoidance of a stress-provoking situation. He has not resolved his symptom, which remains essentially unchanged, but its impact has been mitigated in three ways: (a) resignation from the orchestra has meant that he is no longer under the domination of a large organization in which he has to play what he is told; (b) becoming free-lance has meant that he can now tell himself that he can refuse to play particular pieces that might give him special trouble (though he has never actually done so); and (c) playing chamber music has meant that he can now use any bowing that helps him to avoid his symptom, rather than having to conform to that used by everyone else. He did not say that there had been any freeing in his playing, but he has clearly done very well, and his symptom must interfere very little with how his playing actually sounds.

As far as his main *symptom* is concerned, therefore, it seems clear that it is essentially unchanged, but that he has rearranged his life in a thoroughly constructive way so that is interferes as little as possible.

Drinking was not mentioned at the follow-up interview.

As far as *problems of aggression* are concerned, there have thus been two instances of constructive self-assertion over major matters. Moreover, the therapist also said that there was a major change in the way in which the patient spoke and held himself; previously he had given the impression of being a "little mouse," now he radiated a quiet confidence. On the other hand, it also became clear that aggression in minor matters still gives him a great deal of trouble. He said that he avoids rows, and when he does have them they intensify his symptom.

3. Sex. He said that his sexual life was very satisfactory, but we do not know to what extent this represents a change.

4. Increased Involvement With His Wife and Family. Here the situation was very interesting. The fact that he has become free-lance means that he travels around the country a great deal, and also goes abroad, so that he has achieved a considerable degree of freedom from his family. However, this has meant in turn that when he *is* at home he feels much more involved and more contented. His wife has her own activities, and he much enjoys the free-and-easy atmosphere at home, with children popping in and out.

5. Freedom in Making Contact With People in General. He still maintains a certain solitariness but also has many friends. There did appear to be considerable freeing here also.

DISCUSSION

There seems to have been a marked change away from passive acceptance toward active dealing with major situations. On the other hand, there seems to be little freeing of aggression in less major matters, his symptom remains basically unchanged, and it is exacerbated by rows. In relation to his wife and family and people in general he seems to have achieved a greater involvement by also allowing himself greater freedom.

SCORES

Team 1	1.5	2.0
Team 2	2.0	2.0
Mean	1.875	

Mrs. Craig

SUMMARY

Category: Long, favorable (76 sessions, outcome 2.875).

A long and complex therapy of a woman of thirty-seven complaining of frigidity. An initial period of therapy resulted in a marked improvement in the sexual situation, but the story then developed into tragedy, with the patient's deeply felt desire to have a baby thwarted by repeated miscarriages. Moreover, it soon became clear that this was a marriage between a frigid woman and a man who had little interest in sex and little interest in changing the situation. The final result was that the patient's feelings were freed and deepened in a most striking way, but her husband then withdrew, and she had to settle for a celibate marriage.

CONTRIBUTION TO THE CORRELATIONS WITH OUTCOME

Motivation. Neutral (moderate motivation, favorable outcome).
Focality. Strongly positive (high focality, favorable outcome).
Transference/Parent Interpretations. Positive (high score, favorable outcome).

DETAILS OF PATIENT AND THERAPIST

1. Patient

Sex	F.
Age	37.
Marital status	Married.
Occupation	Editorial assistant to a publisher.
Complaint: what seems to bring patient now	Severe distaste for intercourse.

2. Therapist

Code	E
Sex	M

PSYCHIATRIC DIAGNOSIS

Depression and frigidity in an inhibited personality.

DISTURBANCES

1. Difficulties With Men. (a) *Sexual difficulties.* Distaste for sexual intercourse. She has never obtained any satisfaction. She freezes up as soon as any sign of passion appears in herself or her husband. She and her husband only succeeded in starting their sexual life after several months of marriage. When they did start they had intercourse only rarely and finally gave it up because her vagina always went into spasm. They have now had no sexual contact for three years. She is contemptuous of her husband's weakness in letting her be frigid, but feels guilty about this because of his kindness. (b) *More general difficulties*. She has experienced great difficulty in getting beyond superficial contact with men. She gets a feeling of tension in her stomach whenever anyone gets emotionally close to her.

2. Possible Depressive Problem. She appeared depressed and hopeless at interview. There were several items concerned with loss in the ORT.

ADDITIONAL EVIDENCE

1. Her mother was a Welsh Methodist, very strict and puritanical. She was rather vague about her father, but seemed to have a fairly good relation with him. Neither parent was demonstrative.

2. She married five years ago after several years of hesitation. Her husband is considerably older. She described him as very understanding and considerate.

3. In her childhood her mother had made a great scene on more than one occasion when she asked questions about sex.

4. Both her interviewer, the psychologist who tested her, and her therapist repeatedly emphasized their impression that she was extremely afraid of sexual and aggressive feelings that were very intense.

5. There was an important moment in the initial interview when the patient mentioned that between the age of seven and nine she slept in her parents' bedroom. She remembers an occasion when her father got on top of her mother, her mother said, "No, no," and then the recollection breaks off. The interviewer said that exactly the same pattern appeared in her own sexual life. He wrote that at this point it was "as if she had seen some light," and they immediately began to discuss possible therapy.

6. The psychologist wrote that beneath the Oedipal anxieties there was probably a depressive basis to her problems.

HYPOTHESIS

She is afraid of her sexual impulses (1) because she feels her mother forbids them, and (2) because they contain an element of intense aggressiveness toward the man.

CRITERIA

1. Relation With Men. Ability to enjoy a relation with a man, including the sexual relation, which must include in addition: (a) ability to have orgasm; (b) ability to enjoy her husband's potency, with loss of the need to denigrate him; (c) ability to enjoy an aggressive element in sexuality; and (d) ability to feel emotionally close to him without signs of anxiety. She should feel more confident in herself as a woman.

2. Depression. She should not be subject to continuing depression.

REASON FOR ACCEPTANCE AND THERAPEUTIC PLAN

The psychiatrist and psychologist agreed that she had a good personality, was under great pressure, had high motivation, and a good capacity for insight. The plan was simply to interpret sexual anxieties.

SUMMARY OF COURSE OF THERAPY

It is only possible to give an overall impression of this extremely long and complex therapy.

The main theme in sessions 2–4 was the resemblance between her behavior with the (male) therapist and with her husband, and the different kinds of feeling involved (i.e., the different aspects of the transference/"other" link). In session 2 she agreed that she had "frozen up" as soon as she entered the session. In session 3 she started inhibited and intellectual, and the therapist interpreted that she was *angry* with him for "wading in" last week, with which she whole-heartedly agreed. With help she was then able to speak of great *envy* of men and suffragette sympathies (nowadays we would use a different term!). In session 4 the therapist interpreted that she was *afraid she had damaged him* by her aggressiveness of last week, which again improved the atmosphere of the session. She then on four or five occasions went so far with a topic and then abandoned it, and the therapist related this to her sexual freeze-up. Her response was to say that her husband was a good man, and to express her despair that anything could be done. The therapist in turn responded by *direct advice and encouragement,* suggesting that they have a go at intercourse again, even after all these years, with open acknowledgment that they would not necessarily succeed.

In session 5 she reported an unsuccessful attempt at intercourse in which she had frozen the moment there was any contact with her husband's penis, and in addition he had suffered from premature ejaculation the moment she touched his penis (the usual pattern for both of them). The therapist suggested that she needed to keep "on top" and to retain full control, and he went on to make a link with the past, suggesting that this was based on identification with her mother. She agreed and went on to tell of her childhood with an ailing, dominating mother, and a father who was not interested in her, in a house where all sex matters were taboo.

In session 6 she reported the first successful intercourse for a long time, in which her husband had achieved full penetration and she had had vaginal pleasure but no orgasm. However, the next time he tried she had put him off, and he now was ignoring her even though she had told him to pay no attention to her resistances. The therapist wrote that he was worried about the husband's ineffectiveness.

In session 7 she reported further attempts at intercourse but no vaginal sensation. For the first time she spoke of her mother's death, of feeling guilty at having been to the cinema just before, and of having been unable to cry. After this she had had to nurse her broken-down father and to do the housekeeping in her mother's place. This again involved a link between the past and the present, for it followed her speaking of her husband as if he were crippled and she were looking after him like a nurse.

The climax of the first stage of therapy came in the transference in session 10. In the previous session the therapist had interpreted that sexual anxieties were being concealed. During the week she panicked at the thought that she was seeking a closer relationship with the therapist than she had allowed herself to admit, and she rang up and was given an emergency session. The therapist's main interpretation was that she was afraid he was as hostile to her as she was to her own sexual wishes. She left much calmer.

Session 11 brought out very clear Oedipal material: The patient was shocked to find herself wishing that a very dear woman friend, who was dying, would leave a television set to her. The therapist pointed out an important parallel, namely that she had benefited from her mother's death by being enabled to enjoy the relation with her father.

During the next six sessions a number of improvements became clear. She arrived brightly dressed and for the first time did not look like a woman in mourning. She and her husband were now having intercourse two or three times a week, and he was now able to last out for up to ten minutes and to give her some pleasure, though she still did not have orgasm. There was an important moment in which she openly became angry at a phrase in one of the therapist's letters, "I am *willing* to see you," and he managed to bring out her feeling of humiliation at wanting a man. They agreed to terminate after session 17, much of which she spent in tears, acknowledging the importance the therapist had for her (score for *importance of termination* was already at a maximum at this point).

She was then seen for a follow-up interview, plus an independent assessment, two and a half months after this first termination. The sexual situation was maintained, and the whole relation with her husband was improved; he was now more confident and would take the lead in matters that formerly he would have left to her. On the other hand, she said that her social anxiety was little improved, and she now wanted further treatment for this, and to help her "feel joy and grief more profoundly."

Three months after the first termination she rang up and asked for another appointment (session 18), revealing that her menstrual period was overdue and she thought she might be pregnant (which in fact she was). She was then seen for six more sessions, in which the two main themes were (1) the feeling that she didn't need men any more because she had now something inside her that was as good as anything they could give her; and (2) further work on guilt in relation to her mother. Her husband soon became reconciled to the fact that the patient was having a baby. However, this whole period was somewhat undynamic, until finally in session 24 the therapist interpreted that she didn't feel she needed him now, but didn't want to lose the relation with him. This was clearly exactly right, and they agreed not to meet for the time being.

The birth of the baby was the beginning of tragedy, for it died within twenty-four hours. Almost the whole of the rest of therapy was now concerned with her repeated attempts to have another baby, all of which ended in failure, because although she became pregnant on two further occasions she miscarried each time. The therapist's main efforts were directed toward helping her to face her anger and grief about this. During this period there were a number of transference/ parent interpretations, mostly of the therapist as *mother*—either as a good mother in alliance against the bad mother, or as the bad mother who did not wish the patient to have babies.

There was a break of six months in treatment after thirty-five sessions, and it is possible to make a tentative assessment of the situation then and to give a score. During this six-month break she became pregnant for the second time, and had her first miscarriage. The therapist then saw her again and continued to see her irregularly for a total of about five years since the initial interview. Inspection of the therapist's diaries then indicates a gap of two years, followed by three more sessions just before the final follow-up. The total number of sessions since the beginning appeared to be seventy-six.

FOLLOW-UP

(A few weeks after the last session of irregular therapy; 7 years 3 months since the initial interview)

The patient was seen by the therapist, and her husband was then seen by him at her request three weeks later. Five months later she wrote a letter describing the latest situation and her feelings about it.

At interview, she said that she and her husband had reached deadlock—she wanted intercourse far more often than he was willing to give it. In his own interview he appeared as a quiet, gentle man, who felt that there were more important things in life than sex, and who was adamant in wishing to leave the situation as it was. In her final deeply felt letter, she wrote that she was far too fond of her husband to leave him, and that she had to accept a celibate marriage. "We have talked about it and I have told him I will no longer press him on the intimate side of our marriage, but neither can I accept the possibility of being expected to behave like a wife about once every three months."

Our assessment of the final follow-up was as follows:

1. Relation With Husband

(a) Ability to Enjoy the Relation, Including the Sexual Relation. There has been a very marked change in her in that, whereas before she used to freeze up at any sign of passion, she now wants sex very badly and can enjoy it, though without orgasm.

(b) Ability to Enjoy Her Husband's Potency, With Loss of the Need to Denigrate Him. At one time her husband showed a marked increase in potency, and also became able to take the lead in other ways, and she enjoyed this. This has not stood the test of time. It seems that there was always a reluctance in him to meet her sexual needs fully, and until recently she handled this in an extremely mature way, encouraging him so that he responded. Her final decision to give up sex altogether rather than to accept being a wife once in three months is one that can only be respected.

On the surface it appears that now all the sexual difficulty is in him rather than in her; but we cannot necessarily accept this at face value. No final decision is possible on the evidence.

At one time she was able to enjoy her husband's increased

forcefulness; and now she is angry with him but respects him and wants to make the best of their relation. It would seem, therefore, that the need to denigrate him is not longer present.

(c) **Ability to Enjoy an Aggressive Element in Sexuality.** The therapist states, "She wants her husband to be aggressive in sexuality but he is not." We must assume this criterion to be fulfilled.

(d) **Ability to Feel Emotionally Close to Him Without Signs of Anxiety.** The therapist wrote that this criterion was fulfilled. "Sometimes the closeness is only that of a mother with a child (or a daughter with an ailing father) but on the rare occasions when they have intercourse she feels very warm, close, and happy."

(e) **Confidence in Herself as a Woman.** All the evidence suggested that she now feels complete as a woman but feels it is too late.

2. She Should Not Be Subject to Continuing Depression
This also is completely fulfilled. During the whole period covered by therapy she has never had a serious attack of depression. On the contrary she has reacted with an entirely appropriate sadness and grief to the loss of her pregnancies and the final deadlock with her husband. It is worth noting that the wish to "feel joy and grief more profoundly" was one of her reasons for continuing treatment beyond the first seventeen sessions. This has clearly been fulfilled.

3. Problems Not Known at Initial Assessment

(a) **Social Difficulties.** At the beginning of the second course of treatment she made a new complaint: an inability to get close to people socially. The therapist said that this was much improved; she was able to get on better with people at work, and to quarrel with her in-laws in a way that improved the situation.

(b) **Difficulties Over Aggression.** These seem to have considerably improved, as shown by (i) her wish for an aggressive element in sex, (ii) the above-mentioned example of constructive aggression with her in-laws, and (iii) her ability to assert herself sufficiently with her husband to persuade him to come for an interview.

(c) **Inability to Bear Children.** The cause of this is, of course, entirely unknown, but it may possibly have a psychologist element.

DISCUSSION

Team 1 felt that there had been a major resolution in her main problem; Team 2 were more cautious, feeling that some of the *inner* aggression toward her husband's masculinity (as opposed to her legitimate anger against him) was unresolved, indicated by fears of damaging him and wearing him out. Team 1, however, also expressed doubts, because of her inability to have orgasm and the possibility that she still contributes toward the unsatisfactory sexual situation. They added that this seemed to be a typical case of a frigid woman marrying an impotent man, and they questioned how much further improvement was possible when the husband was not willing to be treated.

SCORES

Team 1	3.0	3.0
Team 2	3.0	2.5
Mean	2.875	

The Dress Designer

SUMMARY

Category: Long, unfavorable (>200 sessions, outcome 1.25).

A married woman of twenty-six presenting a crippling agoraphobic condition of acute onset. She was misdiagnosed as suffering from a disturbance at the hysterical level, but was later found to be suffering from a very severe and primitive disturbance involving fear of loss of identity.

Hers was the most dynamic of all our therapies, being given high scores for all three important dynamic factors. The poor outcome thus caused strong negative contributions to all the important correlations.

DETAILS OF PATIENT AND THERAPIST

1. Patient

Sex	F.
Age	26.
Marital status	Married.
Occupation	She works in a dress designer's office.
Complaint: what seems to bring patient now	Panic attacks (about three months). Seven weeks ago the attacks became so bad that she felt she could not go out of the house.

2. Therapist

Code	B
Sex	M

PSYCHIATRIC HISTORY AND DIAGNOSIS

Family History. Her mother is described as chronically depressed; and she has three sisters, all of whom have shown evidence of difficulties in personal relations.

Previous Personality. Until the present illness she had appeared to be a very stable person, always able to cope with difficulties.

Present Illness. Within the last three months there were two premonitory anxiety attacks. These consisted of the need to go out and pass water when she was in the presence of a number of other people, and when she returned, feeling frightened of everybody. Her present illness proper began dramatically seven weeks ago with attacks of panic at home accompanied by palpitations. She became too frightened to go out of the house or to meet people. She was unable to concentrate and she could not sleep without hypnotics. One month ago, while eating her dinner, she suddenly had the passing thought that she might cut her own throat. Soon after the beginning of these attacks, she and her husband went to live at her mother's house so that she could be looked after. Since then she has spent most of her time in bed.

Mental State. She arrived at the interview in an agitated state, but settled down, made very good contact, and spoke about herself seriously and with considerable insight.

Diagnosis. Acute anxiety state.

DISTURBANCES

1. Symptoms. Anxiety state as above.

2. Difficulties in Relation to Men. Although she likes and respects her husband, she has never been able to express herself sexually with him. She has never had an orgasm. Two years ago she fell in love with a younger man at the office who was in trouble. She felt that she would be able to express all her sexual feelings with him; but in fact the relation didn't go beyond his kissing her once. She now feels this was a "fake" love affair. Discussing this with her husband recently has improved their sexual relation.

3. Difficulties Over Her Own Needs and Other People's Needs; Difficulties Over Aggression. The initial assessment material contains the recurrent theme of setting aside her own needs in favor of those of others, feeling extremely resentful about this, but being unable to express her resentment.

ADDITIONAL EVIDENCE

1. She is the second of four girls. She said that her mother was never demonstrative, but worked extremely hard and expressed her affection for the children through material things. The only way the patient knew to win her mother's love was by doing well at school. Her father was very retiring and hardly played any part in the family at all. He was disappointed at not having a boy. Two of her sisters suffered from a good deal of illness when she was a child, and consequently got more attention than she did.

2. She has been married for four years. One year ago her husband

gave up his job in advertising, and started an advertising business of his own. While he was working this business up, they lived on her salary.

3. She said that members of the family always came to her when they were in trouble. About six months ago she had had to cope with an emotional crisis in which her younger sister, Liz, had thought she was pregnant. Since this theme of attending to other people's needs rather than her own ran throughout the whole of the initial interview, the interviewer (Therapist F) interpreted that she must really feel resentful about this, must be guilty about feeling so resentful, and then perhaps—in compensation—felt that she could not go out and enjoy herself at all. Her response to this was to say that that would explain why her breakdown occurred when it did. Recently her husband had said that his business was now doing well enough for her to think of giving up work and to have a baby. It was just at this point, when at last she could sit back and relax and have what she wanted, that her breakdown had occurred.

4. In the projection test (ORT), the psychologist was impressed by her accurate perception of the cards. She told real-life stories, but with a tendency at first to gloss over feelings of resentment and aggression, and to present a rosy picture of family life. The psychologist commented on this, and later stories became much more aggressive. The dominant fantasy, which ran through the whole of the material, was of a situation in which her needs are not being satisfied, but she must cover up her resentment and hatred about this and show a smiling face to the world. This theme applied particularly to men. The man is seen as someone very superior whose every whim she is expected to satisfy. She is supposed to be content with swallowing her own resentment and devoting herself to a life of service to him. Later there was a theme of lynching, and later a funeral scene in which the people were not really mourning, but feeling sulky and angry. Women seemed less useless to her than men, but the basic theme appeared in relation to them as well.

5. Between the initial interview and the projection test a fortnight later, she had a relapse and spent most of the time in bed. In session 2, much more conscious aggression emerged, which the therapist concentrated on interpreting. She had been haunted by the image of a knife at her throat. When her mother brought her a meal in bed, she looked up and all she could see was her mother's wrinkled neck. She said she knew that she was bottling anger up inside her, but only once or twice in her life had she ever really given way to it and then she was terrified by what happened. As a little girl she had chased one of

her younger sisters around the garden and really felt that she could murder her. This was followed by the theme of remaining calm and uninvolved while her sisters threw tantrums, and also while her husband became sexually excited with her. The therapist interpreted that in this way she expressed triumph and contempt.

HYPOTHESIS

There seems clear evidence that both her mother and her father have failed to recognize her emotional needs. Her lifelong defense against admitting her murderous resentment about this has been to deny her needs and to attend to those of others.

She is now faced with a situation in which she (1) has to give up looking after her husband and become dependent upon him; and (2), if she has a child, will have to give to it the maternal care she feels she has missed herself. The result has been a complete breakdown of her defenses.

CRITERIA

She should be able to strike a balance between her own needs and those of others. This should result in:

1. Loss of symptoms.

2. Evidence of enjoying both (a) her dependence on a man as an adult woman and (b) his dependence on her as an adult man.

3. Ability to assert herself constructively where appropriate.

4. Enjoyment of the sexual relationship with a man and valuation of his masculinity.

REASON FOR ACCEPTANCE AND THERAPEUTIC PLAN

This patient was in the midst of a severe crisis and it would have been difficult to refuse to help her. The initial interview and projection test both emphasized the same theme, which could clearly be made into a focus: the feeling that her own needs were not being met, and that she must cover up her anger about this by attending to those of others. Both interviewer and psychologist were impressed with her capacity for insight and her apparent ability to face her true feelings, the psychologist writing that there was "strong evidence for a basically sound ego." The only reservation was the severity of her symptom, and the extreme degree of dependence expressed by it, for which the material available did not offer any satisfactory explanation.

The therapist wrote as his plan: "To enable her to express her resentment and hatred of people. Presumably this would mainly be done in the transference."

SUMMARY OF COURSE OF THERAPY

With hindsight we should have been warned by the severity of her main symptom. Therapy took the course typical of a very severe hysteric: de-repression of intense and violent feelings, intense ambivalent sexual transference, "false" sexuality, desperate crises, the dramatic acquisition of apparently genuine insight that failed to lead to the expected therapeutic effects—those improvements that did occur being followed by relapse to a position as bad as ever—the emergence of considerable overdetermination and of a fundamentally pre-genital disturbance much severer than originally suspected (involving deep-seated identity problems), and in the short term little therapeutic effect accompanied by the impossibility of considering termination.

It is important also that this basically unsuccessful therapy with an unrealistically chosen patient was the *most dynamic* of our whole sample—high motivation, high focality, the emergence of early transference, many transference/parent interpretations, and much work on termination—and it thus made a strong negative contribution to all the important correlations.

Precipitating Factors. In the initial assessment it seemed that the original precipitating factor had been the fact that her husband's business was now doing well enough for her to think of having a baby. In session 3 she mentioned that her breakdown occurred shortly after her husband had passed his driving test, and perhaps this meant that she felt no longer in control and resented it.

However, in session 18 a precipitating event emerged that cast an entirely different light on her symptoms. As already mentioned, a few months before her first panic attack she had had to help her younger sister, Liz, over a crisis in which Liz thought she was pregnant and in a state of desperation had come to stay with the patient. In fact Liz had then had a rather heavy menstrual period, and it was never quite clear whether or not this was a miscarriage. It had already emerged in therapy that Liz was the one who rebelled against her parents and in addition seemed to get more attention than the patient did. The therapist suggested that the patient must have envied Liz her pregnancy, and felt very guilty about the wish to triumph over her and kill her baby. The patient went on to describe the first occasion on which her panic had occurred—she was taken to the theater by a male friend as a substitute for his wife who was having a miscarriage. Eventually it emerged that the patient had consciously thought that she deserved to have a baby whereas Liz didn't. She went on to admit that when her elder sister suffered a tragedy she had felt it served her right.

This event also appeared to be the essential factor in the major crisis of the whole therapy, which occurred after session 19 and will be considered in the next section.

The Main Theme of Therapy: the Transference, Relation to Men, Triangular Relations. In session 3 she mentioned that she had previously tended to choose men who appeared strong but were really weak, as a result of which she always had felt compelled to remain the strong one, but that her husband really was strong.

However, in session 3 she said that "perhaps she had not allowed her husband to be strong with her." The therapist linked this with her weak father, saying that she had never felt she had a proper man as an ally against her mother. To this she said, "Are fathers really important for girls?"

In this session she had reported some improvements, but in session 5 she arrived in a panicky state. She said, "My husband has been having intercourse with me quite a bit recently," but she added that she had not been satisfied. The therapist suggested that she really wanted to have a "flaming row" both with her husband and himself, because like her mother and father they were being nice and kind and considerate and helpful, but she felt nevertheless that they were useless (transference/parent interpretation). At this she seemed to become calmer. The therapist then added that both with him and with her husband she was bottling up her intense sexual needs, which were threatening to overwhelm her. Soon after this she asked if she could go to the lavatory.

A theme that emerged in session 6 was how for the whole of her life she had put off the hope of satisfying her own needs and had patiently waited for better times. The therapist interpreted that as soon as she was faced with the possibility of giving up this waiting and getting something for herself, it seemed like "opening the floodgates" and she became overwhelmed by the intensity of her needs and the expectation that no man would be strong enough to satisfy them. He related this both to the precipitation of her symptoms, to the transference, and to her feeling of hopelessness about getting anything from such a useless and remote father.

In session 9 she said something that shed light on the problems of her childhood, namely, that she had been looking through old photographs and she had found that there were many of them featuring her sisters but very few of her.

In session 12 she reported that she had been furious with her husband for taking female clients at his office after all the rest of the staff had gone. She had never felt such an intense feeling—it was as if her whole head was red and bursting. The therapist remarked on her anger both that her husband should attend to other women and that he should get satisfaction while she didn't, and he linked this with the feeling that her own loving offers toward him (the therapist) had been rejected. She accepted this interpretation immediately. Later in this session therapist and patient provisionally agreed that they should have six more sessions.

Typical of this hysterical patient was that in the next session (no. 13) she said, "For five months people have been telling me that my trouble is repressed anger and I haven't really felt it yet"(!). The therapist said that at all costs she had to prevent him from making any impact on her, and thus could demonstrate her contempt for him. He did not link this with the termination issue brought up in the last session, which he perhaps might have done.

As has already been mentioned, in session 18 the possible miscarriage of her younger sister, Liz, emerged as an important precipitating factor in the patient's symptoms. In session 19 the therapist interpreted that because the patient's early childhood experiences were contaminated by hatred and rivalry, she had come to mistrust entirely her capacity to love, and that love had become inextricably mixed up with hating and killing. He linked this both with the patient's mother and with her husband. Later he asked her what in her imagination would be the greatest triumph over Liz, to which she said it would be to seduce a boyfriend away from her. The therapist interpreted that becoming a complete woman was the most frightening thing of all, because it represented achieving this kind of triumph over her mother. At this point the patient came to life and told a dream in which Princess Margaret had told the patient that her husband, Antony Armstrong-Jones, was impotent, and suggested that it might be a good idea for him to sleep with the patient. They tried, but he failed. She then told of another dream in which she was carrying a head on a tray and trying to get rid of it. These dreams were told at the very end of the session, and the therapist interpreted only that her frigidity was a defense against rivaling her mother.

Session 19 was on a Friday. On the Monday morning her husband rang to say that the patient had been having shivering fits and attacks of panic over the weekend, and that the G.P. had recommended admission to a hospital. The therapist said that it would be better if the situation could be dealt with in therapy and offered to see her daily during the crisis period.

The patient managed to come and said that she had begun to get anxious on Friday evening, and that by Sunday morning she was experiencing fear that was absolutely indescribable. The name of the man in the office with whom she had had an idealized and abortive relation kept coming into her mind, and especially the thought of his indifference to her. The therapist linked this with the theme of termination, and the patient replied that last Friday's session had reminded her of the very first therapeutic session (no. 2), in which she now said that she had been so swamped by physical desire for the therapist that she could hardly hear what he was saying.

In sessions 23 and 24 there was much further discussion of her sexual feelings for the therapist, her need to keep control, and her fear of being overwhelmed. At one point in session 24, however, he suggested that in the recent crisis she might have been reliving Liz's experience during her possible pregnancy and miscarriage. The patient brushed this aside.

Nevertheless, in session 25 she said that she had been thinking about this interpretation and suddenly it had all slipped into place. She realized now that many of the details of her own crisis were identical with those of Liz's crisis; e.g., her own fear of dying of hemorrhage. Moreover, the most extraordinary thing of all was that when she looked in her diary she found that her own crisis had occurred over exactly the same weekend this year as Liz's crisis last year. The therapist interpreted that her reliving of Liz's crisis must be a punishment for the feelings of triumph she was having a year ago.

In sessions 34 and 35 there emerged for the first time the breakdown of the idealization of her husband. She described him as silent, unresponsive, and infuriatingly detached. She said that she had never felt the marriage to be satisfactory and for years she had pretended to herself that everything was all right. She felt hopeless; she cannot remain a baby forever, yet to become an adult again is equally unrewarding because it means being lonely and having to pretend again. Attempts to link this with the transference met with the reply that she felt it much more in relation to her husband. In the next session (no. 36) she said that he had never aroused her physically and nor had any other man.

In session 37 she said that she had tried to show her husband how she wanted him to make love to her, but he just said that he was going to do it his way and she must submit. She got angry and seriously thought of leaving him. She said she cannot go back home and pick up the same pattern of life as before. She then said that the reason why she dare not go out and mix with people may be the fear that she may lose control of herself and show the world how frustrated and resentful she is. She even thinks that the reason why she may have chosen to marry this particular man is exactly because he was not capable of arousing strong feelings in her and thus breaking down her control. She again denied an attempt to link this with the transference, and said that treatment had done a lot for her; she does not feel the same person, and she has been put in touch with feelings that were entirely hidden previously. The session ended with her reiterating that she cannot go back home to the previous impossible situation, with her husband unchanged and her going back to the apparently good-tempered person that she was before.

The Course of Therapy in Terms of Time Limits and Attempts at Termination; the Relation With Her Mother; Further Therapy. The original plan put to the patient was that she should have twelve sessions; i.e., (adding the initial interview) therapy would end at session 13. By the time session 12 came around she was in the middle of intense feelings and termination was nowhere near in sight. Therapist and patient then agreed to have six more sessions (i.e., to end on session 19). However, by session 14 this seemed to have been forgotten and the therapist suggested that they should decide on a termination date within the next few sessions, though he would be able to see her irregularly according to need thereafter. Her response was bewilderment—how could she possibly know how many more sessions she needed?

What happened in the next session (no. 15) was quite unexpected. There was an outpouring of resentment against the therapist, not for suggesting termination, but for failing to see that her problem was not with her husband but with her mother. Her mother is convinced that her own way of life is the right one and that she knows what is best; and the patient, ever since she was a child, has refused to become like her mother and sisters and has tried to be a separate person in her own right. Her account of her feelings was at times almost incoherent, and the therapist had difficulty in making effective interpretations. He tried suggesting that she felt that he pretended to know what was best for her, like her mother, and would not allow her to assert her independence and find a solution that was true to herself (transference/parent interpretation). He brought up the question of termination. She again said that she had no idea how many sessions she wanted, so he fixed a time limit of eight more sessions, which she accepted with a shrug.

In session 16 the therapist expected anger about termination, but this was not so. She said that during the week she had decided to make a real effort to visit her home, but she had begun imagining that she might find a body hanging from the ceiling there, and she had not managed to go. During the session she started shaking as if she was terrified. She went on to say that her mother interfered in everyone's lives, and she was frightened of finding the same traits in herself. The therapist interpreted that despite her efforts to be as unlike her mother as possible, she was afraid that her mother had got inside her and was swamping her personality, and her only way of breaking free from this would be to kill the mother inside her. (In her fantasy the body hanging from the ceiling was that of a man, which possibly did not fit in with this interpretation, though of course it might have represented the therapist himself.) However, the patient gave the impression that this interpretation was meaningful, and her trembling stopped fairly early in the session.

The termination issue seems also to have contributed to the crisis of sessions 20–25, already described. In session 21 the therapist suggested that the crisis expressed her rage about termination and was for the purpose of getting everybody rallying around and attending to her—since he was now seeing her daily she had achieved what she wanted. In fact in the next session (no. 22) it emerged that the immediate cause of the present crisis seemed to have been that the patient's G.P. (a woman) had told her she was going away for a fortnight. The patient eventually said that though it was important to be able to see the therapist daily, it would be even more important to know that she could ring him at any time, and she pressed him to give her his home phone number. Though doubtful about the wisdom of doing this, he gave it to her.

In session 28 there was a further discussion of the termination issue and it was agreed that they would re-assess the situation after the therapist's holiday in a month's time. In the next session (no. 29) she brought the important piece of insight that she had never terminated a relationship in her life with a feeling of something having been successfully completed. She felt it was essential to try and break this pattern in her relation with the therapist. The therapist felt that she was closer than ever before to a sincere acknowledgment of what she was feeling in a relationship.

In session 32 she reported that she had been home with her husband for the first time and while there had burnt some papers concerned with the man at the office. She went on to say that the relationship with this man never came to anything, nor could she get rid of him. The therapist pointed out that this was identical with the situation with him, to which she replied, "Exactly."

In session 36 she suggested that after the therapist's forthcoming holiday they should meet twice in the first week and thereafter once weekly, perhaps tailing off after a little while. This was the first time that she had ever volunteered anything about what she needed from the therapist.

However, when treatment was resumed after the holiday, the therapist abandoned all hope of a quick termination and discontinued writing up individual sessions. Two months later the therapist wrote a report in which he said that termination was still not in sight. She was still living with her husband in her parents' home, and she continued to take heavy doses of drugs. Recently he interpreted to her that this meant keeping him impotent, and she responded quite dramatically with most violent feelings of anger toward him.

Lengths of time given in the following paragraphs date from the initial interview. The above note was written at nine months. She continued to be seen at the rate of once a week. Work was fairly steady, interspersed with minor crises, and she made slight symptomatic improvement. After about two years she at last managed to move back home out of her mother's house.

At three years two months she gave birth to a baby boy. She had a very bad confinement and this was followed by a serious relapse. Her anxiety became severely exacerbated, so that she was in a constant state of panic and unable to go out of the house. She again began to feel the need to cling desperately to her mother, while suffering from severe anxiety in her presence. She felt unable to take a maternal role with her baby, feeling instead that she wanted to be a baby herself. She was admitted to the hospital with her baby.

During her stay in the hospital, she and her husband were given psychotherapy in joint interviews. Her husband was now revealed as quite severely emotionally restricted, though of course much of this may have been a reaction to the desperate situation caused by his wife's prolonged and crippling illness. The result of this treatment was that she gained some symptomatic relief, and her husband became more in touch with his feelings. The question arose of continued psychotherapy especially for her husband after discharge, but he did not seem to be very interested in this. She was eventually discharged, after a stay of fifteen months, at four years seven months. She was then seen irregularly by the therapist again until five years one month.

Total number of sessions (estimated)   200
Total time   5 years 1 month

FOLLOW-UP
(6 years 1 month since initial interview; 1 year since termination)

1. Symptoms. Whereas, when she first came, she was confined to bed at her mother's house, she is now able to be left alone at her own home, to go out alone a few hundred yards and much greater distances accompanied, and to go out to meet people socially. This is, however, only a very limited improvement, as her life is still seriously restricted by severe agoraphobia. The actual feeling that she has seems to have changed from one of anxiety to one of confusion, accompanied by the loss of her sense of identity. There has also, however, recently been one severe attack of panic.

2. Evidence of Enjoying Mutual Dependence With Her Husband as Adult Man and Woman. Although it may be true that she would *like* to have this state of affairs between her and her husband, their relation is so restricted that there is no possibility of its being fulfilled in practice. How much of this is due to her neurosis, and how much to her husband's, is impossible to say.

3. Ability to Assert Herself Constructively. She seems to be more able to feel anger consciously, and the interviewer elicited a single situation in which she was able to assert herself with her mother. But it is quite clear that the ability to assert herself is still severely restricted. Her mother has recently behaved in a most unreasonable way toward her, and she has been quite unable to do anything about this.

4. Enjoyment of the Sexual Relation With a Man and Valuation of His Masculinity. Here there has been limited improvement. Whereas previously sex made her feel tense, now she is able to enjoy it much more than she used to, though probably without orgasm. She is also able to handle her husband's severe difficulties over sex in a very tolerant and mature way. But the situation is made utterly unsatisfactory by what appears to be her husband's own sexual difficulties. How much she may contribute to this is, as before, impossible to say. Her husband now appears to have little masculinity, so the part of the criterion referring to valuation of masculinity cannot be applied.

5. General: Ability to Strike a Balance Between Her Own Needs and Those of Others. It is quite clear that her original defense of putting aside her own needs and looking after other people's has completely disappeared. The present situation is that she fully recognizes her own needs but can find nobody to satisfy them. In other words, there has been a major inner change that results in her being more of a real person, but that she is not at the moment able to make any use of in her relations with people. From her account it seems probable that a great deal of this is due to the neurotic difficulties of the people close to her.

The evidence suggests that she is still at least able to recognize other people's needs, and partly to meet them. She seems to look after her child quite well, but she said that she still could not feel herself to be a mother.

The follow-up suggests that her problem went far deeper than was originally realized.

EHR emphasized that the giving up of the previous false personality must have enabled her to have become much more *real*, and that even though this has resulted in exposing problems not evident before (e.g., her lack of a sense of identity) it can only be a gain.

All judges agreed that the result was extremely difficult to score.

SCORES

Team 1	1.5	1.5
Team 2	1.5	0.5
Mean	1.250	

The Gibson Girl

SUMMARY

Category: Short, favorable (28 sessions, outcome 2.875).

A very successful brief therapy with an unsophisticated agoraphobic girl of eighteen, highly transference- and transference/parent-oriented—though the response to such interpretations was never clear—in which the psychopathology turned out to be concerned with sexual anxieties, triangular relations, and hostility toward the parents.

CONTRIBUTION TO THE CORRELATIONS:

Motivation. Negative (unsophisticated in her attitude to insight, highly satisfactory outcome).
Focality. Poor agreement between the judges.
Transference/Parent Interpretations. Strongly positive.

DETAILS OF PATIENT AND THERAPIST

1. Patient

Sex	F.
Age	18.
Marital status	Single.
Occupation	Shop assistant.
Complaint	Fear of losing consciousness, especially in places where there are a lot of people (5 months).
What seems to bring patient now	Her father has taken her to a number of doctors, who told her there was nothing physically wrong with her. Finally he took her to a Tavistock-trained G.P. who referred her to us.

2. Therapist

Code	I
Sex	F

PSYCHIATRIC HISTORY AND DIAGNOSIS

Family History. Her mother had a "nervous breakdown," requiring admission to the hospital for a few months when the patient was eight. Her mother is described as a nervous person now.

Present Illness. The onset of her illness was sudden, while she was fetching a coat of her mother's from the cleaners. She suddenly got the feeling that she was about to have a blackout. These attacks have persisted. The fear is of losing consciousness, though she has in fact never done so. She becomes panicky, her back begins to twitch, and she feels compelled to keep shrugging her shoulders. These movements seem to be partly an attempt to fight off the loss of consciousness that she fears. When the attack is really bad she seems to drag her right foot. The attacks are worse the more crowded the place where she is, and tend to occur especially in the subway. They also occur if she has to wait for anything, especially in lines. She has several times had to take a taxi home. She feels less frightened if she is accompanied, especially by her boyfriend. She is less secure with her mother because her mother herself is nervous. She has been unable to work since the onset of her illness.

She also previously suffered from severe headaches, but these no longer occur.

She has seen a number of doctors, including a neurologist. Nothing abnormal was found. Her blood pressure was normal, and she has had her eyes tested.

Diagnosis. Phobic anxiety-hysteria.

DISTURBANCES

1. Symptoms. As above. She was also very restless at interview.

2. Superficial Relationships. The relationship developed with both the (male) interviewer and the (female) therapist was superficial, and we have made the inference that this applies also to her relationships outside.

ADDITIONAL EVIDENCE

1. The therapist thought she looked like a "Gibson girl"—hence the pseudonym.

2. Little information could be got from her about the home atmosphere. She said that her father was kind and understanding about her illness. Her mother's nervousness, she said, did not appear obviously; but she, the patient, could always sense it. She said her mother and father have rows at times like anybody else, usually when he comes home a bit merry with drink.

3. Her boyfriend was also described as kind and understanding.

They plan to get married one day, but are not yet engaged. The parents approve of him and do not interfere with their relation.

4. She seemed relieved when the interviewer asked her about sex. She said quite spontaneously she knew some girls had intercourse before marriage, but she thought it was wrong. She and her boyfriend have discussed it and he doesn't seem to mind, though she had been afraid that he would think her a bit old-fashioned. She very much likes being kissed.

5. Nothing could be got from her about why she had begun to get these attacks when she did.

6. In her projection test (ORT); she gave, quite unself-consciously, some very dramatic stories about being followed by men in the street. In addition to these stories containing aggressive men, there were a number that contained protective men. It seemed that the protective man was, however, not sexually exciting. There was very limited ability to integrate these two different aspects of men, and the psychologist made the comment that this did not augur very well for a satisfactory adjustment in marriage. Many of the other stories were concerned with happy family scenes in which everybody loved everybody else. There was a consistent tendency to retreat from sexual anxieties to a clinging dependence on a mother figure. The therapist also wrote that he felt that sexual guilt would be an important issue. There was excessive emphasis on situations in which parents have absolute trust that the daughter will not get into mischief.

7. Although she was able to talk fairly freely about herself, little real contact could be made with her either in the initial interview or the first therapeutic session. After the latter, the therapist wrote: "There was no feeling of any developing relationship. She remained factual, showing no change of manner, either warmth or coldness. She had presented herself for treatment, about which she knew nothing, and she would do her part."

HYPOTHESIS

She is anxious about the strength of her wish to be sexually overwhelmed by a powerful man. She defends against this by gross denial and by avoiding, both actually and symbolically, the anxiety-provoking situation.

CRITERIA

1. Loss of symptoms, without substitute symptoms.

2. Ability to enjoy both tenderness and some degree of aggressiveness in her relation with a man, including full sexual satisfaction.

3. There should be a general freeing of all feeling.

REASON FOR ACCEPTANCE AND THERAPEUTIC PLAN

Everyone was very doubtful about this patient on the grounds of experience with similar agoraphobic patients who were little in touch with their feelings. On the other hand, it was clear that she was more in touch than many such patients, and since the symptoms were of relatively recent onset and also were potentially crippling, we felt we ought to try. The (woman) therapist—mistakenly, as it turned out—had the idea that this patient's father may have been away during the war. She had previously treated three agoraphobic girls whose fathers had returned from the war when the patients were about five, and said that the fantasy of the father attacking the mother was common to such patients. She therefore had a special interest in treating this girl and volunteered to take her on.

The therapist wrote: "My immediate aim will be to try and break through her idealization, and to help her become more aware of and more tolerant of her aggressive feelings toward her mother, father, and boyfriend.

SUMMARY OF COURSE THERAPY

The style of this particular therapist was to interpret the transference wherever possible, and in addition to make the transference/parent link, the woman therapist naturally being usually interpreted as representing a mother. Although this was true, two of the three crucial passages in therapy involved little or no transference interpretation.

The first crucial passage occurred in session 4. The patient arrived looking apprehensive, and the therapist eventually suggested that there was something the patient wanted to keep from her and from her parents. This therapist/parent interpretation was not entirely accurate, since what the patient came out with was something the parents already knew perfectly well, namely, that the father was an alcoholic. Nevertheless, the patient now revealed this, which was something she had never told to any doctor before. She said that she and her mother wait in growing apprehension until they hear her father come in. Sometimes he shouts, and once he pushed her mother and tore her dress.

This led during the next eight sessions to a series of criticisms of both her parents, of whom she spoke with increasing contempt. It emerged (session 8) that her mother had been for two years in a sanitarium with TB when the patient was two, and that during this time—though the patient herself was looked after by an aunt—her father had lived with another woman. Her mother blamed her father for causing her own breakdown when the patient was six. The patient tended to be involved by her mother in quarrels with her father, and she spoke with further contempt of her mother's inability to stand up to the father herself.

Toward the end of session 10 she spoke again of the awful life her mother had with her father and his drinking; and finally of her own fears as a child when she was left alone in the house, and particularly of her childhood fantasy of a man who came out of the wardrobe, drawing a black hood over his head. The therapist reminded her of her fear of having a blackout, with a feeling that darkness would come over her head from the back; and made a reference to the possibility that the patient had seen her father and mother in intercourse or her father's erect penis. The patient denied this very matter-of-factly, as hitherto she had repeatedly denied all anxieties about sex.

Whether in consequence of this or not, in session 11 the patient for the first time reported improvement. She had rung up her boyfriend and told him not to call for her and had then gone round to his house alone.

The second crucial passage then occurred in session 13. She started by reporting a relapse; she had been very bad all the week and in fact was jerking badly in the session. Attempted exploration of the cause of this got nowhere until she mentioned her boyfriend's brother's wedding, which was due the following Saturday. Her boyfriend was best man and couldn't accompany her. She described how she would be worrying all the time about passing out, the fuss there would be as she was carried out of the church, and the anger of the bridal pair—particularly the bride. The therapist forcefully interpreted her envy of the bride and fury at her for separating her from her boyfriend. The patient accepted this and for the first time in the whole therapy added an interpretation of her own, that she was angry at the bride for being the center of the picture. This was said very sadly and with real feeling. She added that she had never thought she could be like that, because she really did want them to have a nice day. It is a measure of her increased motivation that although she then raised the question of whether she ought to take tranquilizers, she ended by deciding she would rather try and manage without.

In session 14 she reported that after a week of increasing apprehension she had enjoyed the wedding and had not worried about having an attack during it. She spoke animatedly about the reception and dance afterward. She was immensely proud of her achievement.

Her improvement was maintained in the sense that she felt less anxious in general, though she was not symptom-free. In session 16 she reported having tried to go down into the subway and at least travel for one stop, but she had had to come up without doing so, very quickly.

The third crucial moment began in session 22. In the early part of the session she spoke of how her mother makes much of her boyfriend and thus irritates her father and makes him jealous. She went on to say, with anger, that her mother insists on being the only one who knows how to cook, and thus humiliates her in front of her father and boyfriend. She is afraid she will know nothing of cooking or cleaning when she gets married. The therapist related this to the patient's jealousy of her mother's relation with her father. She denied this, but she went on to speak of her dissatisfaction with her boyfriend, who, she feels, is not exciting to her. The therapist suggested that although she always says she doesn't enjoy lovemaking, she really resents the fact that her boyfriend accepts this. She agreed with this and went on to speak of her girl friends who all "do it," and that she always says she does it, but of course she doesn't. The therapist here made what may or may not have been an important transference/parent interpretation, suggesting that the patient was angry with her, as with her mother, for keeping all the sexuality to herself.

In session 23 she told how a friend had recently got married, and she had gone round to her to try and find out what had happened on the wedding night. This led to a discussion of her fears about sex, which she now admitted openly for the first time. She was afraid of penetration, of being hurt, and she admitted that she wanted reassurance from the therapist as a married woman, and she then admitted that she was ignorant of her genital anatomy. Finally she openly and honestly asked for information about what really happens. The therapist in turn gave her the information she wanted, and it then emerged that *at the time when she had first become ill her boyfriend had begun pestering her for intercourse.* She then for the second time gave an interpretation of her own, saying that what she really wanted was to continue as a child while enjoying having her boyfriend dance attendance on her. She saw that she was behaving unfairly to him; and she now admitted—in total contradiction to the position she had maintained previously—that she had never really felt she would make a good sexual partner for him.

Dramatically she announced at the beginnng of session 24, "I've got a job."

This was the beginning of the final phase of therapy. Both patient and therapist vacillated about whether to go on with therapy or not; and after a workshop discussion in which the consensus was that the patient still needed to work through her own violent sexuality, the therapist tried to press the patient to stay for another six months. In fact the patient gradually withdrew from therapy, first failing to come for an appointment (after session 27), and then writing to say she felt so much better that she would prefer not to come any more.

Finally she was seen for session 28, two months after session 27. The main news in this session was that her parents have bought a caravan and go there every weekend. She enjoys the weekends without them and has no fears when she is left at home on her own. She added that she felt it was good for them to be together without her being there all the time, and that she felt they were more united than ever before in her memory. The therapist suggested that the patient also felt free from her and was enjoying being grown-up. The patient was amused, but agreed that she had been afraid that coming back would make her anxious, though in fact it had not done so.

Total number of sessions   28
Total time   10 months

FOLLOW-UP

8 Months

The patient was cheerful, friendly, and quite eager to speak of herself and how she had changed. She had found a new job, better-paid and farther from home, necessitating changing buses. The only residue of her original symptoms is that she is still afraid of traveling by the subway and does not do so. She not only enjoys her work but is also happier at home; she gets on better with her mother and is less concerned by her mother's depression and anxiety. She and her boyfriend go out often and especially join groups of friends to go dancing. She travels about alone. Rather gaily she said that she watches anything on TV and goes to horror films again. She was reticent about her sexual relation. The impression was that although she and her boyfriend had the opportunity to sleep together, they did not do so. She said she was looking forward to getting married next year, and that at the same time her parents will be moving away and she expects to see much less of them. Of her boyfriend, she conveyed the impression that he was reliable but perhaps somewhat unexciting.

5 Years 8 Months

At the follow-up interview she appeared to be considerably changed. She was much calmer, more self-confident, and more poised, and the restless movements seen when she originally came had entirely disappeared. She was less "glamorous" and much more attractive. She spoke with warmth and sincerity. She had now been married for four years and had two children.

1. Symptoms. She is almost entirely symptom-free but not quite. The exceptions are: (a) a very slight feeling in the back of her neck that apparently tends to occur after she has seen her mother; and (b) the fact that she still avoids traveling on the subway.

At interview she also mentioned that when she first came she had suffered from fears of illness, and she said that these had also disappeared.

2. Ability to Enjoy Both Aggressiveness and Tenderness in Her Relation With a Man, Including Full Sexual Satisfaction. All the evidence suggested that the relation between her and her husband contained warmth, companionship, and sexual satisfaction. She can criticize him, quarrel with him, and make it up. She made clear, however, that she did not enjoy forcefulness in her husband's making love to her.

3. Freeing and Deepening of Feeling. Within the limits of her cultural background, this seemed to be entirely fulfilled. The area where most warmth was shown was when she spoke of having children. The happiest moment of her life was when she saw her husband's face and her father's immediately after having her first baby.

4. Relation to Parents. There has been a very considerable change here, although this was not included in the original criteria. Her attitude toward her parents has become reversed. She now feels much of the trouble between them was due to her mother rather than her father, and that her father had had a lot to put up with. Both parents visit her, but they come separately and not together. She feels very much closer to her father—even perhaps idealizes him—and she feels that her mother is jealous of their relation. With her mother, on the other hand, there still seems to be a suppressed running battle going on. The symptom mentioned in 1. (a) above occurs after her mother's visits.

General. All four judges had reservations about this result. EHR emphasized (1) that there is still trouble between the patient and her mother; and (2) that her father appears idealized. Another fact that underlines the doubts about her is her inability to enjoy male aggressiveness. In this connection it is interesting to note that she described her son as totally lacking aggressiveness.

It therefore seemed possible that the exciting and violent man who appeared in the ORT stories had been entirely avoided, meaning that this particular sexual conflict might not have been resolved at all.

SCORES

Team 1	3.0	3.0
Team 2	3.0	2.5
Mean	2.875	

The Indian Scientist

SUMMARY

Category: Short, favorable (12 sessions, outcome 3.5).

An extremely successful brief therapy with an exceptionally highly motivated unmarried man of twenty-nine. The focus was Oedipal and therapy was highly focal, but little work was done on the transference and none on the transference/parent link. There was a dramatic moment of insight in session 4, followed immediately by clear improvements. Initial termination was followed by a return for more sessions. The final termination was unsatisfactory.

CONTRIBUTION TO THE CORRELATIONS WITH OUTCOME

Motivation and Focality. Strongly positive (near-maximum scores, highly favorable outcome).
Transference/Parent Interpretations. Strongly negative (score zero, highly favorable outcome.)

DETAILS OF PATIENT AND THERAPIST

1. Patient

Sex	M.
Age	29.
Marital status	Single.
Occupation	Scientist working in industry.
Complaint	Premature ejaculation (six years).
What seems to bring patient now	It is only within the last two years that he has become aware that this is a problem, since a girl complained about it.

2. Therapist

Code	F
Sex	M

PSYCHIATRIC DIAGNOSIS

Anxiety state.

DISTURBANCES

1. Attacks of Premature Ejaculation, With Anxiety About Them. He has had intercourse with several girls since the age of twenty-three, and as far as he knew there was nothing wrong. About two years ago, however, one of his girl friends told him that he ejaculated prematurely, and said that there was something seriously wrong with him and that he ought to see a doctor. In fact he used to ejaculate about ten seconds after penetration. He then took up with another girl, who didn't complain, and the result was that after the first two occasions he was able to function normally. However, on one occasion when he was in a hurry, his trouble returned.

He showed considerable anxiety about this at the interview.

2. Problems Over Aggression, Especially With Authority. He often says rude things to people and then worries about it for a long time afterward. He tends to take an intense dislike to people who try to exercise authority over him.

3. Difficulties Over Achievement. He has not attained his potential academically, nor has he found a job that satisfies him. He did extremely well in an intermediate exam, but later he did not want to work and he did badly in his finals. He has no interest in his present job.

ADDITIONAL EVIDENCE

This is best presented by means of an account of the initial interview. In the early part of the interview a number of facts were elicited, without the feeling of much contact between patient and therapist. These facts included: (1) that the patient and his family are Hindus; (2) that his father is a lawyer; (3) that the patient is the eldest in his family; (4) that the competition for Indian girls in England was too strong, and he had always concentrated on European girls; and (5) that his potency, though sometimes normal, was adversely affected when the conditions in which he had intercourse were not quite right. The therapist, feeling that there was not really very much wrong with him, tried to reassure him about this, adding that it would probably be perfectly all right if the patient got the right conditions. The patient completely rejected this reassurance, saying that he knew there was nothing physically wrong with him but he wanted to know what the real trouble was. He then suddenly started to communicate, and spoke about how up to the age of about seventeen he used to get into a lot of fights with other men, but that he had completely stopped this since he got into a fight with a man who gave him a really good thrashing. The therapist interpreted that the patient was afraid of competing with other men, and when the patient said that this was true, suggested that the man that he was really in competition with was his father. It turned out that his father was an extremely successful and pugnacious man. The therapist interpreted that the patient felt he had to fight his father in order to become a man, felt guilty about this, and when he had been beaten in a fight, felt he had been punished and did not want to try again. This interpretation brought out (1) that the patient often felt he wanted to rebel against authority; and (2) that, when he was a boy, his father often used to thrash him and he was always determined not to cry.

HYPOTHESIS

His rivalry with and hostility against his highly successful and aggressive father has left him with anxiety and guilt. He has tried to cope with this by getting away from his father and coming to England; but this makes no difference because he still carries with him the fantasy of his father, which he meets in new situations. This results in difficulties over attaining masculinity in sex, work, and relations with authority.

CRITERIA

The essential change required is that he should lose his anxiety and guilt about attaining any form of masculinity. This should lead to: (1) ability to attain full sexual potency, together with a mutually satisfactory sexual and emotional relation with a woman; (2) ability to be self-assertive or aggressive where appropriate, in a constructive way, without either irrational guilt or compulsiveness (he should be able to get on easily with authority); and (3) ability to do well, in accordance with his ability, in a job that satisfies him.

REASON FOR ACCEPTANCE AND THERAPEUTIC PLAN

He was accepted on the basis of: (1) his high motivation for insight, as shown by (a) his refusal to accept reassurance, followed by (b) an openly stated wish to understand the root of his problem; (2) his striking unconscious communication and response to interpretation, and (3) the therapist's ability to make a clear therapeutic plan. Although the patient was considerably handicapped by his difficulties, he appeared to be without deep pathology.

The plan was to interpret Oedipal problems forcefully, in the transference to the male therapist where necessary.

SUMMARY OF COURSE OF THERAPY

Early sessions were remarkable for the rapid progress toward ever more explicit Oedipal interpretations.

In session 2 the patient found difficulty in talking; but he eventually managed to speak of his tendency to take a dislike to people in authority, and by the end was talking quite animatedly. The therapist interpreted that he himself represented authority, and that the patient became able to speak more freely when he could admit his rebellious feelings.

In session 3 the patient again did not know what to say, and the therapist interpreted himself as the older man with whom the patient had to compete. The patient started talking, gradually getting deeper, and eventually said (1) that at one time he had daydreamed a lot about being a hero, until one day he saw someone have a fit and go mad, which frightened him so much that he stopped his daydreaming altogether; (2) that he had a constant feeling of guilt; and (3) that in his teens he had become interested in a girl cousin, which was absolutely forbidden in India, and had been told off for this by his father. The therapist interpreted that the patient seemed to need to keep both sexual and aggressive feelings under strict control, since he was frightened that either he would be punished for them or else he would be overwhelmed by them and go mad.

This kind of work led to a climax in session 4. The patient spoke of (1) how he sometimes thought that his father might die, but was afraid of the responsibility of taking over as head of the family; and (2) how he had borrowed money to come to England, refused to pay it back, and his father had had to pay it for him. The therapist said that this was really like stealing his father's money, which in turn probably represented stealing his father's sexual power. Any form of achievement—e.g., in work or with women—meant the same, and because he felt guilty he couldn't go through with it. In answer to this the patient spoke first of his difficulty in writing home; then of an intense anxiety attack with difficulty in breathing, in which he felt he hadn't written all he should in an exam; and then of going around all day with a sort of lump in his throat, which he eventually traced to guilt about something he had recently done. The therapist said that it looked as if guilt was at the center of his trouble and that it probably had something to do with his father. To this the patient suddenly said, "Yes, you know, once I read his love letters to my mother." He spoke of his great love for his mother, which more recently seemed to have been blunted. The therapist suggested that father and son could be rivals for the mother's love.

In session 5 the patient arrived ten minutes late, having lost a book on the way in his hurry. He said he was always losing things—was it normal? Later he spoke of masturbation in his teens, of having been suspected of tuberculosis, and feeling that the two were connected. The therapist suggested that he felt he had harmed himself with these sexual impulses, and this was why he was now preoccupied with whether he was normal or not, especially sexually. The patient spoke of a friend who, after an exam, had "gone quite potty" and shouted rude things in the street. He then said that he had built a shell around himself. The therapist suggested that the patient was afraid therapy would take off his shell and his primitive feelings would get out of control. Yet, he had seemed to be relieved after the last session. The patient immediately said, "Yes, you know, I felt quite peculiar after the last session—I felt I wanted to jump in the street from relief."

This was followed by two not very intense sessions, in which the patient reported (1) that he had decided to go back to India, and (2) that he had broken with his current girl friend. Patient and therapist agreed to meet again in a month's time. Session 8 then became a follow-up session, in which the following emerged:

1. The patient had not put his potency to the test.

2. The guilt-laden anxiety attacks reported in session 4 had not recurred.

3. He seemed no longer worried that there was anything physically wrong with him.

4. He felt, unexpectedly, that the therapist had not come to represent an authority for him. He then reported an improved relation with two older men at work, with one of whom—a man with a chip on his shoulder—he had suddenly found himself, to his surprise, being quite cooperative. It was agreed that he would stop coming, but would return for a follow-up before going back to India.

He was then seen five months later (session 9). The position was basically the same, except for the following: (1) He had postponed his plan to go back to India; (2) the anxiety attacks had not recurred; and (3) he now had a girl friend with whom he had not attempted intercourse.

There were four more sessions at irregular intervals. In these he reported that his improvement in relation with men was maintained, and he also now had been having intercourse. Here there were certain important improvements, especially that a feeling of detachment from which he used to suffer had now disappeared, and he also could manage at times to have intercourse three or four times in a night; but he was still occasionally suffering either from premature ejaculation or sudden loss of erection, and moreover he seemed to have the same kind of anxiety about this as he had had at the beginning of therapy. The therapist tried to explore feelings of hostility against women, which didn't seem to be right. Therapy petered out in an unsatisfactory way, the patient then failed to answer several letters, and the therapist lost touch with him.

It is worth noting that although the transference interpretations that were given during this therapy were all on the same theme as those about the patient's father, there were in fact no interpretations recorded that explicitly made the T/P link (and almost certainly none given). There were also no interpretations about termination. It seemed that the great majority of the work, and particularly the therapeutic climax in session 4, occurred outside the transference.

Total number of sessions	12
Total time	1 year 1 month

FOLLOW-UP (7 years 4 months)

A letter to his last English address produced a long and extremely helpful reply from a country to which he had emigrated. Condensed quotations from this letter are as follows:

"The complaint I saw you about does not exist now, in fact I got over my difficulty a few months after I last saw you. Two years later I got married to the then girl friend. The insatiable physical want that I had to begin with, these resulted to satisfaction of both the partners, gave way after marriage to limited but regular intimacies. On the second year of marriage we had a child and we are expecting a second one at the end of this month. I am very happy in marriage both physically and mentally. There is no clash of personality, and though our backgrounds are very different, our likes and dislikes are similar.

"If I remember correctly, you suggested that I had Oedipus complex resulting in a feeling of inferiority. It was true and I always used to think that I am destined to mediocrity, which I could not accept logically. That's why I was quite satisfied with the job I was doing for five years. In the second job, due to departmental reorganization, the position of group leader was forced on me and I had to guide others and to take responsibility, which I managed to avoid till then. The third job I took was more senior and I was compelled to make decisions on the spot. These went a long way to boost my self-confidence. Lastly in my present country, where I moved two years ago, my branch of science has a much better status, and I recovered the professional pride. I studied in a European college with the sons of colonials and this gave me a complex that manifested as hate. Living in England, of course, did not help. The position of group leader was a great help in that respect. It was the first step toward racial equality. As I went up the professional ladder I slowly got over the hate. Luckily I was not ostracized either by my wife's family or by their village, a beautiful village in Switzerland. In my present country the color is no problem at all.

"Well, here is the whole picture. I am very much in peace with my surroundings. If there is something else I could tell you, do let me know.

"By the way, it might interest you to know that my wife is a practicing Catholic, and as she is not a fanatic the religion does not pose any question. As I think that the holiness has been invested only to *Indian* cows, food is no problem either!"

CRITERIA

General

The general criterion that he should lose his anxiety and guilt about attaining any form of masculinity appears to be almost entirely met. We note that the main residual area of anxiety lay not so much in sex but in his problems over his work and his color. Here he has been helped by having promotion thrust upon him, and by moving to a country where his branch of science is more respected and where the color bar is no problem. An important feature of his letter is the honesty with which he describes his anxiety about these two problems, and how it has been overcome; in other words, there are no neurotic denials and it looks as if we can trust what he says.

1. Relations With a Woman. (a) *Sex.* In the three last therapeutic sessions his potency seems to have improved somewhat, and his previous indifferent attitude to sex had given way to a genuine desire for it; but his anxiety when sexual failure occurred was unchanged. In the final letter, the sexual difficulties seemed to have entirely disappeared. His description sounds absolutely normal. (b) *General.* In the last three therapeutic sessions his attitude toward his girl friend was still very immature, and he admitted that he had never thought about her feelings for him. The whole tone in the final letter is much warmer, and on the limited evidence available his relation with his wife sounds excellent.

2. Ability to Be Constructively Self-Assertive: Ability to Get Along With Authority. In the later stages of therapy his attitude toward older men seemed to have become much freer and easier, and he was able to disagree with them without trouble. He was, however, subject to attacks of rage, though admittedly from the great provocation resulting from color prejudice against him. He now says that the "hate" against this attitude has disappeared.

In his job he has now assumed a position of leader, and he seems eventually to have been able to cope with this. The only reservation is that he apparently twice had to have leadership thrust upon him.

The obsessional anxiety that was revealed during therapy, and that almost certainly was concerned with his anxiety about his relation with authority, had disappeared toward the end of therapy. We have no later evidence about this.

3. Ability to Do Well in a Job That Satisfies Him. This criterion seems to be entirely fulfilled.

SUMMARY

There are two reservations: (1) that the only recent information we have is by letter; and (2) that he had to have leadership thrust upon him. Otherwise the criteria seem entirely fulfilled.

SCORES

Team 1	3.5	4.0
Team 2	3.5	3.0
Mean	3.5	

The Military Policeman*

SUMMARY

Category: Short, unfavorable (4 sessions, outcome 1.375).

An extremely able married man of thirty-eight whose lifelong intolerance of strong feeling had broken down into anxiety fourteen years ago. He now suffered an acute exacerbation and seemed in danger of total breakdown. In a therapy of four sessions the main therapeutic factor seems to have been his discovery that one of his brother officers suffered from similar anxieties. He made an extraordinary—but largely symptomatic—recovery and treatment was terminated by mutual consent.

CONTRIBUTION TO THE CORRELATIONS WITH OUTCOME

Motivation and Focality. Variable.
Transference/Parent Interpretations. Strongly positive (score zero, poor outcome).

DETAILS OF PATIENT AND THERAPIST

1. Patient

Sex	M.
Age	38.
Marital status	Married.
Occupation	Officer in the Military Police.
Complaint	Tremor of head and hand, attacks of anxiety, fourteen years.
What seems to bring patient now	A recent attack of extreme nervousness while giving evidence at a court-martial.

2. Therapist

Code	F
Sex	M

PSYCHIATRIC HISTORY AND DIAGNOSIS

For the history of his symptoms see below. He was investigated by a neurologist six years ago and again recently, and on both occasions was told there was nothing organically wrong with him.

---

* The reason why this patient was referred to a civilian psychiatrist is not given for reasons of discretion.

Diagnosis. Chronic anxiety state with a recent exacerbation; writer's cramp.

DISTURBANCES

1. Symptoms

(a) Tremor of Right Hand. This developed fourteen years ago after he had been in the hospital in Cairo with malaria and dysentery and was just due to go back to his unit in the Western Desert. Since his return to England at the end of the war, this has become very much worse and his hand becomes fixed after a short time if he tries to write, so that writing becomes impossible. The tremor makes his writing look uneducated, or like that of a very old man.

If he goes to pick something up and nearly misses it, his whole body jerks in an attempt to correct the mistake.

(b) Nodding of Head, Anxiety. This has developed since his return to England, and occurs when he is required to speak at courts-martial and before senior officers. He feels very apprehensive before any such ordeal, and he is entirely concerned with trying to prevent any appearance of nervousness. This has sapped his self-confidence and he cannot perform his duties efficiently.

There was a recent exacerbation when he had to give evidence at the court-martial of a sergeant, and he behaved in such a nervous way that it looked as if he himself were guilty.

2. General Intolerance of Strong Feeling

Whenever he touched on any strong feeling at interview his jaw tensed. He says he can't "be sloppy the way women want you to be." He is not very interested in sex, feels there is something lacking in it for him, and only has intercourse once in three weeks. He would not lose his temper with subordinates as this would be weakness.

3. He is over-neat in the house, and has never been able to relax.

ADDITIONAL EVIDENCE

1. His father was a private in the Military Police all his life. He was retiring and unambitious. He retired from the Army twelve years ago, became more withdrawn, and "sat around the house moping" until he died three years later. He was self-centered during this time and caused the patient's mother a lot of trouble.

2. His mother is still alive but was little mentioned.

3. The father had always encouraged the patient to follow in his

footsteps. The patient has done extremely well, and became the youngest sergeant in his unit. Two years ago he was commissioned from the ranks.

4. Unlike the patient, his wife is quick-tempered. She complains that he doesn't show her enough affection.

5. His commanding officer is a bully who rules by fear. The patient had a showdown with him two years ago and now gets on better with him.

6. Neither he nor his wife wants children and they have none.

7. At interview with the ex-workshop (male) psychiatrist he showed two sides of his character: He presented a rocklike exterior, and often spoke through clenched teeth, and this became intensified whenever emotion or weakness were touched upon; on the other hand, he showed obvious anxiety, and the tremor of his head was periodically noticeable throughout. He tried to give his history as if he were making a report to a superior. The interviewer interpreted how frightened he must be of any weakness being discovered in him. He was extremely grateful for a tentative offer of treatment and left the room almost in tears.

8. In his projection test (ORT), he completely avoided triangular situations in his stories. The psychologist (a woman) wrote that he heroically maintained his idea of himself as a strong, manly, considerate person, at the cost of rigidity and repression of strong feeling. Strong emotion—whether anger, depression, or sexual desire—is for him a sign of weakness that he must avoid. The level was described as "pre-Oedipal." "There is a danger that his rigid defenses may fail to yield adequately in treatment, or alternatively may crack and expose helpless dependency."

HYPOTHESIS

He is desperately defending himself against identifying himself with his broken-down father. The need for this identification arises (1) because of his guilt about triumph over his father, and (2) because it represents a real part of himself, namely, a person full of needs. We suspect that these include the need to be looked after like a child.

CRITERIA

1. His symptoms should disappear without the emergence of substitutes.

2. He should be able to tolerate all kinds of strong emotion without feeling it as a weakness. He should be able to express his own

needs, particularly with his wife. This should include warmth, tenderness, and sexual feeling, with evidence that she is happier and more satisfied. At the same time he should be able to retain and make use of the strength and determination he has developed.

3. He should retain his ability to deal with superiors, and there should be no evidence of irrational guilt or excessive hostility.

REASON FOR ACCEPTANCE AND THERAPEUTIC PLAN

This patient was taken on after prolonged hesitation, because of his urgent need and the mute appeal of a strong man threatened with breakdown. The danger was clearly foreseen that therapy would weaken his defenses to the point of his breaking down completely. The therapist formulated his intentions as: to go very gently, to interpret the patient's defenses against strong feelings, and to try to reach the Oedipal problems presumed to lie underneath.

SUMMARY OF COURSE OF THERAPY

This very brief therapy showed a clear pattern: tentative communication in session 1 (not counting the initial interview, which was with a non-workshop member); quite intense communication about the past in session 2, with the emergence of highly significant new information about the patient's father; further intense communication in session 3, mainly about the present; and symptomatic improvement plus emotional withdrawal in session 4.

In session 1 the therapist tried to make contact with him by interpretation—e.g., that he was more angry with his C.O. than he had admitted to himself, and felt guilty about it, and that his writer's cramp had to do with the fact that his C.O. would read the reports he had written—but whenever some contact seemed to be made, the patient would quickly come up to the surface again. Toward the end of the session, however, he began to show some feeling for the first time, speaking with contempt of the "archaic" system of discipline in the Military Police, and how much time had been wasted over the court-martial that had brought him to therapy, when all that was needed was to have given the accused a good telling-off. In session 2 the atmosphere gradually became one of much greater communication. He spoke of the first time that he had got writer's cramp, when he had had to sign a charge sheet eighteen years ago. The therapist suggested that since this consisted of accusing somebody else of something, it might give him anxiety if his own conscience was in some way uneasy. The patient went on to speak of hating to admit weakness, and the therapist first introduced the word "manliness," and then suggested that the patient might feel that in the sessions he was forced to reveal his own weakness. The patient said that he did not mind admitting his weaknesses to the therapist. He went on to say that he had been talking to one of his fellow officers who had had attacks of anxiety in crowds, and this man had said that after seeing a psychiatrist for a few weeks he felt much calmer. From this he went on to speak spontaneously about his father. He started by mentioning that his father had done a great deal of writing, and he wondered if his father had been trying to overcome a writing difficulty like that from which he himself was suffering now. He spoke of how his father had always encouraged him to go for promotion. He went on to say that he had always been a good father, but it then emerged that about five years before his death his father had become ill and had then become increasingly critical and cantankerous, especially with the patient's mother. Also, on one occasion his father had actually cried—"he was in a terrible state." The therapist emphasized that there must be some connection between this breakdown in his father and the patient's fear of breakdown now. Perhaps there had been a lot of resentment against his father that he had been unable to express, and about which he felt guilty, because he knew that it had not been entirely his father's fault. There was no direct response to this, but it kept the atmosphere one of tentative communication. In session 3 this atmosphere was deepened, and he spoke particularly about the situation in his unit, caused by the C.O., which he described as the "unhappiest" unit he had ever been in. The way he spoke about this was very moving, and the therapist emphasized that the patient must really be a very sensitive person despite the rocklike exterior he presented to the world. During this session the patient also mentioned that he had spoken to a number of other men who had had difficulties similar to his own, from which he had clearly derived a good deal of reassurance.

In session 4 it became clear that there had been a considerable recession of his symptoms, although the background of anxiety was still there. His writing difficulty was better and the tremor of his head was completely absent during the whole session. The therapist immediately felt that it would be unrealistic to try and break down his defenses further, and he suggested that they might stop therapy there and allow the patient to come back in a crisis if he wanted to. The patient readily accepted this. One of his later communications was to tell of a sergeant in his unit who was always "flapping" and seeking guidance from a superior. The therapist said, "Surely you're trying to tell me that you don't want me to think you're like the sergeant who had to come running to me for help whenever anything goes wrong?"

The session came to an end and the patient left with the words, "Well, in a way I hope I don't see you again." There was no work on termination and there were no transference/parent interpretations in this therapy.

Total number of sessions	4 + interview with ex-workshop member
Total time	3 months

FOLLOW-UP (7 years)

The interview was extremely uneasy, so much so that the therapist at no time felt able to ask searching questions, and in particular never had the courage to ask the patient about sex at all. An important communication was when the patient asked about the test that he had had, and said, "I suppose you put people into classes, A3 and B2 and so on." This might have been evidence that the patient felt he was coming up to be judged, but if it was so, the therapist felt so uneasy that he totally missed interpreting this. The patient gave the impression throughout of a considerable conflict between not wanting to talk about himself and wanting to but not knowing how.

An important event since therapy was that six months ago the patient had finally left the forces and had obtained a civilian job of comparable earning capacity that also made use of his experience.

CRITERIA

1. Symptoms

At interview the therapist noticed an occasional nodding of the patient's head as if he were acquiescing unnecessarily. This was less noticeable toward the end of the interview. Apart from this, the patient reported that the writer's cramp, the tremor of his hand and sometimes his body, the anxiety on giving evidence, and the anxiety in the presence of authority, had all completely disappeared. It is very important that on two occasions he had had to arrest fellow Military Policemen and given evidence against them, and under this specific stress his symptoms did not return. He seemed more able to relax, though his tendency to be tidy and conscientious seemed unchanged. When asked when it was exactly that his symptoms had disappeared, he was quite unable to say.

2. Intolerance of Strong Feelings

As far as superficial things were concerned, he and his wife seemed to have quite a full life together. Any more searching questions were parried with the answer, "I am sure we are very happily married." There was considerably less ability to communicate real feeling than there had been at the height of therapy.

He had done well in his career and had clearly retained his strength and determination. He knew that if he had stayed in the forces he could have been promoted further, but he said on more than one occasion that he had no regrets about leaving.

3. Ability to Deal With Superiors, Etc.

He had clearly retained this, and there was no evidence for excessive hostility or irrational guilt.

DISCUSSION

The two judges of Team 1 agreed that assessment was very difficult because of two unanswered questions: (1) Was the massive inability to express feelings at interview mainly a transference phenomenon, or did it affect him just as badly in his life outside? (2) It was not at all clear how his position compared with that *before* his breakdown and it is on this that scoring must depend.

Two two judges took opposite views on both these questions, hence the discrepancy.

Team 2, who had emphasized anxiety about competitiveness in their hypothesis, noted that he had made things easy for himself by leaving the forces.

SCORES

Team 1	0.5	2.0
Team 2	1.5	1.5
Mean	1.375	

Mrs. Morley

SUMMARY

Category: Short, favorable (9 sessions, outcome 2.25).

A woman in her sixties wishing to improve the relation with her grown-up daughter, in which the disturbance was clearly mainly due to the patient's possessiveness. The therapist deliberately kept to relatively superficial, entirely nontransference work, and the patient responded dramatically.

CONTRIBUTION TO THE CORRELATIONS WITH OUTCOME

Motivation and Focality. Negative (low scores, relatively favorable outcome).
Transference/Parent Interpretations. Strongly negative, (score zero, relatively favorable outcome).

DETAILS OF PATIENT AND THERAPIST

1. Patient
Sex	F.
Age	60.
Marital status	Widow.
Occupation	None.
Complaint: what seems to bring patient now	She came wanting to improve the relationship between herself and her grown-up daughter. Her request for help was precipitated by a particularly bad quarrel with her daughter two weeks ago.

2. Therapist
Code	A
Sex	F

PSYCHIATRIC DIAGNOSIS

Character disorder with underlying severe depression.

DISTURBANCES

Unsatisfactory Relation With Her Children. As she sees it, she tries to do her best for her children but only meets ingratitude and deteriorating relationships. It seems that she does not leave the initiative to her children but tactlessly does things for them. She seems to be unable to let her daughter go.

ADDITIONAL EVIDENCE

1. Her husband died about ten years ago.

2. The best evidence about the psychodynamics came from the ORT report: She absorbs people into herself as a way of keeping her depression at bay. She is constantly feeding on intense relationships with people, whom she gets emotionally embroiled with her. She unconsciously lives in dread of being left alone, which means not being needed, and without the constant stimulus of relationships she feels faced with utter loneliness and depression. She seems to have little awareness of her intense need to control other people, and she is puzzled and confused by other people's ingratitude toward her.

3. In the initial interview (which was with the therapist), the patient repeatedly said she only wanted to know how to help her daughter. To this the therapist said that perhaps she needed help in order *not to have to help her daughter.* Quarrels between mother and daughter seemed to be brought about when the mother showed preference for a rival of her daughter's. Toward the end of the interview the therapist risked asking what the patient thought *she* did to cause the trouble. The patient was startled, but tried to be honest, and said that she found herself not leaving the initiative to the children but tactlessly doing things for them. Finally, the therapist said that it looked as if the patient wanted help to find out how to let her children go. The patient agreed, and then told a transparent dream: She was in a car that she let her daughter drive, although her daughter was a bad driver. There was an accident and all four wheels of the car came off. She wanted to help her daughter to put them on again but her daughter wanted to do it herself.

HYPOTHESIS

She has some very powerful emotional need that she expresses by having to keep people close to her. This is also used as a defense against loneliness and depression.

CRITERIA

1. She should be able to experience her own fear of loneliness, and then to solve this by finding a life for herself in relationships that do not have the intense possessive quality of the present relation with her daughter.

She should allow her daughter to live her own life, and at the same time, if possible, she should maintain a good relation with her.

2. We note the possibility of a depressive breakdown. If this occurs, she should recover from it and show the changes under 1. above.

REASON FOR ACCEPTANCE AND THERAPEUTIC PLAN

The therapist had seen the patient for consultation and had made remarkable contact with her, with very clear response to interpretation. She felt able to formulate a clear therapeutic aim, and wanted to try to put this into effect. She wrote as follows:

"The patient knows she has gone wrong, and it might be possible to help her control her behavior enough to allow her children to escape from her. It is a superficial aim, but I feel that if an attempt were made to go deeper, one would get too involved and do no good. It will be necessary to concentrate on behavior rather than on the dynamics behind it."

SUMMARY OF COURSE OF THERAPY

The therapist carried through her plan with remarkable consistency. The patient's response was to alternate between recognizing her own problems in the relation with her daughter, and denying them. Toward the end of this very brief therapy, there was a crisis and a threatened depressive breakdown, which was successfully handled by the therapist with remarkable flexibility and skill. The whole therapy was characterized by a total absence of transference interpretations, being the only case in which no single transference interpretation was recorded.

In session 2 the theme was the patient's jealousy of her daughter's men friends. The therapist linked this with the triangular situation between the patient, her husband, and her daughter. The patient discussed this triangular situation in quite a useful way, but ended up by emphasizing that all the jealousy was in her daughter and not in herself. In session 3 she began by saying that she was now convinced the therapist had been right in what she said last time, and she brought some important confirmatory material linking the two situations. She went on to say that she felt her children took advantage of her, to which the therapist said that she somehow got herself into this position herself. The patient agreed; but toward the end of the session she went on to take back all she had said about the therapist being right.

In session 4 the pendulum again swung the other way. She said she had been thinking over what the therapist had said, and it was a terrific indictment. She could see that the therapist was right—she found herself influencing her children's lives, and though what she did seemed all right it seemed to have terrible effects. She was trying hard to keep away from them.

In session 5 she said that she was very much better and the relation with her daughter was quite different, and she and her daughter were enormously grateful. In fact she spoke as if the original focal aim of letting her children go was already accomplished. It was left that she would ring the therapist if she felt she needed help again.

There were then four more sessions at irregular intervals, mainly concerned with the patient's feelings about the relation between her daughter and a man. The therapist handled this flexibly, at one time giving advice about how the patient should handle the situation, at another linking the daughter's feelings with the patient's own feelings when her mother had tried to interfere between her and her husband. In sessions 8 and 9 the patient reported a major crisis, with the feeling that she was near to breaking point, which the therapist handled partly by interpretations of the patient's ambivalence toward her daughter, partly by reassurance, and partly by suggesting that the patient should rest for a week in bed. There seemed some evidence that the patient was now transferring her feeling about her daughter to another young person. It was again left that the patient would ring up if she needed more help, but in fact she did not do so.

Total number of sessions	9
Total time	5 months

FOLLOW-UP (5 years 4 months)

External Events. Four of her children are now married.

1. Ability to Experience the Fear of Loneliness. The therapist says that the patient has been able to do this.

2. Ability to Allow Her Daughter to Live Her Own Life, Maintain a Good Relation With Her, and Find Relationships that Do Not Have an Intense Possessive Quality. The therapist wrote, "The patient is trying to live her own life and is very aware of the need to do so." She pursues her own interests with enthusiasm. She tries to leave her children alone, and on the whole succeeds, though not always. She seems to be on good terms with all her children, but the therapist says that this is only maintained with considerable strain, and there is an anxious quality in it.

2. Depression. The therapist mentioned that there were "marked depressive features" in the patient's story, but there has been no question of any breakdown.

SUMMARY

It is clear that the patient has been made aware of the need to allow other people to live their own lives, and is trying hard to do so and is partly succeeding. This is an important advance, and must make an enormous difference to her children. It is very difficult to know how deep this goes, and hence the score depends to a considerable extent on inference. Team 2 took a more optimistic view than Team 1.

SCORES

Team 1	1.5	2.0
Team 2	2.5	3.0
Mean	2.25	

The Oil Director

SUMMARY

Category: Long, favorable (46 sessions, outcome 2.0).

A married man of forty-nine, with a lifelong pattern of compulsive self-driving, breaking down into acute anxiety. Therapy was largely directed toward enabling him to accept the passive side of his nature. This was initially highly successful and his anxiety disappeared. At follow-up, however, there was some degree of relapse to the original patterns.

CONTRIBUTION TO THE CORRELATIONS WITH OUTCOME

Motivation and Focality. Neutral (both variables rapidly rising to maximum values, but only moderate outcome).
Transference/Parent Interpretations. Strongly positive (intermediate score, intermediate outcome).

DETAILS OF PATIENT AND THERAPIST

1. Patient
Sex   M.
Age   49.
Marital status   Married.
Occupation   Director of an oil company.
Complaint: what seems   A breakdown into anxiety during the last
  to bring patient now   year.

2. Therapist
Code   B
Sex   M

PSYCHIATRIC HISTORY AND DIAGNOSIS

He had had no previous psychiatric illness. The present illness occurred four months after the death of his mother.
Diagnosis. Anxiety state with depression in a compulsive character.

DISTURBANCES

1. *Symptoms.* (a) Stupidity over details at work; (b) obsessive preoccupation with work, to the extent of being unable to work; (c)

insomnia, due to work problems racing through his mind; (d) indecisiveness; (e) anxiety; and (f) depression. He feels that he is going to die soon, is finished at work and at home. With this in mind, he has started to put all his affairs in order.

2. He has had a lifelong *compulsive need to drive himself* and others. He cannot allow any rebelliousness in his children. He has always had a compulsive need to seek adventure.

3. He has always had an *intolerance of all kinds of softer feelings* in himself and others, which are felt as weakness. He could not mourn his mother's death, and continued to work until the day of the funeral. He has never been able to cry. His children are apparently not allowed to show any dependency, pining, or even affection. At the same time, there were signs of *dependence* in his relation to the interviewing psychiatrist, e.g., he rang up twice between sessions seeking instruction.

4. He seems to insist that his wife must obey his every whim and the children must take second place to him.

ADDITIONAL EVIDENCE

His father was very hardworking but not very able, and there was little money in the family. His mother was extremely ambitious for him, and he greatly enjoyed her admiration for his successes. He did well at school and very early became a leader, despising weakness, bookishness, and dependence. His parents wanted him to stay in this country, but he rebelled against them and joined his present company. He hoped to be sent abroad where he could find adventure, and could "bring civilization to the dark places."

He was largely responsible for building up a big oil refinery in the Middle East. During all this time he worked furiously hard. He enjoyed going out into the desert in order to help protect the pipeline from saboteurs.

He was surprised to fall in love when he thought he was a confirmed bachelor. His children were sent to boarding school in England from an early age, and he does not seem to have been able to feel any sympathy for their loneliness.

At one point his employees in the oil refinery complained about being driven too hard, and he only just avoided being transferred to another job because of this. He learned his lesson, treated his juniors more sensibly, and eventually came back to England and was made a director.

HYPOTHESIS

From childhood he has developed an intense wish to succeed and to prove his manliness and strength. This seems to have been developed through praise from his mother who also drove him hard. His drive for success was probably spurred by Oedipal rivalry and a wish to triumph over his father.

This character defense operates against the recognition in himself of:

1. His wish to be looked after as a very small child, and his mourning for the care and protection that he has had to give up.
2. His angry and rebellious feelings, particularly against his mother.
3. Also, since we believe that his ability to be a successful rival to his father must imply strong guilt, we think that his need to succeed has become the more compulsive so as to hide this guilt from himself.

CRITERIA

He should be able to recognize the feelings that he has been defending himself against, and to use them appropriately in his adult life; and at the same time he should lose the compulsive quality of his defensive maneuvers while retaining those aspects of them that are useful. This should result in:

1. Loss of symptoms. In particular, if he has been depressed, he should have recovered from this and not suffer from serious depressive episodes.

2. Loss of the compulsive and self-driving character of his work, without loss of effectiveness. Ability to tolerate rebelliousness in others, e.g., people at work and his children.

3. Ability to admit his weakness and dependence when appropriate and to tolerate this in others. Ability to mourn where appropriate. Evidence that he can express softer feelings, especially with his wife.

REASON FOR ACCEPTANCE AND THERAPEUTIC PLAN

This was an acute problem in a basically good personality, where it was possible to see fairly clearly the kinds of feeling that he had been defending himself against all his life. The plan was to see him twice a week and to support him in the task of making painful discoveries about himself, mainly concerning his fear of dependence.

SUMMARY OF COURSE OF THERAPY

The initial assessment had taken three interviews and the patient was then transferred to Therapist B. In session 4 he reported that he had gone daily into the room where his mother died in order to try and recapture the feelings that he had not allowed himself to have at the time. This was evidence of a marked increase in motivation. With the therapist's help he then (session 5) produced a crucial piece of insight: that he was driven by two opposing forces, (1) an almost frantic drive for achievement, and (2) a feeling of laziness, that he didn't want to bother with anything, which was entirely new to him. It emerged that his mother had had an extreme ambition for him, and that his self-driving had started after a quite unexpected failure in an exam.

In sessions 5 to 7 the therapist concentrated on interpreting the self-driving as a *defense* against *guilt*, which was caused by the *impulse* of *anger* against his mother, which in turn was caused by her driving him and rebuffing his need for tenderness from her. The realization of his compulsive efforts to satisfy her was very meaningful to him; and he now mentioned a source of anger with her, namely, that for some time before she died she had been staying in his home and had been the source of considerable tension.

In sessions 8 and 9 there was a return of defenses, typified by his quoting Churchill's speech, "We will fight on the beaches," etc., which the therapist interpreted as his saying that he must never surrender to weakness. The patient answered yes, he must never surrender to tears.

This work was accompanied by certain noticeable improvements: He felt more relaxed and began to envisage going back to the office, he noticed an improvement in the relation with his wife, and he found himself more tolerant of failure in one of his daughters.

An important moment in his therapy was reported in session 12, when he said that while watching a play in which a family deserts a mother he had actually cried (note the link with his response to the interpretation of Churchill's speech, quoted above). His wholly changed attitude was revealed by the fact that he regarded this as an almost unbelievable achievement. He went on to say that he had recently had the feeling that he was now cured, and he had felt elated. But this had been followed by several periods of tension, all associated with thoughts of going back to work. The therapist interpreted that he was afraid he would not be allowed to carry through to the end the period of dependence that he needed. He put forward a plan for returning to work for a limited time each day, as an experiment, and reported in the next session that this decision had taken a great weight off his mind. In session 15 he spoke of the insight about his "side no. 2," i.e., the passive, dependent side, capable of soft feelings, as a turning point. This had emerged particularly in connection with his tears at the play.

There was then a two-week break in treatment. During this time he went to work daily, gradually increasing the number of hours, but there was some return of his anxiety. The therapist intrepreted the fear as being concerned with loss of support, to which the patient said, "Yes, that's right—I was at my worst when my assistant, whom I rely on a great deal, was away—and of course you were away, too." In the next session there was a temporary return of the old patterns: He had been angry with the lazy side shown by his children. Interpretation of this led in session 18 to greater sympathy for them, and to gratitude for having this pattern interpreted.

In sessions 20 and 21 the therapist brought in a new kind of interpretation, suggesting that the patient needed his newfound "potency" to be accepted by men, including the therapist representing his father (the first transference/father interpretation—there had been two previous transference/mother interpretations). The patient agreed, saying, "After all, that is the test, isn't it?"

This therapy was remarkable for a number of moments in which the old patterns began to return, only to be relieved by insight. One of these was reported in session 22: At the beginning of the week he had experienced a general feeling of uneasiness that had continued for four days. He then quite suddenly felt that he didn't want to be bothered with work, and he experienced a great sense of relief. He was calm for the rest of the day, and much to his surprise managed to work well. A few sessions later he reported having been able to relax during weekends, something he had *never been able to do all his working life* (this is direct evidence for a major improvement due to therapy itself).

Not long after this the therapist stopped recording therapy session by session, but wrote a final summary at the end of the total of 46 sessions. During this period there was a weekly cycle: The patient would often feel bad at the beginning of the week, at times feeling that he could only just carry on, that he was a broken man, etc. This would get better as the end of the week approached, and indeed his sessions were usually on a Friday. Therapy consisted of consolidating the kind of work already reported. Toward the end, interpretations centered on the patient's reluctance to give up a secure dependent relation with the therapist, until he had taken into himself enough of the "good feeding experience" that therapy gave him. By that time he was doing a full day's work, and the cycle of depression had disappeared.

Total number of sessions   46
Total time   1 year 2 months

FOLLOW-UP

The follow-up on this patient afforded a very clear example of a peak reached soon after termination, followed by a gradual, but only partial, return to the old patterns; and thus also an excellent example of the application of psychodynamic assessment to outcome.

6 Months

The weekly cycle of depressions has now disappeared and he is now symptom-free. Whereas before his illness he always approached work with enthusiasm, he now approaches it as a necessary thing to be done, very much as he thinks anybody else regards it.

The family regard him as cured and are very pleased with him. He feels he is functioning again as head of the family rather than an invalid. He said he thought he had given up attempts to control his children: "I find that they can be responsible for themselves—e.g., switching off the fire at night, etc.—so I just go off to bed." He said the sexual relationship was good.

He said that he felt happier and better off than before his breakdown, probably better than he has for the last fifteen years.

1 Year 7 Months

The situation was much the same as at six months. The one change seemed to be a re-establishment of some of the old patterns with his children. He spoke of being able to *command* at home and the therapist felt that he was quite unaware of his children's needs and unrespectful of their individuality.

The therapist also felt that the patient was wanting to keep him at a distance, so he suggested that he would not get in touch with the patient again, to which the patient agreed. It was left that the patient could get in touch if he felt the need.

3 Years 10 Months
1. Loss of Symptoms. He said that his mental state had continued to improve until six months ago, when he had had a partial relapse. He now had enough insight to say that the cause of this had been excessive work and responsibility, resulting from the fact that his

former boss had been replaced by a man who was weak and ineffective. The symptoms that recurred were: anxiety about keeping up at work, insomnia, and thoughts of death. They were not as severe as in his original breakdown. The compulsiveness and excessive preoccupation with work did not recur; he was still able to leave work at six P.M., only took work home in emergencies, and was still able to relax in the evenings. This was a striking difference from the original illness.

He had not wanted to commit himself to the time involved in going for psychotherapy, and had been treated with drugs by his G.P. He has now been symptom-free for about three months, but is still on Largactil.

2. Ability to Admit Weakness and to Tolerate This in Others. He still felt that the "new me" that arose from treatment was valuable. At the six-month follow-up he had left with some moisture in his eyes. Against this can be set his attitude to his children (see below); and perhaps his unwillingness to return for psychotherapy.

3. Ability to Tolerate Rebelliousness. It is clear that he has continued to be rather authoritarian and driving with his children. He does not like the fact that his daughter does not work very hard and prefers going out with men, but he has given up any attempt at influencing her. We felt that his inner feelings here have probably not changed.

4. Loss of Compulsive and Self-Driving Character of His Work, Without Loss of Effectiveness. Apart from some presumed loss of effectiveness during his relapse this criterion was completely fulfilled.

5. Evidence That He Can Express Softer Feelings. He managed to put the therapist off from inquiring too deeply into the relation with his wife. He said the marriage was "fine," but the therapist felt that it somewhat lacked deep emotional contact. The sexual relationship remained satisfactory. See also 2. above.

SUMMARY AND DISCUSSION

Two major changes are (1) the loss of compulsiveness and (2) the complete loss of symptoms apart from his relapse. The relapse shows, however, that some of the original conflicts remain unresolved. This is confirmed by the fact that those criteria that refer to the release of feelings that he has been defending against seem to remain largely unfulfilled.

He is definitely better than before his breakdown. His whole attitude toward work has changed. On the other hand, there is little evidence for a change in his human relations. It looks as if he has got as far as being able to admit weakness to himself, but not to others.

SCORES

Team 1	2.0	2.0
Team 2	2.0	2.0
Mean	2.0	

The Personnel Manager

SUMMARY

Category: Long, favorable (62 sessions, outcome 3.25).

A long but highly successful therapy with an unmarried woman of forty who had a special gift for psychotherapy. The initial Oedipal focus quickly gave way to one based on dependence and maternal deprivation, in which interpretations of depressive mechanisms were given at a very deep level. Changes found at follow-up appeared to have a deeper quality than those in any of our other patients.

CONTRIBUTION TO THE CORRELATIONS WITH OUTCOME

Motivation. Strongly positive (extremely high motivation, highly favorable outcome).
Focality. Negative (poor focality, highly favorable outcome).
Transference/Parent interpretations. Strongly positive (very high score, highly favorable outcome).

DETAILS OF PATIENT AND THERAPIST

1. Patient

Sex	F.
Age	40.
Marital status	Single.
Occupation	Personnel manager in a large industrial firm.
Complaint: what seems to bring patient now	Panic about driving a car (few months).

2. Therapist

Code	D
Sex	M

PSYCHIATRIC HISTORY AND DIAGNOSIS

She originally went to her doctor complaining of lethargy and drowsiness, was diagnosed as incipient hyperthyroidism and treated with thiouracil in decreasing doses for three months. This treatment temporarily relieved her symptoms, but the drowsiness then returned and she complained of increasing frustration with life. She then attended a group at the Tavistock Clinic for about two and a half years. The therapist spoke very highly of her in his reports, saying that she was very intelligent and thoughtful, and had a considerable flair for insight into her own reactions and those of others in the group. One of the themes of group treatment was attempted interpretation of sexual fantasies about the therapist, which were repeatedly denied by the patient but eventually met with some success. There was at least one confirmatory dream, with partial realization that these fantasies concerned her father. The eventual result was that her drowsiness disappeared and she felt better adjusted to life.

Diagnosis. Phobic anxiety (see below).

DISTURBANCES

Panic Attacks

1. One to two years ago she had had a rather special boiler installed in her house, and soon after this had got into a state of panic about it. She had tried to analyze her feelings about this and had come to the conclusion that altering the house meant "coming between her father and her mother." This had relieved the panic.

2. A few months ago she decided that she wanted to drive, and had started driving lessons. Her instructor had told her that the trouble with her driving was that she *did not have herself under control*, which had worried her because she had always had a reputation for great calmness. When she signed a contract for buying a car she had got into an absolute panic, and had had to cancel it. She was then completely calm during the driving test and succeeded in passing.

Two weeks ago she bought a car. At first she was able to drive it, but she got panic attacks in bed at night, turning her feelings about driving over and over in her mind. Eventually she couldn't drive at all, though she felt all right in the car if someone else did the driving. She said that her fear was of *getting into a difficult situation while driving and being unable to cope with it.*

3. She felt that any major alteration in her life (such as getting a job abroad or getting married) would have brought on a similar panic.

ADDITIONAL EVIDENCE

1. She was one of the middle children in a fairly large family. She had come to realize under treatment that she was an unwanted child.

2. She relied on her father, but felt her mother—with whom she now lived alone—to be difficult and moody. Her father and mother

"were in love all their marriage," and she felt that her mother's whims were more important to her father than the children's needs.

3. The following information seemed relevant to a possible understanding of the car phobia: (a) She had learned to cope with her feeling of insecurity by having everything under control and "going ahead along a narrow path without paying attention to what might be on either side." (b) She felt inferior, being unmarried, and needed status symbols to impress other people with. These included her job and her car. (c) She felt she had no right to the status of having a car and that other car owners wouldn't accept her. (d) Cars were associated with her father in that her father used to take the children for drives in the country; and one of the reasons why she wanted a car was so that she could revisit the places where her father had taken her.

4. At interview she was full of genuine insight clearly derived from her preceding therapy, but the interviewer found himself unable to make interpretations that would carry her beyond this.

5. The psychologist wrote in his Rorschach Report that she suffered from great masculine/feminine conflicts and was trying to masquerade as a man. "This defense is falling to pieces and she is left at the mercy of severe depression." She in fact had a rather masculine appearance with an air of great efficiency.

6. Whatever the nature of the underlying disturbances, she is in fact extremely efficient and her job involves a great deal of responsibility. She said she had learned in the group to stand up to directors.

HYPOTHESIS

1. There seems to have been considerable deprivation in her early relation to her mother. This has probably left her with a mixture of anger with her mother and longing for her, which is essentially a depressive problem.

2. She then turned to her father as compensation. Although she loved him and relied on him, this in turn was not satisfactory because of the way in which he "put her mother's whims before the children's needs." She was then left with mixed feelings about her father as well and conflicts over jealousy in addition.

3. She has defended herself against the whole of the above by developing a masculine identification, a careful control of feelings and situations, and an essentially false competence and efficiency.

These defenses are now breaking down.

CRITERIA

1. (a) Loss of car phobia without the development of any substitute symptoms. Ability to enjoy driving (or any other "masculine" activity) without anxiety. (b) She should feel free to be adventurous, and she should react with pleasure rather than anxiety to those changes in her life that represent improvements. (c) If she became depressed during therapy or soon after termination, she should have recovered and should not now suffer from serious depressive episodes. In particular she should not become seriously depressed at the menopause.

2. She should become *genuinely* self-confident, lose the feeling that she needs to impress people, and feel that she has a place in life.

3. As far as moving in the direction of femininity is concerned, we feel that she should at least be able to admit her own weakness and her longing for a man, without anxiety. She should drop any excessive masculine identification, and should show no irrational jealousy of men or resentment against them.

4. Since, before her illness, she seems to have been able to cope perfectly well with people and things, the essential change in a really successful therapy would be that she now realizes that this was at least partly false, and is now able to feel that she can cope in a way that is really *her*.

REASON FOR ACCEPTANCE AND THERAPEUTIC PLAN

She was taken on as an acute problem in a patient who had a good basic personality and had responded well to previous psychotherapy. The dangers of breaking down her defenses were clearly seen, but it was thought the risk was worth taking.

The discussion of a therapeutic plan was confused. It did not seem clear what the car phobia meant, nor how much disturbance lay beneath the defenses. It was tentatively suggested that the therapist should work with the patient's aggression against men.

SUMMARY OF COURSE OF THERAPY

In sessions 2–4 the therapist made a conscious attempt at guiding the patient toward her relations with men, making a number of interpretations about Oedipal problems and linking these both with her father and the transference (transference/parent interpretations). However, during this phase there had already appeared a number of references by the patient to her mother; and it soon became clear that she suffered from a deep feeling of insecurity and deprivation. She told of an incident in her childhood when she had cried and been comforted by a stranger, and it had been a surprise to her that tears could bring help. She also now realized that she felt anxious not only in the car but in various situations away from home; and the therapist made an interpretation in terms of a conflict between a wish for independence and a wish for dependence on her mother.

In session 7 the patient spoke of her feeling of being left out in her childhood, an outsider with no rights of her own, and how she had had to master her rebellion and rage at having to settle down to an apparent conformity. From this had begun her feeling that she had to manage on her own; it was no use relying on anyone else.

Thus, with hindsight, it is possible to see how the patient's great independence and efficiency were revealed as at least partly a *defense*. With the interpretation of this defense a quite new and unforeseen focus crystallized, namely, her feeling of deprivation in relation to her mother and her anger about it, and her defensive withdrawal resulting in a vicious circle. The focus of her relation to men was entirely forgotten from session 5 onward, and the many transference interpretations became exclusively concentrated on the therapist as mother (transference/parent interpretations). Moreover, her car driving, instead of being seen as concerned with Oedipal problems or an identification with masculinity, became seen as concerned with her defensive needs for *independence* and *control*; and her phobia became seen as the breakthrough of anxiety when these defenses were threatened. Various incidents in connection with the car were interpreted in this sense, e.g., (session 5) one in which she had got lost after following her mother's directions and had felt resentful about giving in; and one (on the day following session 8) in which she had allowed the car to get out of control and had mounted the pavement, and she spoke of *how badly she had needed the therapist* but how she felt she had no right to ask for an earlier appointment. The therapist's basic interpretation was then that when she felt abandoned by him, she could only feel destruction and anger against him, and thus could not carry within herself the experience of him that she wished, which would enable her to function effectively away from him. In sessions 9, 10, and 12 she spoke of how the problem (temporarily in fact) no longer seemed to center on her car. She no longer felt compelled to take it out in order to prove herself, but could take it out or not as she felt, and could enjoy driving it. At the same time she began to report (sessions 13 and 15) a mounting sense of panic and dread as the time for coming to the sessions drew nearer. She was able to recognize that these feelings were connected with her early experience with her mother—needing her but finding her failing to respond. The theme of the therapist's interpretations was her fear of the repetition of this experience with him, which would result in her turning away from him in hate and anger and then being plunged into a state of despair. Each time an interpretation of this kind was made she would feel calmer, but would then relapse. During this period her ability to drive her car fluctuated according to her state of mind.

The climax of therapy came in session 32, which followed a three-week break between sessions 29 and 30. As the break approached she felt depressed, muddled, and unreal, but was able to speak openly of her resentment at being left alone for such a long period. In session 30 she spoke of not wanting a relation with a friend, and the therapist interpreted that she was denying her relation with him (defense) in order to escape from her feelings about being left. In the next session she reported a relapse—during the night she had felt terrified of the idea of taking the car out, though in fact she did so perfectly well the next day. She went on to recall how when her father died she had been left to clear up the estate; and she linked this with her childhood in which she felt she was always left with the responsibility. The therapist interpreted that she was re-experiencing much of her past life in her relation with him; that she turned away from people in hate and anger; that she felt unwanted and unloved, but contrived by her behavior to exclude herself from relationships.

Part of the therapist's account of the therapeutic climax in session 32 reads as follows:

"Last week on leaving here she felt very unsettled and disturbed. This feeling increased as she approached her office, and having arrived there she realized that she wanted to talk to me. It seemed terribly important to be able to do this, though the things she wanted to say were much the same as what she had told me in the session. She then realized that all this had to do with feeling herself to be UNWANTED. She thought of this for a while and felt very disturbed, but this was followed by a feeling of great peace and content. Since then this feeling has persisted. She described it 'as if a great load had been lifted off my mind.' "

She went on to say that she felt there had been pleasurable experiences with her mother, but that she had been made to pay a high price for them. She added that she now feels that she has received something very precious and important from her therapist.

This was the last session that the therapist recorded. He gave a summary of the next five months' work as follows: The patient's contributions continued to center on anxieties about car driving, with the fear that the car would break down and let her down. There were many references to anxiety about separation. The session after the summer break gave her the opportunity to realize how intense her feelings of hostility to the therapist had been. She was very aware of the approaching termination, and her main anxiety was that there would not be time enough in which to accomplish all the things she would like to. The therapist recorded that his own contribution was to confront her again and again with her dependence on him, her resentment arising out of this dependence, and the possibility of emerging from this experience with increased ability to deal with life. The importance of the T/P link may be gauged from his statement that "repeatedly it has been possible to show her that there is a close parallel to her mother in her relation to me; insofar as I am setting a limit to treatment, I am experienced as the mother who is depriving her of something she wants."

Total number of sessions   62
Total time   1 year 6 months

It is worth noting that this patient had already had two and a half years in a group before she came to the therapy recorded above. It is clear that the main theme of her group therapy had been Oedipal problems, and we may suppose that these had already been suffi- ciently resolved to enable her individual therapy to concentrate on the much deeper problems concerned with her relation with her mother. If this had not been so, it seems probable that individual therapy would have had to last much longer.

It is also worth noting that once the final focus had crystallized in session 5, this was a highly focal therapy of medium length in which depressive problems were dealt with in depth with a patient possess- ing great inner strength.

FOLLOW-UP (6 years 9 months)

Subsequent Medical History

A few months after termination she consulted the physician who had treated her for hyperthyroidism. There is no record of her actual complaints, but these were probably feelings of dizziness, lethargy, and unreality. The physician made a diagnosis of incipient *myxoe-dema*, probably brought on by the beginning of the menopause, and treated her with thyroid. However, these symptoms have persisted up to the present, and moreover she has continued to have her periods regularly. It seems probable, therefore, that the symptoms are psychological rather than physical. Her G.P. continues to treat her on and off with thyroid, estrogens, diuretics, stimulants, antidepressants, and tranquilizers.

Follow-up Interview

This will be presented in some detail because of the extraordinary degree to which the patient showed certain qualities—qualities that could not have been included in our criteria, but which, when found, cast a shadow by comparison on almost all the other therapeutic results reported in this book. At the same time the patient illustrates how, when a case is properly assessed at the beginning, the criteria can be made extremely specific; and when the result is a good one, how close the fit can be between the criteria and the findings at follow-up. Yet, since at follow-up she was not entirely symptom-free, nor were her personal relations free from disturbance, many objective scales might give her a lower score than, for instance, the Military Policeman.

It is first necessary to establish a base line. It is clear that she was always potentially a person with deep feelings. Before she came to us she had had over two and a half years of group treatment, beginning ten years before she came back to us. Her group therapist wrote: "She appears to have been one of the most profitable investments in the group. She is very intelligent and thoughtful and contributes effectively almost every session. She has a considerable flair for insight into her own reactions and those of others in the group."

Although this was so, there seems to have been considerable loss of feeling between then and when she first came to us. The interviewer at that time wrote of how she was able to speak of previously acquired insight, but how he was unable to make any interpretations that might carry her beyond this or lead to a deeper relationship with her. He also made the judgment that she had built up a powerful mask of efficiency and capableness that "almost amounts to an obsessional defense" against her dependence.

Very fortunately, the follow-up interview was tape-recorded, so that the quality of her feeling can be conveyed by verbatim extracts.

A crucial factor in her life emerged of which we had been quite unaware at initial assessment, namely, that she had been living alone with her mother, who had to have everything on her own terms and had become increasingly difficult, demanding, controlling, and progressively crippled with rheumatoid arthritis. No other member of the family would help. She described most graphically the feeling of almost suicidal despair that she went through, though she never actually contemplated suicide:

". . . as if everything was against me, everything I touched would go wrong; and that no matter what I did, how hard I worked, how much I planned and resigned myself to everything, there was nothing and nobody who would lift a little finger to get me out of it. It was like climbing out of a well, and getting your fingers over the top, and the world at large walking past and treading on your fingers heedlessly— 'Well, too bad, chum, we're too busy to give you a helping hand.' "

She spoke of the resentment that she met from her mother if she went out for a few hours, and in answer to the question whether she allowed this to restrict her life, she said:

"Yes, I'm afraid I did. But, at the same time, because I knew that three years was about as long as she had to live, I planned and worked on what I should do. This sounds terribly callous, but it's the only way you can live. I spent my time thinking out how I would have my own home, and thinking of what sort of things I would take up when I had got on my own and was able to live freely."

Reading between the lines, however, we felt there was some evidence that she allowed her mother to control her life unnecessarily severely, and did not stick out enough for her own rights.

During this period she was able to drive her car freely by day but was still somewhat anxious at night.

Three years ago her mother died. This led to a remarkable moment of enlightened self-interest and constructive self-assertion:

"And it seems as if I was very calculating, but I said to my doctor, 'Look, I want three weeks sick leave from you. I'm not sick but I want three weeks sick leave. I'm going away because I want to make the break, completely free to adjust myself to starting my new life.' He understood this, he was a very good friend at that time."

She added here that only after her mother's death was she able to appreciate some good things about her, and to understand something of the quality of her parents' relation with each other.

Not long after her mother's death, most of her residual anxiety about driving disappeared:

". . . when I got the wheels in motion to get my own house and so on, I found I could drive quite without bothering. I had only the normal qualms of a person driving at night—a little bit nervous about it, but no more than that; and I could get into the car at the drop of a hat, and just go off."

At the original interview she had made clear that she suffered from phobic anxiety about any major change in her life, and we laid down in our criteria that she should react to favorable changes with pleasure rather than anxiety. At follow-up she described going to stay with friends after her mother's death:

"They said, 'Well, look, we've got a dinner party on Saturday, why don't you stay over?' And the feeling—it wasn't pleasure, it was a feeling of combined pleasure with satisfaction, contentment, even a sort of gloating—that I could do this and I didn't have to ask anybody's permission, or overcome any ill-feeling."

It may be remembered that in our initial assessment she had been judged as defending herself against femininity and dependence by control, intellectualization, and masculine identification. The criteria included that she should "at least be able to admit her own weakness and her longing for a man, without anxiety." In this connection a crucial new fact in her earlier history emerged, which was unknown at initial assessment. This was that when she was quite young and the first man had paid attention to her, she had experienced the *same kind of panic as she had later when driving,* and it seemed clear that this had caused her to keep men at a distance until now. The information about her relation with men emerged in the follow-up interview in a dramatic and unexpected way. The interviewer asked her if she still felt she needed her car as a status symbol, to which she answered as follows:

"Yes, well, of course it was one of those curious twists of fate; a couple of months after my mother died, a man came into my life. We started going round together, and of course this has developed into an affair; so that the car has receded into the background. And now I have got my status, because though I can't broadcast it around as you can a husband, I know in myself that I am just the same as other women."

Later this subject led into one of the most moving moments of any interview:

"I have also had an experience of sex, which to me was always a loss—as, if I had to go to my grave without having been to bed with a man, I had missed out on something. It was something I felt was my birthright, just the same as that I feel if I really let myself that I am going to have a child. In fact, this is one of the things: If I can only hold this man's child in my arms, I would be quite happy. I would take whatever came, even if we were not married."

The above passage is clearly relevant to the part of the criterion quoted above that refers to admitting her longing for a man. The passage below concerns the part referring to admitting her own weakness. She spoke of her relation to her man friend during her mother's illness:

"All I wanted, really, was somebody's shoulder to lean on, and say, 'Well, look, talk to me about it. I might not be able to help you but talk to me about it'; and even somebody to say, 'I think you're handling this beautifully, aren't you clever?'—some sort of contact with somebody else, the feeling that I wasn't alone in doing this."

The relation with her man friend is by no means perfect. Coincidence or not, he—like her mother—suffers from rheumatoid arthritis; and, also like her mother, he is difficult, often says hurtful things to her unnecessarily, and has to have everything on his own terms. She described one such hurtful occasion, and went on:

"Eighteen months ago I would have been deeply hurt. But this time I thought rather more deeply about it; and I thought the best thing to do was virtually to take no notice of it, and just learn to try and understand him. I think he is more involved with me than he wants to recognize, and I realize that in a sense he wants me, but doesn't want me to want him because this would be too much involvement. If I let things go on like this, maybe things will go the way I want them to go; and we will both reach a better understanding of ourselves and our relationship."

Was she able to get angry when appropriate? Her answer was as follows:

"I very seldom get angry. This is something, I suppose, that I've been conditioned to. I *have* been angry in my time and it's practically lethal; I don't usually stop until I get my own way, and I think any of my friends will tell you this."

The sexual relation with her man friend is not entirely satisfactory as he suffers from difficulty with his potency and she does not get orgasm in actual intercourse, but only when he masturbates her afterward. Nevertheless it is extremely enjoyable to her.

The interviewer asked her if any of the original panic had been repeated, either when she met this man, or at any of the other important events of her life:

"When I started this relationship with this man, I thought, 'No panic, no difficulty whatsoever.' It just slipped into place. And I think it was the same when I took on this new job—there were no difficulties at all." (Interviewer:) "No, nor over moving into the new house?" "No, none whatever. In fact, no, there was none at all. It was all a kind of exhilaration. *No, absolutely none.* It seems as if I had thrown it all off when I moved."

One of our criteria was that she should feel that her ability to cope was really *her*. Much of the above evidence will surely confirm that this criterion was fulfilled. In addition, she has continued in the same work, has done very well, and gave evidence of using her extreme sensitiveness to other people's feelings in a constructive and effective way.

It should be added that she showed a most extraordinary intuitive capacity to understand feelings in her therapist as well, the full details of which cannot be given here for reasons of discretion. Perhaps the following brief extract will give a sufficient impression of this:

The interviewer felt it was right to reveal to her that her therapist had since died. When he asked her what she felt, she replied:

"It's a kind of sorrow for him. I think he had a sad life, and he probably struck a note in me of loneliness, you see, which is something I know a lot about; and I think I would have liked him to know that he had helped me because I think he probably had the feeling that he hadn't."

Finally, in discussing how she had been helped, she made a statement that sums up, from her own experience, all that any therapist could ask to be said about his therapy:

"I have realized the value of letting your feelings overwhelm you, so that you know what they are."

If we wish to relate the quality of this therapeutic result to any foregoing factor (apart from the enormous potential of this very remarkable woman), then I think we should refer to the great depth with which her depressive feelings were faced and worked through in the transference during her therapy. This is epitomized by the account of session 32, described above.

ASSESSMENT OF FOLLOW-UP

This patient provided the most fascinating and rewarding exercise in follow-up assessment.

Both teams agreed on the assessment in all essentials. We had three reservations: (1) the residual somatic symptoms, which appear to be psychological; (2) the part played by an external event, namely, her mother's death, in her final recovery; and (3) the fact that, in her relation to her man friend, she seemed to be repeating a pattern present in her relation with her mother.

Apart from this, not only were all the criteria fulfilled, but the criterion concerned with relations to men was far exceeded. It is important that she responded to the three important new events in her life—that is, the new freedom provided by her mother's death, the new house, and the relation with a man—without panic and with evident enjoyment, just as our criteria required. There seemed no question that her self-confidence was now genuine rather than defensive. The most striking feature of all was her depth of feeling, and the extent to which she appeared to be not only in touch with feelings of all kinds, but could use these constructively both in her work and private life.

SCORES

Team 1	3.5	3.0
Team 2	3.0	3.5
Mean	3.25	

The Pesticide Chemist

SUMMARY

Category: short, favorable (14 sessions, outcome 2.5).

A married man of thirty-one in a crisis resulting from the breakdown of obsessional defenses. His problems involved an inability to demand his rights either at work or at home. His motivation was distinctly ambivalent but therapy was highly focal and highly therapist/parent oriented. The outcome was a marked improvement at work but limited improvement in the relation with his wife.

CONTRIBUTION TO THE CORRELATIONS WITH OUTCOME

Motivation. Negative (ambivalent motivation, favorable outcome).
Focality. Strongly positive (high focality, favorable outcome).
Transference/Parent Interpretations. Strongly positive (high score, favorable outcome).

DETAILS OF PATIENT AND THERAPIST

1. Patient
Sex	M.
Age	31.
Marital status	Married.
Occupation	Industrial chemist.
Complaint: what seems to bring patient now	Sudden uncontrollable outburst against his wife (four weeks).

2. Therapist
Code	B
Sex	M

PREVIOUS PERSONALITY AND PRESENT ILLNESS

At interview the following reconstruction was made of his outburst:

1. He has always been perfectionist and overanxious at work. He worries that the materials he develops may not have been tested properly, and that this may result in a large claim against his firm. He is not able to relax at home because thoughts about work keep occupying him.

2. He has been upset about the way his boss has not shown appreciation of his work and has been critical of small things instead.

3. He has always suffered from premature ejaculation. In recent months this has been worse and he has been unable to satisfy his wife.

4. One morning he went to his doctor complaining of loss of energy during the last few months. He returned home and his wife suggested that he might stay at home for the day. (He said that it had been a "good-humored joke" between him and his wife that his work is more important to him than his home.) Despite his wife's remark he started off for work. His wife said that in that case perhaps she might get on with treating the house for woodworm. (He had been doing this slowly over the last year. The first job he did wasn't satisfactory and had caused some staining.) This remark of his wife's enraged him. He got out of control, tipped a gallon of anti-woodworm solution down the sink, and when his wife tried to prevent him he hit her. He then cried for three hours.

DIAGNOSIS

A sudden attack of rage in an obsessional personality.

ALL KNOWN DISTURBANCES IN PATIENT'S LIFE

1. Work. (a) Loss of energy (six months); (b) perfectionism and overanxiety (see above); and (c) takes criticism hard.

2. Relation With Wife. (a) Premature ejaculation. This has been better since his outburst; (b) recent outburst as above; and (c) he regards his marriage as "a pleasant background for what he does in life."

ADDITIONAL EVIDENCE

1. He described his father as a self-made man who worked from eight A.M. to eight P.M. six days a week and Sunday mornings as well. He remembers no warmth from him.

2. On the other hand, he described his mother as a very motherly person.

3. He regarded himself as having had an ordinary background and as having done ordinarily well, with a grammar school and night school education. His job involves considerable responsibility.

4. The psychologist who gave him the ORT wrote: "A man who is unconsciously quite intolerant of his sexual wishes and who has formed an adjustment on the basis of obsessional controlling mechanisms, together with an extremely severe superego."

HYPOTHESIS

1. He has to be continually appeasing a sense of guilt, which is presumably about sexual and aggressive impulses. Since this defense makes him compulsively preoccupied with work, it only increases his guilt toward his wife, whom he does not satisfy.

2. When his wife complains he breaks down because of his dilemma between these two areas of guilt.

CRITERIA

1. He should feel able to work hard without undue fatigue.

2. He should feel able (a) to tolerate imperfections in his work without anxiety, and (b) to relax at home without being preoccupied with work.

3. He should be able to tolerate criticism but stand up for himself when appropriate.

4. He should enjoy sexual intercourse without premature ejaculation and should enjoy satisfying his wife.

5. He should enjoy home life for its own sake and not simply as a background to his work.

6. There should be more warmth and companionship between him and his wife and evidence that she is more contented.

REASON FOR ACCEPTANCE AND THERAPEUTIC PLAN

He was taken on as an acute problem that was partly understandable, in a patient with a good basic personality. At discussion there was much emphasis on the interpretation of his tipping the anti-woodworm solution down the sink as a wish to express his rage by making a mess with feces. Nevertheless, there was confusion about whether the focus should be in terms of this, or his problems in relation to men (his boss), or sexual anxieties. No clear plan was formulated.

SUMMARY OF COURSE OF THERAPY

Both judges agreed that *motivation* was highly ambivalent. On the one hand, the patient genuinely tried to cooperate in understanding himself, and on the other he kept attempting various defensive moves such as trying to rearrange his life so that there was less strain, without looking at what the strain consisted of.

During the initial period the therapist rapidly gained an understanding of the situation, the sequence being as follows: (1) the patient said that he thought his outburst had to do with criticism he had been receiving from his boss (probably for being slow); (2) the therapist made the link between the impossibility of being angry with the *boss* and the impossibility of being angry with the patient's *father*; (3) the patient agreed, saying that though his father was never at home this was because he was doing so much to support the family; (4) the therapist then suggested that there must be some link with the angry outburst against his *wife*; (5) this brought out that he had been criticized by his wife for putting more energy into work than home, which was of course like his father in his childhood. In session 3 the patient then tried to escape by saying he was "cured," and the therapist made a major interpretation of *defense, anxiety* and *impulse*: that he had based his life on control of feelings, that the feelings of which he was afraid were violently *aggressive* and *soiling*, and that he was dealing with the situation by clamping down even tighter than before. In session 4 the patient adopted a passive attitude toward the therapist, which the latter interpreted both in terms of fear of being left unsupported, and as a defense against defiance, as with his father (*transference/parent interpretation*). Thus, there appeared an interpretation about hidden aggressiveness, which was the main focus of therapy. The patient now took all these interpretations as *criticism by the therapist*, and the latter interpreted (session 5) that the patient was angry with *him* for making impossible demands, and that this was like his childhood in which he was expected to suppress his feelings and grow up. It then emerged that he had had hardly any home life as a child, his father being constantly away. This led to important understanding of recent events, which the therapist gave to the patient in the following interpretation containing *impulse* and *defense* and completing the *triangle of insight*: that the patient had denied his rage and despair at being unloved by his father, that he unconsciously wished to rebel and attack his father, and that it became the last straw when his efforts to control this part of himself (e.g., by being overconscientious in his work) themselves became the object of criticism by his boss, his wife, and the therapist. This rapid progress toward what appeared to be the central issue gained maximum scores for *focality* from both judges.

This approach was confirmed when the patient in session 10 first acknowledged the impossibility of being able to satisfy everybody, and then went on to describe his marriage in terms of *demands* by his wife for affection and sexual satisfaction. He then reported two *therapeutic effects*. The first (session 11) was an increased ability to be spontaneously angry at work when unreasonable demands were made on him; it just seemed to happen, and only in retrospect did he see what he was doing. The second started with his having a showdown with his wife about her lack of enthusiasm for sex. This resulted in an argument and he felt the result was a catastrophe. However, two days later she herself initiated lovemaking and it ended up by being satisfactory to both of them. Nevertheless, his underlying resistance was shown in the fact that he was not as pleased about this as one might expect, and he was still afraid that he might do something that destroyed the solid basis of his marriage. He finally (session 14) made the highly inconsistent statements (1) that he was being more "open" both at work and at home, (2) that he was dissatisfied with the time that his treatment was taking, and (3) that he wanted a test period away from treatment. The therapist could only agree. There was thus no work on feelings about termination.

Total number of sessions   14
Total time   5 months

FOLLOW-UP

2 Months

There now appeared to be very marked improvement in work and considerable improvement in his home life. At work there have been two occasions on which the boss has criticized him unjustly. On the first he became depressed; but on the second he was able to stand up for himself. The quality and quantity of his work have improved, he feels more relaxed, he can now shift from one job to another without obsessional worries, and his fear of making costly mistakes now appears to be no more than normal.

At home the tension has been considerably relieved and he feels more relaxed and confident. There is no longer the urgency to get out of the house during weekends, and he and his wife are content to be at home together without the compulsion to be always doing something. As for sex, his needs seem to have been moderated, while his wife's have increased, so that they are more evenly balanced; and moreover, she now gets orgasm "75 percent" as opposed to a former "10 percent" of the time.

He made clear that he wanted to go ahead on his own and felt confident that he could do so.

1 Year 2 Months

His position at work has been maintained and he has made further progress. He said his former pattern had been to allow things to slide because he was unable to express his own opinion, with the result that he was criticized. He now prevents trouble from developing. There was one setback eight months ago when he started to get depressed, but he understood what was happening to him—i.e., that he was trying to do too much without letting his feelings out—and he had gone to the boss and talked about his difficulties in the lab and all had been well again. He is shortly to receive greatly increased responsibility. He no longer takes worries about work home with him.

At home the situation seemed to remain improved as in the last follow-up. He said that the reason why his own sexual needs have moderated is that he is now less tense about work and therefore needs sex less as a compensation for external dissatisfactions. The problem of premature ejaculation seems to be still present to some extent, but he can usually wait long enough for his wife and, as before, she reaches orgasm "75 percent" of the time. There is far more shared family life than before.

He felt that the improvements were due to his not expecting too much of himself and being able to express his feelings more openly both at work and at home.

3 Years 10 Months

There has been further progress at work, where he is earning more and has much greater responsibility. He achieved his raise in salary by going to the boss and saying that he was underpaid and was looking for another job. Not only this, but there was a recent incident in which something had gone wrong and the boss complained, referring to the imminent collapse of the department that he (the boss) had given so much effort to in the past. To this the patient said that he did not require the boss to add to the department's difficulties by his own personal reminiscences. This is a clear example both of constructive aggression and of a new way of handling emotional difficulties (see Sifneos).

However, at home there has been a deterioration. His wife had gone through an emotional crisis concerning one of the children and had lost interest in sex. The patient had therefore had to "discipline" himself; and although his wife has now recovered, the discipline has remained; he now has little sexual drive, and his wife is sexually frustrated. Intercourse is once a week to once a month, but when it does occur it arises from good feeling between them. Also, although he feels he does still suffer from some degree of premature ejaculation, his wife reaches orgasm most of the time. He thinks this is because he has encouraged her to be more active sexually.

The total relationship in the marriage is not really satisfactory. His wife criticizes him for not giving enough of himself to the family. He has a number of active interests, whereas she seems to have few and not to share his. There is now a good deal of quarreling, in which he is able to be much more open with his feelings than he used to be. However, the therapist made the judgment that he had "not reached the point of being able to satisfy a woman's emotional needs."

He emphasized as good evidence of increased maturity the fact that he had not been thrown off balance by his wife's fairly severe emotional crisis, but had managed to deal with it.

CRITERIA

All the criteria concerning work seem to be entirely fulfilled. The criteria concerning his relation with his wife, however, are only fulfilled to a limited extent.

SCORES

Team 1	2.5	2.5
Team 2	2.5	2.5
Mean	2.5	

The Receptionist

SUMMARY

Category: Short, unfavorable (9 sessions, outcome 1.875).

A therapy with a poorly motivated patient in which the original therapeutic plan was mistaken, but in which the theme that emerged seems to have resulted in some moderate therapeutic effects.

CONTRIBUTION TO THE CORRELATIONS WITH OUTCOME

Motivation and Focality. Positive (low scores, low intermediate outcome).
Transference/Parent Interpretations. Strongly positive (intermediate score, low intermediate outcome).

DETAILS OF PATIENT AND THERAPIST

1. Patient

Sex	F.
Age	21.
Marital status	Single.
Occupation	Receptionist and secretary for an optician.
Complaints	Depression, irritability, fear that she is losing her looks (one year).
What seems to bring patient now	Probably the fact that she is due to get married in two months time.

2. Therapist

Code	G
Sex	M

PSYCHIATRIC HISTORY AND DIAGNOSIS

Previous Medical History. At the age of twelve she had begun to suffer from brief attacks of loss of consciousness, which she described as follows:

She might be sitting talking, and would suddenly "lose herself" for a brief period, although she went on talking and often people did not notice anything wrong. These attacks were preceded by an epigastric aura; and for a brief period during recovery she would be confused, misidentify people, and have the feeling that people were talking about her. She was seen by a psychiatrist who said that apart from these attacks she appeared a normal child, and he could elicit no psychological stresses of importance. There were no abnormal physical signs. Although her EEG was consistently normal, the psychiatrist wrote that he felt very strongly that she was suffering from slight attacks of epileptic automatism. She was treated with phenobarbital. The attacks apparently continued to occur occasionally until she was sixteen, after which they disappeared and have not recurred.

Present Illness. For a year she has been feeling rundown and not herself, mildly depressed, and irritable, especially with her fiancé. She has begun to notice bags under her eyes, and her skin has seemed to become dry, so that she has been very much afraid that she is losing her good looks. Her G.P. referred her for a psychiatric opinion.

Diagnosis. Character disorder with mild depression.

DISTURBANCES

1. Symptoms. (a) Depression, irritability, tiredness; and (b) anxiety about losing her good looks. She is very jealous of other girls who are retaining theirs.

2. Difficulties Over Her Forthcoming Marriage. She is engaged but keeps putting her marriage off for no good reason.

3. Difficulties Over Aggression. She has angry feelings against her fiancé that are strong enough to frighten her. She has always had difficulty in standing up for her rights; she will do so, but it upsets her and she will go away and cry afterward. She is unable to stand violence of any sort, e.g., in plays or films.

4. She needs to be always on her best behavior, and is much preoccupied with what other people think of her.

5. She tends to lie awake and worry about small things that have gone wrong during the day.

ADDITIONAL EVIDENCE

1. Her father died when she was eight, and she is still living alone with her mother. She feels that she can always to go her mother for support; but she also feels that her mother doesn't give her enough sympathy and tells her she worries about herself too much.

2. She could give no real picture of what her father and fiancé were like.

3. Projection test (ORT and Rorschach): In the ORT she conscientiously described the cards but there was very little interaction

between people in her story. There were scenes of fire or accident; and later stories about people waiting to go somewhere but afraid of being seen; or people going somewhere to look at things and hoping to be shown them, but being afraid. The psychologist interpreted to her that she might be afraid of what she would reveal about herself. This led eventually to a story of people going to look at something, but it was doubtful whether it was a palace or a ruin. In the Rorschach there were repeated themes of things destroyed or burned, skeletons, things sticking out, and things cutting. The psychologist also wrote that she was still very preoccupied with her father's death, and was still yearning for him to look after her.

4. She was very eager to be seen by a psychiatrist, and her fantasy was that she would be admitted to the hospital for psychiatric investigation. She seemed vastly disappointed when it was made plain to her that she would only be seen as an outpatient.

5. In the initial assessment period, most interpretations were denied. In session 2, for instance, the therapist introduced the topic of the death of her father, and said that her feelings about this and about killing and destruction seemed to be very frightening to her. To this she only replied that she had got over it now. He later suggested that she had a fear of sexual intercourse because of her impending marriage. Her only reply to this was to say that she had no worries about it, because she had been to her doctor and had been told all about it. The last thing that happened in session 2 was a summing-up interpretation by the therapist, to which he did not wait for a response. This was to the effect that she was frightened that marriage was going to reveal to her fiancé that she wasn't the good, sweet person that she likes to feel she is; and that perhaps some of her bad feelings were concerned with violence, and sexual anxieties derived from her childhood. Despite the poor direct response to interpretation, the therapist felt that there was an indirect response in terms of a gradual deepening of rapport.

6. When this patient was discussed in the workshop the therapist said he felt that this was basically a genital problem, and that the regressive tendencies in the patient were a retreat from sexual anxieties brought about by her impending marriage. Several workshop members disagreed, suggesting that the regressive tendencies were in fact primary.

HYPOTHESIS

The evidence suggests that her approaching marriage has exposed anxiety about losing her image of herself as a "good" person both to men and women: perhaps (1) to men, because of violent feelings against them; and (2) to women because a relation with a man involves her in rivalry and jealousy.

CRITERIA

1. Loss of symptoms, including obsessional anxieties.

2. (a) She should no longer have to be on her best behavior; and (b) she should lose her excessive preoccupation with her appearance.

3. *Relations With Men.* (a) She should be able to make up her mind about getting married; and (b) she should ultimately be able to form a lasting and mutually satisfactory relation with a man. She should be able to enjoy sex without evidence of anxiety or guilt.

4. *Problems of Aggression.* She should lose any irrational resentful feelings; should not be overdistressed by violence; and should be able to assert herself in an effective way when appropriate, without being distressed by this.

REASON FOR ACCEPTANCE AND THERAPEUTIC PLAN

The therapist both felt he had made some contact and thought that there was a clear focus in terms of a retreat from sexual anxieties brought on by her forthcoming marriage. The rest of the workshop agreed that he should try working on this focus for a few sessions, but were skeptical that he would be able to get anywhere.

SUMMARY OF COURSE OF THERAPY

This therapy gives the impression that the therapist did not really know where he was going and that he made interpretations on an *ad hoc* basis throughout. His therapeutic plan was to work on the patient's retreat from sexual anxieties brought on by her forthcoming marriage. In fact the interpretations to which the patient showed the greatest response concerned aggressive feelings, especially against her mother. At follow-up also it was this that she remembered; the way she put it was that she had felt "slighted" because her mother had not looked after her properly after her father's death. In the account of therapy, therefore, it will be this theme that is picked out. The patient's fears about her appearance were eventually interpreted as a guilt-laden identification with her mother, who three years ago, as emerged in session 3, had suffered a physical illness that she had tried to conceal, and had later had to have an operation.

The patient's motivation for therapy was poor throughout, and she repeatedly canceled appointments on the grounds of being unable to get away from work.

Aggressive feelings were first touched on in session 4 when she said that she had recently suffered from irritation of her face at night, which made her want to scratch it. The therapist made interpretations about angry feelings, and she responded by saying that she got irritable with her mother and felt guilty about it.

In session 5 she said that sometimes she could stand up for herself with her boss but sometimes she just cried. The therapist suggested that she could not face her own hostility and felt sorry for herself instead. She later spoke of how she felt that sometimes she could scream, particularly with her mother; and it emerged that it seems a vicious circle is being set up between her and both her mother and her fiancé, in the sense that she punishes them both by becoming irritable and withdrawn, and they retaliate by doing the same to her.

This led in session 6 to the possibility of reaching some real feelings. She said that there was no point in getting married when she had originally planned, because she comes home tired each evening after work and she then wouldn't want to have to look after her husband. This was quickly linked with her actual present situation at home, in which her mother also goes out to work, and the patient comes home before her and is expected to have supper ready for her. This in turn was linked with her strong feelings about the fact that after her father died, her mother had had to go out to work, and was therefore not at home when the patient came back from school. She had felt, therefore, that her mother wasn't a real mother. The therapist linked this to the patient's original wish to come into the hospital, suggesting that she wanted to find the mothering that she had missed. She became thoughtful at this but there was no other response.

In session 7 she reported that she was sleeping better. Later in the session she said that when she first began to feel ill she had blamed her mother; and she went on to ask why she should always have to look after her mother who had recently recovered from an operation, and why couldn't her mother care for her more?

In session 8 she spoke of tormenting herself with worry about her looks, and the therapist suggested that she was in this way repeating a relationship in which she had done the tormenting. He had intended to refer to her mother, but she responded by speaking of the way in which she had treated boyfriends in the past—letting them take her out, liking them for a few weeks, and then dropping them. This led her eventually to speak of the one man who had really become very dependent on her, to whom she had in fact been very cruel. The therapist suggested that she was afraid of becoming dependent on anyone because she felt she would be treated in the same way. She responded by saying, rather thoughtfully, that she had never thought of herself like that, as she has always felt that she does need people, especially for reassurance and advice.

In session 9 she said with greater conviction that she was more settled and more relaxed. She then said that this would have to be the last time she came, as there was going to be no one who could stand in for her at work on this particular day of the week. She went on to describe how over the last two years she has grown more cold toward her fiancé, and has become irritated when he wants to make love to her. This was in contrast to their earlier relation, when she felt very passionately toward him, and he was very "considerate" in not insisting on intercourse. The therapist suggested that really she would have liked him to take the responsibility for her passionate feelings by overwhelming her, and that the fact that she had become cold to him recently was her revenge on him. He linked this with her anger against her mother for never having been the passionately warm person whom she wanted, and instead being the woman who was not at home to meet her when she came home from school. Perhaps she played out against her fiancé her wish for revenge on her mother. Her response was to accept this with much more feeling than she had shown before. The therapist then suggested that out of guilt she was afraid she had become the worn out old woman she had caused her mother to be. He also linked her revenge on her fiancé with the transference in the sense that having raised the therapist's expectations she was now withdrawing. However, she seemed to have little drive for treatment left.

Total number of sessions	9
Total time	4 months

FOLLOW-UP

Re-test (1 Year 4 Months), Interview (1 Year 6 Months)

She was now married to her former fiancé. She said that there had been no hesitation in her about getting married, and no difficulties about leaving her mother. She had at times had attacks of feeling bad about herself but she said she keeps this at bay by being busy. In any case there has been a considerable improvement in her symptoms since she got married. Her attitude toward her husband seems to have changed, in that she now respects him and welcomes him in his various roles, including that of lover. Of sexual intercourse, she said that it was "all that she expected and a bit more." The therapist wrote that the bit more seems to be the capacity to lose control of herself and to enjoy this experience. The therapist also wrote that she was still to some extent tied to her mother, but less so than before. She has been getting some support from a woman doctor at her birth-control clinic. The therapist summed up by saying that he felt the changes consisted mainly in a restoration of her defenses; and that problems connected with her femininity, e.g., maternity, might produce difficulties in the future.

In the re-test there was less preoccupation with disasters and other depressive material, though still a considerable concern about death. Her preoccupation with looking seemed to have shifted to a preoccupation with exhibiting. The psychologist wrote that this seems to be linked with phallic fantasies. She was more in touch with her ambivalence about men. Whereas the first test showed a strong sense of responsibility for her mother, maternal figures seemed now virtually nonexistent.

7 Years 2 Months

About four years ago her husband had bought an interior decorating business, and they had moved into a new flat in the outskirts of London. The business has had its ups and downs, but is now doing quite well, and she helps him run it. She is very contented with their new way of life. She was now eight months pregnant with her first child, and she was visited in her home. She was extremely welcoming and charming, but the interviewer felt that there was a lack of freedom in this that produced a feeling of constraint in him.

1. (a) Loss of Depression, Irritability, Debility. She still has feelings of irritability and wanting to be left alone; and she still gets depressed and worries that she is getting old or looking tired. Her judgment was that these symptoms are now about half as bad as they were before.

The interviewer asked her if she could describe any really bad patch that she had gone through. She said that the only time that this had happened was when they had first decided to start trying to have a baby. When, after six months, she still had not conceived, she had got really worried and had had three or four sleepless nights. She had eventually been sent to a specialist, who had told her there was nothing wrong and that if she worried she would be much less likely to conceive. She had been completely reassured by this, and in fact had conceived shortly afterward. She added that this was the nearest she had got to her previous depressions but that it was different in some way. The interviewer asked her what she meant, and she said that previously the depressions had been about *herself*; now it was still true that she was worried about failing as a woman, but the worry was that she was failing her *husband*.

(b) (i) **Worry About Small Things Going Wrong,** and (ii) **Any Other Obsessional Phenomena.** (i) "I am still the sort of person who worries quite a bit about things." (ii) She does not suffer from compulsions—e.g., after typing a letter she will read it through once to make sure there are no mistakes, but no more than this. If the flat is untidy and she and her husband want to do something else, the tidying up just gets left. On the other hand, the theme of preoccupation with cleanliness recurred several times. This preoccupation is clearly part of her character, which she accepts, and thus cannot be regarded as a symptom.

2.   (a) **She Should No Longer Have To Be on Her Best Behavior.** From her behavior and manner at follow-up this tendency seemed still to be present very much incorporated into her character. It isn't that she *has* to be, she *likes* to be.

(b) **Preoccupation With Her Appearance.** This is still present but not to the same degree.

3.   (a) **Ability to Make Up Her Mind About Getting Married.** She seems finally to have had no hesitation about getting maried, though it appears she did not in fact get married on the date originally planned.

(b) (i) **Lasting and Mutually Satisfactory Relation With a Man,** and (ii) **Ability To Enjoy Sex Without Anxiety and Guilt.** She gave the impression of being very happy in her marriage. Some of her remarks had a touching simplicity and sincerity—"I love him, and I just want to please him, you see." She was also able to admit strains in their relationship and irritation with him. (ii) Owing to the rather strained atmosphere of the interview, less information about this could be obtained than at the earlier follow-up.

4.   (a) **Loss of Irrational Resentful Feelings.** This seems to be fulfilled.

(b) **She Should Not Be Overdistressed by Violence.** She is less distressed than she was, and can now admit that some people must like violence.

(c) **Effective Self-Assertion Without Distress.** She still has some difficulty in getting angry, and cannot say anything that would hurt anyone. On the other hand, she can complain when it is necessary to do so.

5.   Insight. She said that, from the first time she had gone out to work, she resented the fact that when she got home she had to start doing the cooking for herself and her mother. She used the unexpected word that she felt "slighted" by this, by the fact that her father had died, and that she didn't have a proper home life like the other girls.

DISCUSSION

An important gap in the information is that we do not know about the present relation with her mother. Team 1 found this a most difficult result to score. She seems to have made an extremely good adjustment, and her preoccupation with cleanliness and good behavior is something built into her character that causes her no distress. On the other hand she still suffers from symptoms, and the overall impression created by her at interview was of a certain lack of emotional freedom. Despite the apparent fulfillment of some of the most important criteria, therefore, both judges scored low.

Team 2 also had very considerable difficulty over this case. They were unable to agree on a hypothesis: One member felt that this was a very primitive mother–child problem; while the other felt that the main problem was concerned with inability to mourn her father. The emphasis in their criteria was therefore quite different. Despite this, and in substantial agreement with Team 1, their two scores were the same.

SCORES

Team 1	1.5	2.0
Team 2	2.0	2.0
Mean	1.875	

The Sociologist

SUMMARY

Category: Short, unfavorable (29 sessions, outcome 1.25).

A therapy in which the patient's determination to deny her feelings broke down repeatedly, revealing a deprived childhood and extreme recent unhappiness, but this was not enough to lead to major therapeutic effects.

CONTRIBUTION TO THE CORRELATIONS WITH OUTCOME

Motivation. Strongly positive.
Focality. Strongly positive.
Transference/Parent Interpretations. Strongly positive. The scores for all the above factors were low in a therapy with poor outcome.

DETAILS OF PATIENT AND THERAPIST

1. Patient

Sex	F.
Age	25.
Marital status	Married.
Occupation	She has a degree in sociology and is working as a research assistant in this subject.
Complaint	Spots on her neck (5 years).
What seems to bring patient now	She has been told by a dermatologist that her spots are probably psychogenic, and although she is doubtful about this, she has consented to be referred by her G.P. for a psychiatric opinion.

2. Therapist

Code	I
Sex	F

PSYCHIATRIC HISTORY AND DIAGNOSIS

Medical History. She has had these spots for five years and has been desperate to try any remedy for them. She has consulted a number of doctors, but all medical treatment has failed, including X-ray therapy.

Depression. (1) When her husband left her temporarily before they were married, she said she had been "very bad" and had done "some extraordinarily stupid things," but we did not get the details of this. (2) She finds it very difficult to get on with her housework after a day at work, and will sit down and do nothing unless her husband brings her the vegetables to peel, etc. (3) At the initial interview, when she first spoke of her sexual problem (see below), she broke down into bitter weeping.

Sexual History. She had no knowledge of sexuality until the age of seventeen, and no interest in men until eighteen. She never had any boyfriends before her husband. She married at twenty-two, but it was a long time before she could allow penetration. Even now she encourages her husband to make love to her and then pushes him away. She discovered masturbation only after marriage, and can get satisfaction and orgasm only from masturbation, either by herself or her husband.

Diagnosis. (1) Dermatitis, probably psychogenic; and (2) character disorder with frigidity and depression.

DISTURBANCES

1. Symptoms. (a) Dermatological symptoms as above; and (b) depression as above.

2. Sexual Difficulties. See above.

3. Idealization of Her Mother. Although her mother has contrasted her stepsister's beauty with her own lack of good looks, and although her mother spoils her stepsister and treats the patient quite differently, she still says she adores her mother and her mother adores her.

ADDITIONAL EVIDENCE

1. She had a very disturbed and deprived childhood. A number of details are not given for reasons of discretion. Her father and mother didn't get on together, and her father was away much of the time. They were eventually divorced. Her mother remarried a man with whom the patient didn't get on. Her stepsister was born when the patient was nineteen, and the patient has good reason to be jealous of her (see 3. above).

2. At the initial interview she opened with a "sensible" attitude, speaking as one woman to another. She at first presented her spots as her only complaint, though the theme of feeling unattractive was also prominent. Toward the end of the interview she reluctantly brought up her sexual problem, and at this point, according to the therapist's

description, she broke down into "bitter, bitter weeping." She then admitted that she had been terrified to come.

＿3. In her projection test (ORT), many of the themes were clearly about sexual conflicts, e.g., wanting a close relation with a man and then denying this, or being unable to admit as a woman that she had sexual feelings, and hiding them under a cloak of conventional behavior. There was also a story of a sculptor who exhibited one statue only, but was hurt to find that people soon lost interest in it. The psychologist linked "exhibiting" with her spots, with a doubtful response. Later there was a story about a poor girl who lives in a shabby room; a burglar looks in but does not think it is worthwhile to break in and goes away. There was one story of desolation, refugees being evacuated from a doomed town with nowhere to go.

HYPOTHESIS

We emphasized the following factors in her background:

1. Because of her father's relative absence, she was forced to direct all her feeling toward her mother.

2. On two subsequent occasions her mother turned to a rival, first her stepfather and then her stepsister.

3. She was never able to develop her femininity through a satisfactory relation with a father.

She has been left unable to express hostility toward her mother, and profoundly unsure of her attractiveness and her value as a woman.

CRITERIA

1. Loss of symptoms.

2. Full enjoyment of a man's sexual love, with orgasm. Increase in her self-confidence as a person and as a woman.

3. She should be able to express aggressive feelings to both men and women while remaining on good terms with them.

REASON FOR ACCEPTANCE AND THERAPEUTIC PLAN

The main factor leading to this patient's being accepted was probably the deep contact made in the first interview. At discussion, however, there was great uncertainty about what to choose as a focus. The psychologist emphasized the patient's sexual anxieties, while the interviewer (who was also the therapist) emphasized the underlying depressive problem. The final conclusion was really that no focus could be chosen on the material available, and it was agreed to review the situation after therapy had got under way.

SUMMARY OF COURSE OF THERAPY

The recurrent theme of therapy was the attempt to penetrate the patient's denials, which when successful revealed a deprived and unhappy childhood and extremely distressing experiences in her relation with her husband. The transference that developed consisted of half-denied dependence, and many incidental transference interpretations were made, but the times of real breakthrough of feeling were concerned with the recent and distant past. Because the dependence was only rarely openly acknowledged, the therapist was clearly unable to make as many transference/parent interpretations as she would have liked (only 4 percent of all interpretations recorded).

Session 3 illustrated typical denials, as the patient laughed about a recent attack of food poisoning in which she had felt like dying, and described how she enjoyed being left alone in the house as a child. She coldly denied interpretation of this.

In session 4, however, the denials were partly penetrated (outside the transference). After further interpretation she described first a childhood memory of running sobbing after her mother, and then of her mother's cruel teasing of her—pretending she was someone else's child, which made her frantic with anxiety. The mixture of denial and wish for comfort in her relation with the therapist was then illustrated by her final remark, "Are you a proper doctor as well as a head-shrinker, because I have got a nasty pain in my leg?" to which the therapist responded sympathetically.

In session 6, almost crying, she said she couldn't talk about emotional difficulties. "You are the last person I can tell. I really want to try but all I feel is 'anti.' Wouldn't it be better to stop?" The therapist left it that her appointment would be kept for next week if she wanted to come.

For session 7 she arrived late and asked if the therapist was expecting her. Later in the session the therapist made use of this, saying that she felt the therapist didn't want her. This now resulted in a partial penetration of the denials within the transference, as the patient's voice broke and she turned her head away. The therapist suggested that she wanted to be sure of being the therapist's little girl and not the changeling child with whom her mother had tormented her (transference/parent interpretation). The patient smiled, saying she supposed it was something like that. As she went to the door she said,

"I did tell you we're expecting a baby didn't I?" The therapist congratulated her.

In session 8, of course, she spoke of being unable to "knit tiny garments" and having no wish for the "patter of little feet." The therapist related the transference to her frigidity, saying that she needed to keep both the therapist and her husband out. She denied this, though with tears in her eyes, and went on to say that she could give herself more pleasure in masturbation than anyone else could. Again a typical incident occurred as she left: She picked up an ornament of the therapist's, saying "Oooh!" as if it gave her pleasure, and then put it down abruptly, saying, "I don't really like that sort of thing."

In the next few sessions feelings partially broke through on several occasions. In session 13 she said almost in passing that the spots on her neck (the reason for which she had originally sought psychotherapy) had disappeared, and in fact they never recurred. Whether this was due to her therapy or her pregnancy no one will ever know.

The rest of therapy can be described in a series of important moments. The first was in session 14, to which she arrived utterly disheveled and shocked, having fallen down the steps at the subway station. The therapist made her lie down and covered her with a rug. She half-cried as she described the accident, and then half-laughed as she asked if this would mean she would lose her baby. The therapist said this was unlikely, and then pointed out that the baby meant much more to her than she wanted anyone to know. The patient admitted this and said that she had begun making some clothes for it. The therapist suggested that she was afraid to admit she loved the baby, because she feared she was unlovable and unwanted as a baby and unlovable as a woman, too; but that really she was secretly proud of it. The patient denied this, but then said (apparently out of a childlike gratitude), "I am going to tell you how I came to marry my husband"; and again it was typical that she went on to recount numerous affairs at college that made her realize she was not ugly as her mother had brought her up to think, but she never got round to the part about how she got married.

In session 16, after a three-week break, she started full of things that had gone wrong. The therapist suggested that she felt hopeless inside herself and she could not hold on to the therapist's help during the break; but it was also true that she was no longer denying that things were wrong. Rather ruefully she said, "Yes, but I have changed. I am not the same Helen." She asked if the therapist had seen *Woman in a Dressing Gown,* and said that that was herself. The therapist put into words her fear that her husband would leave her. She began to cry, putting her hand into her mouth and biting it; and then gasped out that he had left her once and she knew what it was like.

A few sessions later there occurred the breakthrough of some open feelings of dependence on the therapist, especially in session 23. She said that she could not speak of her difficulties without emotion, and so could never speak of them. The therapist said she was afraid her inner despair was without end, like her tears. Crying quietly, she spoke of her need to watch people she loved—like milk, which always boiled over if you left it. The therapist likened this to her fear of being left— love, milk, and mother suddenly gone. The patient here returned to a memory of being left alone when a baby of two, and her terror. Later the therapist brought in the fact that no mention had been made of the possibility of termination, to which the patient said, "After all, it has to end, doesn't it?"

Then, in session 23 she continued the story begun in session 16. She opened by asking if the therapist was interested in some "deep emotional stuff." This started with her jealousy of her husband's relation with another woman, which led her to start crying in deep despair. The therapist linked her difficulty in giving herself in therapy to her difficulty in giving herself to her husband. The patient went on to describe how her husband had lived with another woman for six months. She became speechless with tears, tearing at her hankerchief and cramming it into her mouth, and then almost shouting, "I hate it, I hate it."

In session 24 therapist and patient considered the question of termination, and the patient herself suggested stopping at the summer holidays, in about a month's time. There were two more sessions recorded, in which some work was done both on termination and on her feelings about her baby, and then three sessions not recorded.

Total number of sessions   29
Total time   8 months

FOLLOW-UP (5 years 3 months)

1. Symptoms

(a) Dermatological Symptoms. The spots on her neck disappeared permanently early in therapy, at about the same time as she became pregnant. We may therefore question whether this improvement had anything to do with therapy.

(b) Depression. There did not seem to have been any clinical attacks of depression since she was last seen. She has in fact been subjected to very considerable stress, and has not broken down. At the follow-up interview she gave the impression of considerable unhappiness, and the tears were never far away, but this is not the same as depression. She still finds it difficult to get on with the housework, but she does it.

2. Enjoyment of Sex; Self-Confidence as a Woman
It was difficult to judge changes in the sexual problem, because she now denied some of the things that she had told us originally. Our conclusion, and the patient's own opinion, was that there was no essential change.

She now says she does feel more self-confident. She has become a mother and she gives the impression that she fulfills this function quite well. Thus, development has been possible here.

3. Ability to Express Hostility to Men and Women, While Remaining on Good Terms With Them
According to her, she avoids the direction expression of hostility altogether. On the other hand the idealization of her mother has completely disappeared, and she has remained on good terms with her under very difficult circumstances.

GENERAL

It seemed that she was not making full use of her potentialities as an intelligent woman. It was also clear that she felt resentful about her treatment, and felt abandoned at the end of it. She may well therefore have wanted to depreciate any improvements that had occurred.

SCORE

Team 1	1.0	1.5
Team 2	1.0	1.5
Mean	1.25	

The Stationery Manufacturer

SUMMARY

Category: Short, favorable (28 sessions, outcome 3.75).

A married man of forty-three suffering from an incipient psychosis. His therapy provides an example of the highly successful use of a deliberately superficial focus. The highest score for outcome in the whole series.

CONTRIBUTION TO THE CORRELATIONS WITH OUTCOME

Motivation. Strongly positive (very high motivation by session 3, very favorable outcome).
Focality. Initially negative, later strongly positive (rapidly rising focality, very favorable outcome).
Transference/Parent Interpretations. Negative (low score—deliberately by the therapist—very favorable outcome).

DETAILS OF PATIENT AND THERAPIST

1. Patient

Sex	M.
Age	43.
Marital status	Married.
Occupation	Co-director with his two brothers of a printing and stationery manufacturing business.
Complaint	Preoccupation with his wife's relation with another man, which happened and was all over twenty years ago.
What seems to bring patient now	His G.P. had referred him to a psychiatrist in his hometown, who wanted to admit the patient to the hospital. The G.P. was unhappy about this and wanted a second opinion.

2. Therapist
Michael Balint

PSYCHIATRIC HISTORY AND DIAGNOSIS

Family history. N.A.D.

Previous Personality. Until he met his wife he had always been shy and diffident with women. Since marriage he has been warm and affectionate, and he and his wife have had an excellent relation. He is now joint director of the family business with his two brothers, under the chairmanship of his father. Everyone accepts that it has been mainly due to the patient's drive and ideas that the business has been so successful.

Present Illness (for further details see chap. 14). The essence of this was that twenty years ago, when he was courting his wife but was away from her on the Burma front, she had had a fleeting relation with another officer, but had eventually chosen and married him. (His wife was Turkish, and he met her in Cyprus). Ever since his marriage, fifteen years ago, he has pondered about this, wondering how it could possibly be that his wife had felt any sort of emotion toward the other man; but this did not make him ill. Six years ago, however, this preoccupation became extremely intense; and he had a breakdown in which he could not go to work, felt extremely tired, and spent much of his time sleeping. This lasted for about four weeks, after which he gradually got better, and after three months was back at work full time.

During this breakdown his preoccupation with his wife's relation to the other man was so severe that he subjected her to constant questioning, trying to extract from her the minutest detail, to the point at which she herself was near breakdown. In trying to pacify him she got herself into hopeless contradictions, which only made the situation worse.

Although much better, his preoccupation continued to be fairly severe until eighteen months ago, when he had a further exacerbation. He now had difficulty in getting to sleep because of his constant worrying. One month ago he had to give up work, and he was referred first to another psychiatrist and then privately to Michael Balint.

When asked if he associated any events in his life with his two breakdowns, he said (1) that a few months before his previous breakdown he had just moved into a new house that he had built, and shortly after this his father-in-law, of whom he was very fond, had died; and (2) that near the time of his relapse eighteen months ago, he and his brothers had finally bought their majority interest in the business from their father.

Mental State. At interview he made very warm contact. At the same time he expressed his ruminations in an inexorable way. There did not appear to be any delusions or hallucinations, and there was no thought disorder.

Toward the end of the interview he was joined by his wife. She was warm and affectionate but clearly at a loss to know how to handle him. Her story tallied with his in every detail.

At the second interview, six days later, he said that after the last interview he and his wife had really understood each other for the first time. That night he had slept without drugs for the first time for some weeks. Nevertheless his preoccupations were still very intense.

Diagnosis. A long-standing paranoid illness with obsessional and depressive features.

DISTURBANCES

The only disturbance elicited was his intense preoccupation with his wife's former relation with another man (for details, see above).

ADDITIONAL EVIDENCE

1. Relation With Close Relatives. He described his father as somewhat old-fashioned and rigid but said that he could get along with him. He did not mention his mother. He gets along well with his two brothers, who complement him in that they are steady and reliable. His children are apparently healthy and well-adjusted and are a source of pleasure to him.

2. Dynamics of the First Two Interviews. In session 1 the therapist brushed aside the endless details of the patient's ruminations, and said that apparently the patient needed a sounding board so that his fleeting ideas and fantasies could be reflected back to him, and instead of vanishing into limbo, could make some impression on him. The patient showed moving gratitude for this small piece of insight and returned to it several times during the interview.

Toward the end of session 2 the therapist again broke into the ruminations, this time trying to direct the patient's attention to the fact that his two breakdowns were associated with particular events in his life that he had already mentioned, and saying that if they could find out what these events meant to him, they might be in a better position to prevent a further breakdown. The patient did not like this attempt to go deeper, and suggested instead that he should come for five or six sessions and simply try to work through what he had already learned. This disagreement was not resolved, but nevertheless at the end he shook the therapist warmly by the hand and thanked him profusely for all he had done.

3. **Rorschach.** This had been given before session 1. The psychologist was a woman. The responses showed a mixture of strength and serious disturbance. The psychologist concluded that large areas of his personality had developed well and were not invaded by his illness. He was able to experience conflict and to show concern for the suffering that his wife was undergoing. He was able to make a number of "popular" responses. On the other hand, there were a number of "original" responses of poor quality, there was an emphasis on parts rather than wholes of human and animal responses, there were an unusual number of sexual responses, four sinister responses, and some indications of thought disorder. The psychologist concluded that he was suffering from an "underlying paranoid state kept in control by obsessional character defenses," that his control was precarious and that he was in danger of a psychotic breakdown.

Psychodynamically speaking, the main anxieties seemed to be doubts about his sexual potency, and fear and envy of a phallic woman who was felt to have a sinister quality. In consequence he either tried to control her, or made primitive and sadistic attacks on her, or else retreated into a position of self-sufficiency. There was evidence for both strong oral and anal impulses.

HYPOTHESIS

We felt that we could only make a partial hypothesis, and that this could not account for the psychotic nature of his disturbance.

1. The external events occurring around the time of his two breakdowns suggested that an important factor might be guilt about triumph over a father-figure.

2. The Rorschach and the account of how he treats his wife give abundant evidence of a sadistic relation to a woman.

We felt that these were two separate problems, and this was all we could be sure of.

The existence of these two problems in no way explains the mechanism behind his main symptom. We felt sure that this symptom involved projection of some part of himself into his wife. One possibility is that his preoccupation with his wife's sexual relation to another man is a disguise for a preoccupation with his own homosexual feelings.

CRITERIA

1. He should be able to weather (a) triumph, (b) rivalry, and (c) threats to his masculinity, without signs of disturbance.

2. He should lose his preoccupation with the other man's relation with his wife, and should be able to accept that this is something that has happened and no longer matters. There should be no other psychotic manifestations.

3. Homosexual manifestations should not be a major feature of his life.

4. In his relation with women he should not show evidence of sadism, but on the other hand he should be able to assert himself appropriately.

REASON FOR ACCEPTANCE AND THERAPEUTIC PLAN

It was clear that the therapist liked the patient and felt he had made contact with him and could formulate a focus, and he also probably was stimulated by the challenge of trying to cope with such a disturbed patient in brief therapy. The other members of the workshop thought the patient was too disturbed and would have nothing to do with it, but naturally Michael Balint went ahead just the same!

At the end of session 2 the therapist wrote that there were two alternative foci: (1) the one chosen by himself, namely guilt about triumph over the "homosexual rival," his father and the other man, to which the patient had reacted negatively; and (2) the one the patient favored, which was to share his wife symbolically with another man, i.e., the therapist (the therapist must have made this inference from his own extensive psychiatric experience, and also from the patient's behavior in the brief joint interview at the end of session 1).

It was left that the patient would talk over the situation with his wife and G.P., and would let the therapist know whether or not he wanted to come for therapy. The marked drop in motivation toward the end of session 2 was further emphasized when nothing further was heard for fifteen weeks, and the patient only returned under the pressure of a severe exacerbation.

SUMMARY OF COURSE OF THERAPY

For a full account see chap. 14.

The chief characteristics of this therapy were:

1. The very high motivation shown by the patient, and the high focality, once regular therapy started;

2. The way in which the therapist's original plan was adhered to throughout therapy, both foci as originally formulated playing their part.

3. The very high degree of selective neglect, enabling the therapist to avoid getting involved in all the complex and primitive pathology indicated by the Rorschach;

4. The relatively sparse use of transference in the form of *interpretation*, as opposed to the *therapeutic alliance*, which was very strong throughout; and

5. The relatively sparse use of transference/parent interpretations, though these were in fact used on two, possibly three, occasions at important moments in therapy.

Total number of sessions   28
Total time   1 year 10 months

FOLLOW-UP (3 years 4 months)

(There were also letters giving news at 8 months and at 2 years 8 months. The tone of these letters was almost effusive in its gratitude, and the reader gets the impression of a good deal of idealization of the therapist.)

1. Ability to Weather (a) Triumph, (b) Rivalry, and (c) Threats to His Masculinity Without Signs of Disturbance

(a) Triumph. Here it should be noted that in session 28 he had admitted to getting a kick out of winning his wife against the opposition of her father and the other man. Since termination, the important event has been his father's complete retirement from the business.

(b) Rivalry. He enjoys good-tempered rivalry with his friend over golf.

(c) Threats to His Masculinity. Since termination his factory has been badly damaged by fire. He took the opportunity to replace some of the out-of-date machinery, the result of which had been a marked increase in efficiency. He has also accepted the idea that when he finally retires his eldest son will take over the business.

(d) It should also be noted that his mother died.

None of these events has given rise to any pathological disturbance in him.

2. (a) He Should Lose His Preoccupation With the Other Man's Relation to His Wife; and (b) There Should Be No Other Psychotic Manifestations.

(a) The questioning of his wife seems now to have entirely disappeared.

(b) There is little evidence for any other psychotic manifestations. The therapist noted some tendency toward projection in the final interview, in the sense that the patient inquired after the therapist's health more than was entirely necessary, but this was not rigid and the patient could easily be turned back to talking about himself. There was also a slight suggestion of hypomania.

3. Homosexual Manifestations Should Not Be a Major Feature in His Life.

The therapist suspected some very slight evidence of latent homosexuality in the patient's close relation with his eldest son. The judges of Team 1 felt that this was entirely within normal limits. In any case, the son has now left home without apparently causing any disturbance in the patient. The only reservation was that the patient's relation to the therapist had a slightly homosexual flavor.

4. Relation With His Wife.

The evidence here was not entirely satisfactory, and the wife was not seen in the final follow-up. In one of his letters he wrote of her with considerable warmth.

DISCUSSION

There are two vital questions that need to be asked in an improvement of this kind. The first is whether the patient's condition is any different from that before his breakdown, or in this case from that in between his two breakdowns. This is not certain. The second is whether he has again been subjected to the same kind of stress that caused his earlier breakdowns, and has survived without developing symptoms. DHM felt that both his father's final retirement and the near-disaster to the factory could be so interpreted. EHR was less impressed with the severity of these stresses.

There is also the following theoretical difficulty: The stresses that precipitated his paranoid illnesses were apparently "Oedipal" in nature and the content of his illnesses was also Oedipal, yet we are sure that the basic difficulty is between the patient and his mother, and through her all women, especially his wife. It is difficult to be sure how deep the warm relation with his wife goes. EHR emphasized the lack of guilt and concern for his wife and all that he has put her through.

A point also emphasized by EHR was that we do not observe any definite widening and deepening of this patient, such as was observed in certain other patients, particularly the Personnel Manager and Mrs. Craig. It must also be said that his attitude toward his improvement appears to be somewhat idealized, and he showed a certain lack of doubt about himself. The therapist himself described the patient's improvement as "precarious," though there does not seem to be any very definite evidence of this.

In the scoring, DHM was much more impressed with the patient's ability to survive stress without pathological disturbance, and—on the grounds that the patient was so much more ill than any others in the series—put him "off the scale" at 5.0, a score higher than any previously envisaged. EHR was much more impressed with the deficiencies and scored 3.5, still a very high score.

Team 2 also had reservations. FHGB wrote: "I am sure the therapist is right to suggest that the balance that has been achieved is precarious, but the result at the moment seems to be a remarkable one."

SCORES

Team 1	5.0	3.5
Team 2	3.0	3.5
Mean	3.75	

Mr. Upton

SUMMARY

Category: Short, unfavorable (5 sessions, outcome −0.625).

An unsuccessful therapy limited to five sessions by what appears to have been reality, in which important work was done on Oedipal problems, but where the patient was revealed at follow-up to be much more severely disturbed than his initial assessment suggested. This was the only patient judged as "worse" at follow-up in the whole series.

CONTRIBUTION TO THE CORRELATIONS WITH OUTCOME

Motivation. Negative, then positive (high motivation, falling; worse at follow-up).
Focality. Negative, then positive (high focality, falling; worse at follow-up).
Transference/Parent Interpretations. Strongly positive (score zero; worse at follow-up).

DETAILS OF PATIENT AND THERAPIST

1. Patient

Sex	M.
Age	18.
Marital status	Single.
Occupation	Junior in an advertising firm.
Complaints	Sweating of palms, insomnia, difficulty in expressing himself, attacks of dizziness and blurred vision, depression. Most of these have occurred only during the last year.
What seems to bring patient now	A few weeks ago he decided to leave his job and he has applied for a similar job near his home in the North of England. He does not yet know whether or not he has been accepted. Shortly after this he suffered from two attacks of nocturnal enuresis. It was this that finally decided him to ask for treatment.

2. Therapist
Code   B
Sex   M

PSYCHIATRIC HISTORY AND DIAGNOSIS

The symptoms enumerated under Complaints have developed during the last year, except for the attacks of depression, which have occurred for a somewhat longer period. He has also lost weight. Physical examination, chest X ray, and blood sedimentation rate N.A.D.

The diagnosis when he was first seen and during therapy was anxiety state with mild depression and latent homosexuality. At follow-up (*q.v.*) the diagnosis was quite different.

DISTURBANCES

1. Symptoms

(a) His first symptoms started at work one year ago, when he suddenly became dizzy and felt he couldn't carry on. These attacks have continued and are accompanied by blurred vision.

(b) Sweating of palms (six months).

(c) Difficulty in expressing himself verbally on and off for one year.

(d) *Depressive phenomena.* Periods of dejection in which he becomes preoccupied with guilt over small things (e.g., not cleaning his shoes); he has on occasions cried without knowing why (but not within the last year); and he talks of the futility of life.

(e) He has wet the bed during sleep twice during the last three months.

(f) He feels sleepy in the afternoon but finds difficulty in sleeping at night.

2. Conflict Over Work, Achievement, and Independence

He wanted to become a singer, but his father persuaded him to take an office job in advertising. Although there are prospects in this job, he is not satisfied with it, and he still wants to sing. He is much preoccupied with the need to do something exceptional, and one of the thoughts that occurs in his fits of dejection is that he hasn't achieved anything. Although he has achieved independence by coming to London, he has now applied for a job back in his hometown.

3. Latent Homosexuality

He had a very close relationship with a friend whom he knew at school. This friend, unlike the patient—who is tall but not strong—is heavily built and does weight lifting. The patient hero-worships him.

4. Inhibited Heterosexuality

The only close girl friend he mentioned was when he was thirteen or even younger. He was halfhearted in speaking about the pleasure he got from kissing a girl. When asked, he said he didn't know if he was homo- or heterosexual.

ADDITIONAL EVIDENCE

1. The situation between the patient and his father over what career he should adopt (see 2. above) repeats a situation between the patient's father and *his* father; the father was in the Army but was persuaded to leave by his father; and he is now in a routine job without prospects.

2. The patient's father was fairly strict with him, and the patient rebelled against this—e.g., continuing to stay out late at night even though severely reprimanded. He added, however, that he got on well with his father.

3. He also said he got on well with his mother. The main thing here was that he said she was on his side, wanting him to go his own way. His idea for putting into practice his ambition of becoming a singer is to support himself by going into business with his friend (see 3. above).

4. The interviewer felt unable to make any deep contact with him despite strong attempts to do so. The most important interpretation given was that he was in conflict about growing up, becoming independent, and becoming a man in his own right; that his clinging to his relation with his friend was a clinging to his school days; and that he now seemed to have given up the attempt to be independent by returning home. The patient's only reply to this was that if he could live at home he could save money, and this might give him some capital with which to realize his ambition of becoming a singer.

5. In his projection test (ORT), one of the main themes concerned rivalry in triangular situations, with accompanying themes of suicide or self-sacrifice. He opened with a story of a man contemplating suicide because his wife, whom he idealized, has left him for another man. In a later story, a man is condemned to die for a murder that he has not committed. The story ends with the condemned man hearing

his wife and mother going away sobbing, while he resolutely prepares himself for his death. One of the other ways of solving this kind of situation was a retreat into a dependent position. In this connection he said in session 2 that going home would mean getting more food, more sleep and comfort, and more security. The psychologist wrote, however, that this regressive theme was not of primary importance and only represented a retreat from the real issue, which was an attempt to reach mature manhood.

HYPOTHESIS

Much of the evidence can be fitted into a hypothesis that this is an adolescent problem of growing up. The evidence suggests that the anxieties are concerned with rebellion against his father, and doing better than his father. The return home is both a retreat from attaining manhood and a fulfillment of the Oedipal fantasy, i.e., a return to a close but dependent relation with his mother.

CRITERIA

1. Loss of Symptoms

2. Ability to Achieve Masculinity

The general criterion is that he should be able to achieve all aspects of masculinity without anxiety or compulsiveness:

(a) He should lose those fantasies of doing something exceptional that are unrealistic; but should finally settle in an occupation that satisfies him, and should achieve reasonable success in it.

(b) There should be a reduction in the intensity of his relations with men, though he should be able to keep close male friends. There should be no evidence that homosexual feelings, latent or overt, play an excessive part in his life.

(c) There should be a marked increase in heterosexual feelings, with the ability ultimately to form a real and mutually satisfactory relation with a woman, including the sexual relation.

(d) All this should be accompanied by an inner feeling of independence and confidence in himself as a man.

REASON FOR ACCEPTANCE AND THERAPEUTIC PLAN

The interviewer made little contact with him, and although a clear focus could be seen in terms of his problems of growing up, was not very hopeful about him. The psychologist, on the other hand, made much better contact, was willing to take him on despite the limitations produced by his imminent departure from London, and wrote: "My aim would simply be to make further contact with him, and start him off thinking about the important issues in his life, particularly his difficulties in becoming a man."

SUMMARY OF COURSE OF THERAPY

The patient's acceptance for his new job came through sooner than expected and as a result therapy was limited to five sessions in all. Its essential course can be described in terms of important work on the main Oedipal focus in sessions 2 and 3, followed by failed communication in session 4, and withdrawal in session 5.

The initial theme in session 2 was concerned with the fact that the patient's paternal grandfather had been wounded in Flanders during the 1914–18 war while doing something rather heroic, and had then forbidden the patient's father to follow a career that might lead him into doing anything dangerous, with the result that the father had ended up in a routine job. Also, the patient's best friend was training to serve in submarines. The patient wanted both to identify with these heroic figures and to express his aesthetic side. The therapist said that if the patient regarded manhood as so heroic, no wonder he had become afraid of the task ahead of him. This interpretation of the *anxiety* led briefly to the expression of the *impulse*, but was followed by a regressive *defense*. The patient spoke of how he had rebelled against his father as a child and his mother had taken his side. The therapist suggested he might feel guilty about coming between his parents. This led eventually to a theme of returning to the security of a childhood relation with his mother. The therapist interpreted the patient's bed-wetting as a plea that he is not ready to use his penis in a manly way. The patient replied that recently he had been living in a hostel and that he feels the need to be looked after properly; hence his need to get a job near home.

This was followed by session 3, full of intense communication on Oedipal themes. The patient began with the communication that his own interests resembled those of his mother much more than his father. The therapist made an interpretation in terms of successful rivalry, namely that he felt closer to his mother than his father was. The patient responded by confirming his close attachment to his mother, and the therapist then made a major impulse interpretation, suggesting that he wanted to attack his father and take his father's place, and he was afraid his father would be weakened by his attacks. This interpretation seemed to change the whole atmosphere of the session, and the patient spoke with much more animation and sincerity than before. He said he wanted to rebel and be better than his father, but his father keeps reminding him that he is not yet twenty-one. He went on to say that when the time came he might fail and end up as useless as his father. This expression of the *impulse* and the *anxiety* was then again followed by a new *defense* (homosexuality), the interpretation of which led to a moment of deep communication about the Oedipal dilemma. The patient said that he was worried that people like himself who had artistic interests might turn out to be feminine. The therapist put it to him that he was worried about becoming homosexual, and that the feminine side was a defense against the threat involved in facing the masculinity in himself. The patient ended by saying, first, that he had recently found himself more interested in girls; and then, "It's rather like somebody who wants to become a king and knows that he can do it, but the trouble is that his best friend is already on the throne."

This was followed by session 4 in which, despite the therapist's best efforts, he felt that both he and the patient ended up muddled. Interpretations were mostly concerned with further anxieties about becoming a man. In his account of the session the therapist wondered if transference interpretations had been missed.

The last session, no. 5, was tense and contained long silences. The therapist made various transference interpretations, e.g., the patient's fear of being humiliated, or his feeling that the demands of treatment would be too great. The patient replied that treatment had been more help to him than the therapist seemed to realize, for he has started to think about many things for the first time. In the end he spontaneously gave the therapist his home address, and said he hoped they would meet again.

Total number of sessions   5
Total time   3 weeks

FOLLOW-UP (6 years 11 months)

1. Symptoms

The picture of his symptoms has radically altered since termination. His history now reveals a distinction between what may be called "major" and "minor" symptoms:

(a) His major symptom consists of attacks of *depression* and *hypomanic* states, with periods of apparent "normality" in between. In the *depressive* attacks he has felt despairing, irritable, tense, has sometimes cried bitterly, and in one attack had suicidal thoughts. He has had at least four attacks, the first of which necessitated six weeks off work followed by six weeks more attributed to a slipped disk. Two later ones have meant about one week off work each. One of these attacks was clearly reactive to the loss of a friend. His last attack was about two years ago. In one attack he was seen by a psychiatrist and put on a waiting list for treatment but when the vacancy occurred some months later he had recovered.

In between attacks he has thrown himself wholeheartedly into a large number of activities, which have been a success. But it seems also clear that at times this goes over into a hypomanic state: He describes himself as becoming tense and excitable, with a great feeling of superiority, and the feeling that he is the only possible intellectual companion for himself. The last of these states was about one year ago.

In addition to this, there has been revealed the suspicion of *psychotic manifestations*. He has become very deep in his fantasy world and when composing has almost thought he *was* the composer on whom he was modeling himself; sometimes the words tumble out of his mouth and what comes out doesn't seem to make sense, as if his subconscious were talking (see Disturbances 1. (c) above); sometimes, just before he goes to sleep, it is as if there is a tape recording of all the voices he has heard during the day going through his head, all talking at once, very loud, but "very much inside."

(b) The position as far as the minor symptoms are concerned is as follows: The tension, sweating, and inability to relax are unchanged. The dizzy attacks recurred up to four years ago, but not since; the guilt over small things, insomnia, and wetting the bed are "recovered."

In balance the two judges of Team 1 felt that he was symptomatically "worse," though he was in a state of remission when actually seen.

2. Other Criteria

(a) Loss of Unrealistic Fantasies, Ability to Find Work That Satisfies Him. One of the activities that he has engaged in has been to produce amateur musical plays and to write some of the music. At this he seems to have been very successful. He has continued in the same work as he was doing when he originally came, until recently. He finally decided to give this up and has now entered a teachers' training college, with the object of becoming a music teacher. The college is in the north of England but he is living away from home. His ambition now is to be a really good teacher.

(b) Relations With Men. (i) He has had a number of overt homosexual relations with men usually slightly older than he is. He invariably takes the passive role, and wouldn't want any other. He always feels guilty afterward. Love and companionship are absent from these relationships. (ii) On the other hand, he has had several very close relations with older men, which are not overtly sexual. In these he has found the love and companionship he seeks. The idea of sex in these relationships would disgust him.

(c) Relations With Women. He has also been able to have a number of sexual affairs with women, in which he is apparently fully potent. However, there is no depth to these relations, and they have always petered out, and the actual sexual act seems to disgust him; though, in contrast to his feelings about homosexual relations, he feels no guilt afterward.

(d) Independence and Confidence as a Man. He now seems to have attained independence, though it is too early to judge how permanent this will be. In view of the marked passive homosexuality, his confidence as a man cannot be high.

SUMMARY

He seems to be "improved" in work and creativity. He is a much more effective and interesting person.

Symptomatically he is probably "worse." He has been revealed as having fairly severe depressive attacks alternating with mild hypomanic attacks, with some possibly psychotic features. Some minor symptoms have improved.

The change in his sexuality seems to be simply that his bisexuality, which was known at interview to be latent, has now become overt. We regard this as "essentially unchanged."

8 Years 7 Months

We received a report from a psychiatrist who had seen him in the town where he was living. He had had an attack of depression that he thought began about six months before, when his teaching was criticized by his tutors. He now feels he cannot cope any more, and has contemplated suicide, but in the end was afraid to carry this through. He has been waking early in the morning. He has had attacks of feeling that people are ganging up on him, and dreams with a similar theme. In a half-waking state he has had hallucinatory experiences at night, e.g., thinking there was a cat sitting on his bed. The hallucination goes as soon as he wakes up properly. He was admitted to hospital and treated with antidepressants and tranquilizers. He improved and was discharged after six weeks.

DISCUSSION

This latest attack has to be taken as part of an overall picture extended over the years. Apart from the mild paranoid features, this attack is probably little different from the worst of his previous attacks.

Three of the four judges felt that he should be regarded as "worse."

SCORES

Team 1	−1.0	0.0
Team 2	−1.0	−0.5
Mean	−0.625	

The Zoologist

SUMMARY

Category: Short, favorable (32 sessions, outcome 2.5).

A young man suffering from a pattern of self-destructive behavior and lack of trust in response to emotional frustration, with extremely high motivation and an ultimately highly focal therapy, who showed striking improvements—with clear limitations—in response to intense work in the transference.

CONTRIBUTION TO THE CORRELATIONS WITH OUTCOME

Motivation. Positive (very high motivation, favorable outcome).
Focality. Negative (although this was a highly focal therapy the focus only crystallized clearly after the eighth contact).
Transference/Parent Interpretations. Strongly positive (high score, favorable outcome).

DETAILS OF PATIENT AND THERAPIST

1. Patient

Sex	M.
Age	22.
Marital status	Single.
Occupation	Zoology student.
Complaint	Conflict over his studies.
What seems to bring patient now	See below.

2. Therapist

Code	F
Sex	M

PSYCHIATRIC HISTORY AND DIAGNOSIS

The patient did his National Service in the Army, where he did well. Two years ago he went to a university, studying zoology and living at home. From the beginning he did not settle down and he had considerable difficulty in studying. Fourteen months ago he began to suffer from indigestion. He had a barium meal that was negative. In a later recurrence of this symptom he was treated with alkalies and Amytal.

Eight months ago he complained of his first attack of depression, of which he had several during the next few months. One of the worst of these followed an episode in which his father reproached him for not enjoying his studies more. On another occasion he was tearful and gave the doctor back his sleeping pills in case he took too many. The doctor gave him about six "long interviews," in which the serious conflict between the patient and his father was brought out. Five months ago the patient decided to give up his studies. Now, however, he wants to go back, but the college requires evidence that he has solved his problem before accepting him. He was therefore referred to the Tavistock Clinic.

Diagnosis. Character disorder with reactive depression.

DISTURBANCES

1. Symptoms

(a) Indigestion (see above).

(b) There are times when he feels extremely tense and cannot eat, for no conscious reason.

2. Problems Over Studying

This started as soon as he went to the university. He found it difficult to settle to study on his own; he couldn't show any interest in the course; he was easily distracted, could not concentrate, and showed little result from hours of study. He passed his first exam with the greatest difficulty, half-hoping to fail. He finally threw up his studies (see above).

3. Tension Between Him and His Parents

At interview he showed much open resentment against his parents for not allowing him a mind of his own. He had the feeling that he was at the university for his parents' sake and not his own, and of being a tool of his parents' ambition. The tension between him and his parents continually simmered but never boiled over. "We never had a row, though one was clearly indicated, as my father has always been determined that there shall be no rows in his house."

4. Difficulties With Girls

He said that his relations with girls just faded out after he had seen them a few times. He had been much attracted by a girl whom he had met on a vacation job, but he hadn't felt there was any point in trying to get to know her because he would be there such a short time. He has never kissed a girl. There were indications from session 2 that he doesn't feel he is man enough.

5. There was evidence from the interviews and the ORT that he has considerable difficulty in expressing his feelings.

ADDITIONAL EVIDENCE

1. The patient described his father as being determined that his son should have a profession. His father doesn't care what profession it may be, but is concerned entirely with financial security and not at all with his son's vocation.

2. The patient's mother was felt to be very much in league with his father over this. It seemed that he didn't really think of his mother as a separate person from his father.

3. With the help of his previous psychotherapist, the patient had come to realize that his giving up his studies had been a blow struck against his father.

4. In keeping with his choice of subject, the patient has a tremendous affection for animals.

5. The course of the initial interview (session 1) was important and revealing. For the first three quarters of the session the therapist was forced to ask questions. The patient answered these readily, and with a good deal of already acquired insight, but there was a marked lack of spontaneity about his answers. The therapist did his best to deepen the rapport by exploring the patient's attitude to his previous therapist and to his referral to the Tavistock Clinic, without success. Finally, noticing a faint "choked" quality in the patient's voice, the therapist said, "You give me the impression of someone who has a lot of intense feeling that can't come out." Immediately the whole atmosphere of the interview was transformed, and the patient began to speak with intensity of a woman of thirty-five in whose house he and other local children used to congregate in an utterly informal way. The therapist suggested that this represented the free and easy family life that he had never had. He agreed, and then said almost with tears in his eyes that when a child had put its hand in his and said, "I like you," it was one of the proudest moments of his life. Patient and therapist agreed that he was talking about his need to get close to *people* and not just to animals.

6. In his projection test (ORT), the patient was once more in resistance. The problem seemed to concern sexual potency and rivalry with his father. There did not seem to be any deep pathology.

7. Immediately after the projection test he wrote a long letter to the interviewer, consisting largely of all the things he had felt but had been unable to express to the psychologist.

HYPOTHESIS

Anxiety about expressing both his loving and his angry feelings to other people. He is very resentful against his parents. One aspect of this is that he feels he cannot express his anger directly but only by self-destruction. As a defense against these feelings he withdraws from human relationships and turns to animals.

CRITERIA

1. Disappearance of symptoms (indigestion, tension, loss of appetite).
2. Ability to return to his studies, to enjoy them, to become a zoologist and enjoy it, or else find some alternative work that satisfies him.
3. Ability to express anger in a constructive way, resulting in an improvement rather than a deterioration in relationships.
4. Ability to form a close and lasting relation with a girl and to express his love to her freely. Mutually satisfactory sexual relation. Ability to feel confident in himself as a man.
5. Greater freedom in social relations.

REASON FOR ACCEPTANCE AND THERAPEUTIC PLAN

The interviewer liked him, felt he had made deep contact with him, felt he understood his problem and could formulate a detailed therapeutic plan, and was eager to take him on. The letter written after the projection test was evidence of high motivation, at least for treatment by the interviewer.

The plan and predictions, written down in advance, were as follows:

"During the first few sessions he will form a very intense relationship. During this time I shall try to deal with his difficulty over expressing his love, and to get him to experience his love in the relation with the therapist. There will then be a period when he will have to experience hate with the therapist because of termination, and on that therapy will stand or fall."

SUMMARY OF COURSE OF THERAPY

See chap. 12.

The therapist originally set a time limit of sixteen sessions in addition to the initial interview (session 1). After initial improvement the patient relapsed, and therapy continued with irregular sessions spread over a further three years.

Therapy was characterized by initial prolonged resistance followed by intense transference work, with many transference/parent interpretations.

Total number of sessions   32
Total time   3 years 7 months

FOLLOW-UP

(3 years 5 months since termination, 6 years 11 months since he was first seen)

He and his fiancée got married a few months after termination. They now have two children. A year after termination he took his final exams and was reasonably successful. His first job involved working closely with a difficult man, and the patient found himself getting his attacks of indigestion again. He determined to leave, and got his present job, which consists of research in mammal ethology combined with teaching. In this job he is left to manage on his own without interference, and he is very happy in it.

Atmosphere of Follow-up Interview

He was interviewed by the therapist. The early part of the interview was notable for its very question-and-answer character. The patient often seemed to get bogged down in detail and to lose sight of the main point, and when strongly emotional subjects were touched on, he clearly could not quite face them and some of his answers were almost evasive. Toward the end of the interview, when he was talking about his children, and particularly when he seemed to identify himself with their bearing suffering uncomplainingly, the feeling became intense in a suppressed way, and he was somewhere near to tears. Nevertheless, the therapist did not really feel that proper contact was made during this interview.

1. Symptoms

(a) The gastrointestinal symptoms did recur during a period of severe strain (see above).

(b) Depressions have not recurred.

2. Ability to Return to His Studies and Enjoy His Work

He completed all his studies, took his finals successfully, has done well, is obviously satisfied, and is able to be creative. This criterion is fully met.

3. Ability to Assert Himself, Resulting in an Improvement in Relationships

(a) It was clear that he could handle superiors and colleagues at work in a thoroughly realistic way; and he has also succeeded in freeing himself from his parents while remaining in touch with them and apparently on good terms with them.

(b) As far as his wife is concerned, his remarks suggested that he handles conflict with her by avoidance, even indifference, and here this criterion does not appear to be met.

4. Close and Lasting Relation With a Woman; Ability to Express Love

Over this criterion there was marked disagreement between the two judges of Team 1. The final judgment depends entirely upon which side of the evidence is emphasized—the progress made or the deficiencies in it. One can only put down the two sides:

(a) When he first came for treatment he had hardly dared to speak to a girl. He is now married, with children, there appears to be a good deal of companionship with his wife, there are no obvious sexual difficulties, and he uses words like "togetherness" and "contentment" to describe their relation.

(b) On the other hand, (i) he and his wife have never really recaptured the enthusiasm of their first relation; (ii) over their sexual relation he spoke of "lack of need" on his part, and he seems to find it difficult to consider his wife's point of view; and (iii) he found it particularly difficult to express any deep feeling when talking about his wife.

(c) *Confidence as a man.* This seemed to be fulfilled as far as work was concerned, probably not fulfilled as far as his relation with his wife was concerned.

5. Greater Freedom in Social Relations

His social life seems very restricted. He used the word "isolationism" about himself. This criterion did not seem to be fulfilled.

SUMMARY

All four judges were agreed that the criteria concerning work were almost completely fulfilled. Three judges emphasized the limitations to the progress he has made in his relations with his wife, while one judge emphasized the progress itself.

SCORES

Team 1	2.0	3.5
Team 2	2.5	2.0
Mean	2.5	

PART IV

The Principles of Brief Psychotherapy

CHAPTER 9

Selection

THE CONVERGENCE OF STATISTICAL AND CLINICAL
EVIDENCE

During a number of recent years I have been acting in two parallel roles concerned with brief psychotherapy: first, as a research worker studying the material provided by Balint's team, and second, as a clinician trying to provide a service at the Tavistock Clinic, by running a unit in which trainees treat patients with brief therapy under group supervision.

This dual role has had some interesting and important consequences. In the brief therapy unit I have operated as a pure clinician, always allowing research findings to be over-ridden by intuition if the two appeared to be at variance. It might be thought that this is yet another example of the divorce between research and clinical practice and the lack of impact of the one on the other (and I have sometimes been deceived into thinking this myself) but it is not so. What has repeatedly happened is that principles reached on purely clinical grounds on the one hand, and those derived from research on the other, even when appearing to differ, are found on closer examination to coincide.

The most striking example of this comes from the relative importance of the two selection criteria, *motivation* and *response to interpretation*, which will be considered below.

In this and the following chapters I shall try to present a distillation of the principles of brief therapy as I see them at the present time after the convergence of these two lines of evidence. The clinical examples will mostly be taken from the Tavistock brief therapy unit, and I should at once like to thank the therapists involved for permission to publish their work, into which they have poured so much of their own dedication and life experience. I have often thought—a sober judgment made entirely without false modesty—that in many cases they have done far better work than I am any longer capable of myself.

INTENSIVE BRIEF PSYCHOTHERAPY

Before we consider the problem of selection, we need to define the form of brief psychotherapy for which the patients are being selected. In chap. 4 I pointed out that there was a continuum between what Sifneos calls crisis support at one end, and what he calls brief anxiety-provoking psychotherapy at the other. The form of therapy described here obviously comes under the latter heading, but we need a term that more exactly describes its essential character. Both Sifneos's term, and Balint's term, focal therapy, describe simply a kind of technique. I want a term that gives weight to the fact that in this form of therapy the aim is really to *resolve* either the patient's central problem or at least an important aspect of his psychopathology. If this seems to involve rather a large claim, I hope I have presented enough clinical evidence to suggest that such an aim is not unrealistic. I would have preferred the word "radical" which of course I have used extensively in *SBP* and in Part II of the present book in connection with the two opposing views of brief therapy; but I have been warned that, as a label, it might have somewhat unfortunate connotations in America. I cannot entirely avoid this word, but in general have fallen back on another—suggested to me by Dr. John Nemiah—namely, "intensive." I should emphasize that I am proposing it for descriptive purposes and nothing else; there are too many terms, coined by various workers in this field, and used as flags for particular schools of psychotherapy.

THE ASSESSMENT OF PATIENTS FOR PSYCHOTHERAPY

Much of what follows will differ little from what many others have practiced or have written on the subject of assessing a patient for psychotherapy. If differences are to be found, they will lie in the emphasis on forecasting and therapeutic planning, but even these features were long ago strongly emphasized by other workers, notably Finesinger (1948) and Alexander and French (1946).

The first steps in selection are—or should be—the same for all forms of psychotherapy: They must start with a *thoroughgoing psychodynamic assessment*, the successive aims of which are as follows: (1) to understand the patient's illness as deeply as possible; hence (2) to be able to make a forecast of what will happen if the patient is taken on for psychotherapy; (3) to decide from this which patients are unsuitable, and which are suitable for which forms of psychotherapy; (4) to assign the patient to the appropriate form of psychotherapy; and (5) to make a therapeutic plan for the form of therapy chosen.

The idea of *therapeutic planning* is central to our form of brief therapy; and I think that an increasing number of therapists are beginning to realize that it needs to play a major part in all forms of psychotherapy, with the exception of full-scale analysis. I hope the days in which patients are taken on "in the hope that something useful will happen," are numbered. At the Tavistock Clinic the following kind of plan for medium-term therapy is becoming increasingly heard: "This deprived patient needs something like six months in which she can learn to trust her therapist, a year in which she can make use of the relationship, and six months to work through her feelings at the loss of regular sessions, with a long relationship after that."

To repeat, the ability to plan depends on the psychodynamic assessment, and this in turn must involve certain elements, each of which is undertaken in the context of trying to forecast what will happen if the patient begins to undergo uncovering psychotherapy. The first of these is a *proper psychiatric history*.

This is something that tends to be neglected, but a few examples will serve to show its importance: For instance, you cannot plan therapy realistically if you do not know (1) that a patient complaining of difficulty in making close relationships was admitted to hospital for two years with tuberculous glands between the ages of one and three; or (2) that a similar patient has one sibling who was once in a delusional state, and another who failed a university degree and is now working as a laborer; or (3) that an apparently mildly depressed patient had a previous attack of depression that was incapacitating, or (4) made a previous suicidal attempt with a large number of tablets, in circumstances in which he was unlikely to be discovered; or (5) once got into a state in which he danced on the desk in his office and did target practice with an air pistol; or (6) that a woman complaining of overeating had an episode in her teens in which she was thirty pounds below her normal weight, missed her periods for two years, and was admitted to the hospital, where her life was in danger; or (7) that what appears to be an agoraphobic patient is in fact afraid of going out because she is afraid that people in the street are talking about her; and so on and so on.

One hardly needs to point out the kind of forecast that can be made on the basis of the above items in a patient's history: (1) that this patient's inability to make relationships is probably based on an inability to face his true feelings about the traumatic separation in his childhood, that getting him to form a therapeutic relation will be difficult, and that if this succeeds he is likely to become dependent in a primitive way; (2) that the disturbance in this patient is probably the consequence of genetic loading and/or some highly pathological family situation, which may have resulted in a much deeper disturbance in this particular patient than may appear on the surface; (3), (4) and (5) that any attempt at working through the patient's central problem will probably result in his becoming *at least as severely depressed or as severely manic as when he was at his worst in the past,* with the result that hospital admission may well become necessary; (6) that this is probably a very deep-seated and primitive condition, that it will require prolonged psychotherapy if it is to be helped at all, and may well involve periods of undereating even with possible danger to life; and finally (7) that in this patient, overenthusiastic interpretation is quite likely to precipitate an overt psychotic state.

I would not necessarily say that any of the above features are absolute contraindications to intensive brief therapy, but they come near to being so, and must make any potential therapist consider very carefully the type of intervention that he is going to make.

The second important feature of the assessment is what may be called the *full-scale psychodynamic history,* which of course overlaps with the psychiatric history in many features. The aim of this is to try to understand the events of the patient's life in emotional terms, and to see how they have contributed to the present illness, and how they give evidence of the patient's ability to cope with difficulties and to face his anxieties. There is one particular type of situation the assessor needs to try and create time and again, and which has an extreme relevance to brief therapy: that the precipitating events leading to the recent onset of symptoms can be seen to have something of emotional significance in common with events leading to the past onset of symptoms, and that these in turn can be understood in terms of the patient's original family relationships. This is the kind of situation that most frequently leads to the possibility of formulating a *focal problem*, and furnishes one side of the triangle of insight, the link between current and past relationships, which will need to be used extensively in therapy.

The psychodynamic history must include a thorough history of the patient's relationships, with particular reference to any clear-cut patterns that emerge. This can lead to an assessment of the depth of disturbance in relationships, and also to the possibility of forecasting the type of transference likely to develop. As an example, a patient may show a pattern of running away from a relation as soon as there is any threat of involvement. If this is severe, the assessor may well conclude that the patient is unsuitable for psychotherapy; and in any case he will know that this inability to become involved is what must be dealt with in therapy, and that the patient's wish to withdraw will probably constitute the main danger to therapy in the early stages.

The quality of the patient's relationships will give one clue to his strength and potential for growth. Other clues will be given by the amount of "good experience" he has had in his early life, his ability to progress and mature in the past, his ability for achievement in the face of difficulties, his work history, his interests, and his capacity for creativeness.

The above history of the patient's relationships must, of course, include an exploration of his current relationships, and indeed of his whole current life situation. In addition to the patient's own internal strength, it is important to know how much support he will receive from the people currently in his life; and, on the other hand, what obstacles such people may put in the way of his improvement. One of our research findings has been that patients who are tied in difficult current relationships tend to have long therapies. (This work was undertaken at a time when it was not routine at least to interview a marital partner, let alone to try and involve him or her in the therapy.) It must always be borne in mind that conjoint marital therapy, rather than brief individual therapy, may be the treatment of choice in such cases. We did achieve occasional successes by treating one partner only, examples being the Maintenance Man (not included in the present book) and to a lesser extent the Pesticide Chemist; but no one can say that these results might not have been better if the partner had been treated as well. Exactly the same considerations apply to patients who are involved in difficult family situations, where it may be possible and right to involve the whole family in the treatment.

The next important feature in the psychodynamic assessment comes from the quality of the interview itself, seen in terms of the interaction between the patient and interviewer. It is important to be able to assess the patient's capacity to speak honestly about himself, to see his problem in emotional terms, to allow the interviewer some degree of emotional closeness. Above all, and *provided there is no contraindication*, it is quite essential that the interviewer should make trial interpretations, carefully thought out and no deeper than is necessary to serve the purposes for which they are intended. These purposes are as follows: first, to deepen the rapport between patient and interviewer, to reduce resistances, to obtain fresh and spontaneous material, to get more honest answers to questions; second, to assess the patient's capacity to use interpretative psychotherapy; and third, to begin to test hypotheses about the origins of the patient's illness, which will be used both in the planning of therapy, and in the therapy itself if this is undertaken. Evidence about the response to such interpretations is thus one of the most important elements in the assessment.

It is also important to note that these trial interpretations may well involve the transference. Much evidence has been accumulated at the Tavistock Clinic in recent years that transference may already be present to an intense degree in the initial interview, and that transference interpretations may have a dramatic releasing effect. The possibility of transference interpretations should therefore be always borne in mind, particularly when the patient is showing obvious signs of finding it difficult to open up. On the other hand, this can of course be overdone, and the routine relating of every interpretation to the transference is something that I regard as artificial and mistaken. It must always be remembered, however, that interpretations may set in train a chain of events that is quite undesirable. This is particularly so where there is potential psychosis, where ill-chosen interpretations may face the patient with feelings that he is not ready to cope with, may make him more disturbed, and may even precipitate a psychosis. The following story, mentioned in passing in *SBP*, may serve as a warning:

A man walked into a hospital where I was casualty officer, complaining of the fear that he might kill his wife. Questioning revealed that while he was serving abroad in the Army during the war his wife had had an affair with another man and had had a child. Being inexperienced and full of enthusiasm for the power of interpretations, I said to him, "So you have good reason to want to kill your wife." He made no clear response to this and went off. Two days later he came back in an exalted state, demanding of everybody, "Do you believe in the Lord?" He was clearly psychotic and had to be admitted as an emergency.

It must also be remembered that correct interpretations, or even just behavior that enables a patient to share his inner feelings, constitute a most potent gift that the patient may never have experienced before, and that carries with it an implied promise of more. If the patient is *not* suitable for psychotherapy, or if there is no appropriate vacancy, the resulting rejection will be all the more traumatic. I once gave a major interpretation to a woman patient, summarizing her life problem. She fell in love with me and was still writing me poems two years later, flattering for me no doubt but not so satisfactory for her husband. Another example is of a severely deprived young man who spent the first half-hour of his interview in silence, and who was eventually led to talk by a combination of sympathetic attention and interpretation deliberately kept as superficial as possible. This was enough to make him write a letter two days later in which he wanted to share his psychotic thoughts. We did have a vacancy to treat him, but if we had not we might well have been faced with an immediate emergency.

To sum up, whereas interpretations are an essential part of assessing a patient whom we accept, they can be used irresponsibly and there should be a constant interaction at interview between the desire to make contact, the severity of disturbance suspected or revealed, and the availability of vacancies for treatment.

At this point the reader may well ask why I emphasize the importance of response to interpretation, when in fact this variable showed only a small positive relation to outcome when judged by Dreyfus and Shepherd on the initial assessment material. The answer is concerned with problems of using statistics on selected samples. The patients whom we accepted in the present series were those who either responded well to interpretation in the initial interview, or else made sufficient contact with the interviewer to indicate that they had a potential for responding. In fact, as has already been mentioned in chap. 7, our assessment of this was 100 percent accurate: In no patient was there any difficulty in obtaining a response to interpretation soon after the beginning of therapy. Thus, the only patients selected were those at the upper end of the scale of contact with the interviewer, and it was within this context that the correlation with outcome did not appear. I can only say that if some of the rejected patients listed in Table 4 had been selected—notably, for instance, Miss L.—the correlation would almost certainly have emerged very clearly.

The fourth important factor to come out of the initial interview is the patient's motivation. My own use of motivation has never been as systematic as that of Sifneos, described in chap. 3. My position can probably be described as follows: I regard very high motivation, such as that shown at initial interview by the Indian Scientist, as being a most encouraging sign for intensive brief therapy: Equally, very poor motivation, such as that shown by some of the patients in Table 4, I regard as a more or less absolute contraindication: On the other hand, I do not regard *moderately* low motivation as a contraindication, *provided other signs, and particularly the ability to see a focus, are favorable.* One must always remember that the therapist has the chance to create higher motivation through interpretation of his chosen focus, the more so the more he is sure that it is correct. It seems that we always intuitively realized this, and the confirmation that it could lead to successful outcome was given clinically by such cases as the Buyer, and statistically by the clear interaction between motivation and focality presented in chap. 5.

At the end of the psychiatric interview, therefore, it should be possible to make a full psychodynamic diagnosis and to see whether there seems to be some circumscribed aspect of pathology that can be made into a focus, and hence whether there appears to be a possible therapeutic plan. These are all aspects of the therapist's role, and thus represent only half of the information that has been provided. It should also be possible to answer many questions to do with the patient's role: to forecast likely events if he undergoes uncovering psychotherapy, and to assess his capacity for insight, ability to respond to interpretation, strength to face anxiety-provoking material, potential for growth, and motivation to carry him through the stresses of therapy.

I am by now convinced, however, by long and sometimes salutory experience, that a single psychiatric interview by itself is rarely enough to be able to assess the patient's suitability for brief therapy. Sometimes the information clearly appears insufficient, e.g., when the emotional meaning of precipitating events is not clear; but even when it appears to be sufficient, in my view the interview should often be followed either by another, or, more frequently, by a projection test. This latter should ideally be given in the context of definite questions asked of the psychologist:

How much is this an Oedipal problem and how much a problem in the two-person mother–child relation? How much dependence is there? How much evidence is there of good experience? What is his capacity to face his primitive impulses? Is there evidence for homosexuality? Is there any evidence for psychotic features? . . . and so on. It may also be possible, if, for instance, a male patient was interviewed by a man, to assign him to a female psychologist in order to highlight both his reactions to women and to triangular situations. With one such patient in our recent experience, the female psychologist has provided the third apex for interpretations about the Oedipal triangle; and he eventually admitted that he was convinced that the psychologist was the therapist's wife, despite the fact that she had an entirely different name.

In several recent cases the projection test has revealed entirely unexpected features and has saved us from making serious mistakes. A particular example was a young man with what appeared to be a simple Oedipal problem; who, on testing by a woman psychologist, revealed an almost psychotically paranoid attitude to women (this patient is considered in more detail in chap. 16).

Of course, even the interview and projection test may sometimes not be enough, and it may save many wasted sessions if the patient is given further exploratory interviews. It is here that the statistical results on motivation and focality become relevant: The patient is regarded as suitable if his motivation increases and the therapist finds himself able to keep interpretations focal. Our recent experience suggests the following recommendations here: that with less experienced therapists these exploratory interviews should be kept as few as possible, as otherwise there is difficulty in rejecting the patient if he appears to be unsuitable; that the number should be left vague, as otherwise the patient may tend to open up falsely in what he knows to be his last session; and that this work should be undertaken by the original interviewer rather than a different potential therapist—it is then more naturally part of the assessment procedure, rather than a clear-cut situation of being on probation, and it is easier to transfer the patient if the final decision is that he is unsuitable.

CRITERIA FOR ACCEPTANCE FOR INTENSIVE BRIEF THERAPY

When the initial assessment has been completed the selection procedure may be described as a series of stages:

1. Elimination of Absolute Contraindications.   In chap. 7 I gave a list adapted from Hildebrand of severe and disabling conditions, the presence of which mean rejection without further consideration. These shade into the next heading.

2. Rejection of Patients With Whom Certain Dangers Seem Inevitable.   These are patients for whom certain types of event are forecast. They have been listed in Table 3, to which the reader is referred. Examples of patients showing these features are given in Table 4.

3. Formulation of a Focus From the Therapist's Point of View. As always, this is some circumscribed aspect of psychopathology, formulated in terms of a basic interpretation, which it seems feasible to try and work through in a short time.

4. The Focus From the Patient's Point of View. It may be easy enough to formulate a focus, but the next essential question is whether there is evidence that it is acceptable to the patient. Ideally, the following conditions should be fulfilled:

(a) The patient has shown a good capacity to think of his problems in emotional terms.

(b) He apparently has the strength to face disturbing material.

(c) Interpretations based on the focus have been given during the assessment period, and there has been a reasonably good response to them.

(d) He appears to have the motivation to face the stresses of therapy.

The statistical results presented in chap. 5 may be incorporated into this selection procedure by considering the balance between motivation and focality. This means that a patient can be accepted either (a) with only moderate motivation but high focality—i.e., it is possible to see a focus very clearly, and the forecast is made that this will generate enough motivation to carry the patient through; or (b) with high motivation but low focality—where it is possible to forecast that the patient's high motivation will lead to the clarification of the focus within a short time. It must always be remembered, however, that in the latter case therapy tends to be longer.

SUMMARY OF SELECTION PROCEDURE

Although the process of assessment is thus very complex, the process of selection can really be formulated very briefly:

A focus can be found, the patient has already responded to it positively, motivation is sufficient, and certain specific dangers do not seem inevitable.

TIME LIMITS

In the brief therapy unit at the Tavistock Clinic we almost invariably set a time limit from the beginning, telling the patient this as soon as he is taken on. Since many of the therapists have only a limited time at the clinic, we often cannot offer the patient the possibility of irregular sessions according to need after termination, though in my view this should always be done where possible. As I wrote in *SBP*, a time limit gives therapy a definite beginning, middle, and end—like the opening, middle game, and end game in chess—and helps to concentrate both the patient's material and the therapist's work, and to prevent therapy from becoming diffuse and aimless and drifting into a long-term involvement. It enables the prospect of termination to be brought in quite naturally as the time for this approaches; and often this enables a therapy that had been in danger of becoming diffuse to become clear and focal again. To adapt Dr. Johnson, being under sentence of termination doth most marvelously concentrate the material.

With trainees under supervision, we now have a standard limit of thirty sessions. This is well above average for the nine short favorable cases in the present series (mean 20.0, median 18), but it gives opportunity to make up for mistakes that may hold up the work for several sessions. In exceptional therapies that are expected to be more complex or more difficult, we have used a time limit up to one year (roughly forty-six sessions, with holidays).

We have also come to realize that in fact it is much better to set a time limit in terms of a definite *date* rather than a number of sessions. This obviates the necessity for both therapist and patient to keep count, which is not easy; and it also removes at one stroke all sorts of complications to do with whether or not to make up sessions that the patient has missed, and having to judge whether his absences were due to reality or to acting out. If he has a long and unavoidable absence, the time can always be made up to him.

CHAPTER 10

The General Aims of Psychoanalytic Therapy

The whole subject of the aims and technique of brief psychotherapy is best introduced by a consideration of the basic principles common to all forms of psychoanalytic therapy.

The *strategic* aim of psychoanalytic therapy is to bring into consciousness and enable the patient to experience his *emotional conflicts*. Of these there may well of course be many, but each is likely to have the same basic structure. Without getting too deeply involved in theory, we can say that this starts as the threatened eruption into consciousness of some intolerable feeling, often an unacceptable *impulse* (not always—grief, for instance, cannot be described as an impulse), which the patient then keeps at bay or redirects by various *defense mechanisms*. This ultimately gives rise to a constellation that can usually be divided into the classical psychoanalytic triad: the *defense*, the *anxiety*, and the hidden *impulse* (or, in Ezriel's terminology—see Ezriel, 1952—which expresses the same in terms of relationships: the *required relationship*, the feared *catastrophe*, and the *avoided relationship*). The aim of therapy is then to clarify all three aspects of this conflict, though the ultimate aim is, usually by interpreting the defense and the anxiety first, to *bring into consciousness the hidden impulse*.

There is, however, also another triad that ultimately leads to what Menninger has called the *triangle of insight*: There are three *areas* or *situations* in which the conflict may be experienced, or three types of *person* toward whom the conflicting feelings may be directed: (1) *current* or *recent past* situations (usually people "other" than parents or siblings, represented in the notation developed in our content analysis by O); and (2) *distant past* situations (usually parents, P); and (3) the *transference* situation (i.e., the therapist, T). In psychoanalytic therapy it is important to clarify the nature of the conflict in all three of these areas and to emphasize the basic similarities in the three. In ordinary clinical terminology, it is important to make clear that the same patterns of defense, anxiety, and impulse occur in the transference as in current relationships, and that usually—again, not necessarily always—each of these is a *repetition* of a pattern that originally arose in the distant past. In the terminology developed here, it is important to make the *linking interpretations*: current/past (usually O/P), transference/current (T/O), and transference/past (T/P). This is the triangle of insight.

The strategic aims of psychoanalytic therapy can therefore be stated relatively simply as: (1) to clarify the nature of the defense, the anxiety, and the impulse; (2) to clarify this in all three main areas: current, past, and transference; and (3) to make the links among the three areas.

This needs to be done, of course, for each of the conflicts that are identified.

The *tactical* aims of therapy are concerned with what type of interpretation to make at any given moment. In terms of the classification given above, this amounts to (1) which of the three components of the impulse–defense triad to interpret, (2) which of the three possible areas to apply the interpretation to, and (3) whether or not to make any or all of the three possible links.

There are some rough general rules as to the sequence in which these types of interpretation should be given. Here the therapist may be partly guided by a general principle always taught by Balint, that an important function of the therapist is to *keep the tension at the right level,* not too little and not too much; or, in other language, to know how *disturbing* his interpretations should be made.

The most *therapeutically effective* but also the most *disturbing* component of the impulse–defense triad is the *impulse*. In general it is found that direct interpretation of the impulse—without the other two components—often leads only to an intensification of anxiety and hence a reinforcement of defenses. It is therefore usually important to interpret the *defense* first, in order to weaken it gradually; and also to accompany any interpretation of the *impulse* with an interpretation of the *anxiety*. The latter interpretation is usually reassuring rather than otherwise because the anxiety is often based on unrealistic fantasy, and the interpretation can be made in such language as to imply this directly—e.g., the anxiety that being aggressive in any way will automatically lead to rejection or to ruining a relationship forever.

An important further consideration is as follows: The interpretation of the link to the past may be *reassuring* because it suggests that the conflict belongs either to the world of fantasy or to an area where it no longer applies, but it may equally be *disturbing*. One of the reasons for this is that the link between the present and the past may involve an *alteration in the character of both the anxiety and the impulse,* which may become more literal, more physical, and more primitive—e.g., the fear of becoming impotent as a consequence of expressing hostility toward a boss may become transformed into the fear of being literally castrated in retribution for the literal impulse to kill the father.

Moreover, of the three *areas* in which the conflict can be interpreted probably not only the *most therapeutically effective* but also the *least disturbing* is the *transference*. It is the *most therapeutically effective* probably because of its here-and-now character—the feelings can be interpreted while they are actually occurring—and it is the *least disturbing* both because of the therapist's attitude of unconditional acceptance, and because, of all types of feeling, transference feelings can be most easily demonstrated to be based on fantasy. This combination leads to the over-riding importance of the transference in psychoanalytic therapy. On the other hand, I very strongly advocate that the therapist should reserve his transference interpretations until the transference has definitely developed, a situation that varies very greatly from one therapy to another. Once the transference has developed, it should be clarified, and then the link should be made with the past; and all the evidence suggests that it is this type of interpretation that is the most therapeutically effective of all.

All these considerations may be summed up in the following general sequence of interpretations:

1. The impulse–defense triad should be interpreted before the triangle of insight, i.e., the components of the conflict should be clarified in one area before the link is made to another.

2. As far as the individual components of the impulse–defense triad are concerned, the *defense* should usually be interpreted first, and the *anxiety* should be interpreted with the *impulse*. One of the main aims of therapy, however, is to reach the *impulse*.

3. When this triad has been clarified in one area, *then* the link should be made to another.

4. There is no general rule as to the sequence in which the triangle of insight should be interpreted. This depends largely on the rapidity with which the transference develops, which is not under the

therapist's control. However, as soon as transference does develop, then it should be clarified in terms of the three components of the impulse–defense triad; and the ultimate aim of therapy is to make the link with the past (the T/P link) many times and in as meaningful a way as possible.

5. Finally, all the above principles converge toward suggesting that, of all the different types of interpretation that it is possible to make, it is the *impulse* component of the *T/P link* that is the most important.

Much of the therapist's skill can therefore be summed up in developing the instinct to know which type of interpretation to make in this sequence, and how deeply to interpret, at any given moment with any particular patient.

It is the ability to formulate the patient's problem in terms of this kind that gives the therapist the opportunity to exert very considerable control over the course of therapy. Because he can foresee the whole sequence, he can choose his own moment both for interpreting each component of the impulse–defense triad and for making links, thus deliberately directing the patient's attention from one area to another. Provided the initial formulation is correct, a good patient will follow these moves actively; that is, having received a partial interpretation, he will go on to complete it; and having received one interpretation in the sequence, he will spontaneously lead the therapist toward the next. This is part of what is meant by the "therapeutic alliance." It is the combination of a simple initial formulation, a responsive and well-motivated patient, and a therapist who intuitively understands these principles, that results in focal therapy.

CHAPTER 11

Planning and Technique

When I was writing *SBP* I was always coming up against the observation that two or more aspects of brief therapy that appeared originally to be separate were really interdependent. Thus, the possibility of using transference interpretations (an aspect of *technique*) clearly depends on the type of patient chosen (an aspect of *selection*). We meet the same phenomenon here: Not only is the ability to make a therapeutic plan an important criterion for *selection*; but a plan means an intention to conduct therapy in a particular way and hence is an implied *prediction*; and the intention to conduct therapy in a particular way immediately involves *technique*—and moreover, the more detailed the planning, the more do aspects of technique need to be described in the plan. Thus, planning, prediction, and technique are best all considered together.

This leads at once to the answer to a question that I am often asked at discussions of brief psychotherapy, How is it possible to keep interpretations focal? I have always found this a difficult question, but the reason, I think, is that the true answer often lies not in technique at all but—before therapy starts—in selection and planning. Put briefly, the best way of keeping interpretations focal is to select focal patients in the first place and then to formulate a correct therapeutic plan.

We may elaborate on this by the description of an ideal type of case, not an idealized case, since approximations to this situation are quite frequently met in practice. It is in cases of this kind that brief therapy can be at its most radical.

In formulating a therapeutic plan, the ideal situation to meet at initial assessment is one in which as many as possible of the following seven conditions are fulfilled:

1. *The Current Conflict.*   There is a precipitating factor that gives a clue to the current conflict.

2. *The Nuclear Conflict.*   There are (a) previous precipitating events, or (b) early traumatic experiences, or (c) family constellations, or (d) repetitive patterns, which give a clue to the nuclear conflict.

3. *Congruence Between Current and Nuclear Conflict.*   The current conflict and the nuclear conflict can be seen to be basically the same.

4. *Response to Interpretation.*   The patient responds to interpretations about aspects of this conflict.

5. *Motivation.*   After interviews in which these interpretations have been given, the patient's motivation remains high or increases.

6. *Transference.*   The conflict is one that is likely to manifest itself in the transference.

7. *Termination.*   The nature of the termination issue can be foreseen, and this in turn can be related to the nuclear conflict.

If most of these conditions are met, it is hardly too much to say that—with a reasonably competent therapist—(1) therapy cannot help being focal, (2) its aims can be clearly defined, and (3) its course, though not, of course, its outcome, can be broadly predicted.

These three statements may be taken in turn. First, therapy cannot help being focal because the patient shows a single type of problem running through his life. It seems probable that any material that he brings will represent an aspect of this problem, and all the therapist will have to do is to interpret each aspect as it arises.

Second, the aim of therapy can be clearly defined in the light of the principles discussed in chap. 10. This will be to clarify the three components of the impulse–defense triad of the nuclear conflict, and then to complete the triangle of insight.

Third, provided the formulation is correct, the course can equally be predicted. The early part of therapy will be concerned with clarifying the impulse–defense triad, working toward deeper and more disturbing material; the middle part will be concerned more and more with making the T/P link; and the later part of therapy will be concerned with bringing out feelings about termination, expressing these in terms of the nuclear conflict, and making the T/P link in this area as well.

This kind of statement may well be greeted with some skepticism, or even (as I have heard in the past) with the epithet "omnipotent." Yet, even at the time of Balint's workshop, some of us tried to formulate such predictions before the beginning of therapy; and in recent years I have been doing the same in the Tavistock brief therapy unit. It is only as I write now, clarifying in my own mind principles that I have been teaching for years, that I see how almost automatic the process of prediction can sometimes be.

In fact the seven conditions listed above could easily lead to the headings of an Initial Assessment Form and a Prediction Form, as will be illustrated in some of the following cases.

We have never in fact formulated our predictions quite as exactly as described in this way, but it is clear that we understood how to do it implicitly, as some of these examples will show. Furthermore, as already discussed, prediction will involve both selection and technique; and this subject will therefore provide an opportunity to illustrate many of the principles that have crystallized from this whole work, clinical and statistical, together with some thinking about the future.

Because most of the examples are fairly recent, follow-ups are relatively short, and it is possible that some of the therapeutic results may be reversed by later events; but I feel I have justification for believing that *over the whole sample,* as in fact happened with the later follow-up of the *SBP* cases, the basic principles would still hold firm.

CHAPTER 12

Clinical Examples

The most successful example of detailed prediction among the second series from Balint's Workshop was the "Zoologist" and the best recent example from the Tavistock brief therapy unit was the "Magistrate's Daughter."

THE ZOOLOGIST

The patient, you will recall, was a young man of twenty-two with a previously successful career, who was studying zoology in order to become an ethologist, but who six months previously had suddenly thrown up his studies. This seemed to have some connection with a conflict between him and his father, and the referring psychiatrist had written that the father's insistence that his son should enter a profession with a high social and financial status "led to constant conflict, the boy's own quite genuine desire to be a zoologist conflicting with the desire to throw the whole thing up just to do down Dad. The struggle between the two ended in an impasse and the boy resigned from college."

The interview (session 1) was marked by extreme resistance. Hard as the (male) interviewer tried, he seemed unable to make contact and often had to fall back on asking questions. The patient expressed a great deal of bitterness against both of his parents for lack of true understanding, particularly against his father who seemed to have no idea of his son's sense of vocation or his deep love of animals. The father was "not the sort of person you can have a row with." It emerged that the patient had never had a close relation with a girl, and that when he tried to start one it "just faded out" after they had met a few times. The interviewer tried linking resentment against the university teachers with resentment against the father, and also tried exploring the patient's feelings about the referring psychiatrist and feelings about being transferred to the clinic, all without avail. The interpretation that finally broke the deadlock was the simple remark, based on a "choked" quality in the patient's voice when he spoke of things that mattered to him, that he "seemed to have a lot of intense feeling that couldn't come out." At this the patient, suddenly opening up, spoke of an incident in which a little girl had put her hand in his and said, "I like you," which he said had been one of the proudest moments of his life.

On the face of it this may seem to be a rather strange story: What is the connection between the interviewer's remark and the story about the little girl, let alone the connection between the latter and the rest of the patient's life and his current problem in particular? Yet, in fact this is an example of the seven conditions set out in chap. 11 being fulfilled; and this was basically seen at the time, though the formulation was not as clear as, with hindsight and much later experience, it is possible to make now.

The patient's *nuclear problem* was that his love for his parents had become spoiled by his parents' lack of understanding and his own anger about it, and that—much as he longed to—he could no longer entrust himself to close human relations for fear that he would be let down again. The *precipating factor* or *current problem* was an aspect of the nuclear problem played out both against his teachers and his father over the question of his studies, with him expressing his anger in a spoiling and self-destructive way. He not only brought the nuclear problem into the *transference* at once, showing an inability to trust the interviewer, but also showed that *this problem could be easily penetrated by interpretation* once the interviewer showed an intuitive understanding of his need to express his love (this was in fact, by implication, an "impulse interpretation"). The story of the little girl who loved and trusted him falls into place immediately.

Both of the triads mentioned above are already present. The impulse–defense triad in terms of Ezriel's three relationships is as follows: the *required relationship* (defense) is of withdrawal and lack of trust, the *avoided relationship* (impulse) is one of trust and closeness, and the feared *catastrophe* (anxiety) is being let down again and spoiling it all with his self-destructive anger. It never became clear exactly when his relation with his parents went wrong, so it is perhaps not correct to speak in terms of a triad involving the distant past; but on the other hand the *triad of person* is clearly present, consisting of (1) his parents, (2) his university teachers and potential girl friends, and (3) the interviewer.

By the end of the interview the patient's *motivation* for treatment by the *interviewer* (not by anybody else!) was exceedingly high. When sent for projection test he was once again in marked resistance; but he then spontaneously wrote a long letter to the interviewer in which he confided the thoughts he could not reveal to the psychologist, and continued with free-associations—some of them quite painful—as if therapy had already started.

Finally, it is of course possible to see how the *termination* issue is likely to affect the therapy: Clearly, it will be crucial because it will be another of the disappointments that will reactivate his nuclear problem.

It is important to note that the interviewer did in fact have a vacancy to treat him.

It should now be possible to predict in detail the issues that will be present in this therapy. There will in fact be at least two impulse– defense triads, which may be formulated as follows:

1. *Before* disappointment there will be (a) inability to trust (defense), (b) fear of disappointment (anxiety), and (c) desire for love and closeness (impulse).

2. *After* disappointment there will be (a) withdrawal (defense), (b) fear of spoiling (anxiety), and (c) self-destructive anger (redirected impulse).

These issues *cannot help* being expressed in the transference (the first triad has already been so), and the aim of therapy will be to clarify them all—probably in the transference first—and then to make the transference/parent link.

Since the therapist has not yet disappointed him, it will be the first of these two triads that will be dealt with in the transference in the initial stages of therapy. The second triad is likely to become prominent over the issue of termination.

I have in fact simplified the story somewhat, though not in any way that is unfair. The projection test introduced a complicating factor, suggesting Oedipal problems; but the material of the interview was so dynamic and so clear that Oedipal problems were swept aside at the time in the formulation and therapeutic plan. The following are quotations from material written after the projection test but before the first therapeutic session:

> [This is a] young man with a good personality, with normal strong love and hate, whose relation with his parents has prevented him from

being able to express these feelings openly. [He is] preoccupied with his
need to rebel and is spoiling his life as an expression of this. [He is]
equally preoccupied with his need to express love.

I feel he needs a deep transference experience of love and hate. Could
this be given by short-term therapy?

The therapist wrote the following prediction of the course of
therapy:

In the first few sessions he will form a very intense relationship.
During this time I shall try to deal with his inability to express his love and
to get him to experience his love in the relation with the therapist [this is
the first impulse–defense triad]. There will then be a period when he
will have to experience hate with the therapist because of termination [i.e.,
the second impulse-defense triad], and on that therapy will stand or
fall.

This formulation includes at least by implication statements of the
following:

1. the nuclear problem;

2. two impulse–defense triads;

3. the manifestation of the nuclear problem in the transference;
and

4. the termination issue.

It does not include an explicit statement of the need to make the *T/
P link*, although the nature of this link is clearly implied, since the
prediction about the transference is based on the relation with the
parents. Also, the third corner of the *triad of person* (namely girl
friends), receives no mention, and in fact it played a crucial part in
therapy, as will be seen.

All this may be summed up in an Initial Assessment Form and a
Prediction Form, which of course are only devised now and will
inevitably contain some hindsight. I always believe that such forms
should be kept flexible and may vary slightly from one patient to
another.

The Zoologist: Initial Assessment Form

1. The Current Conflict (Expressed if Possible in Terms of Impulse,
Defense, and Anxiety).   Anger against his parents (also against his
university teachers) at their lack of understanding, expressed in a
spoiling and self-destructive way. It is not easy to formulate this in
terms of the impulse–defense triad, because the way he expresses his
anger appears to contain both the anxiety (fear of spoiling) and the
defense (redirected anger).

2. *The Nuclear Conflict.* This appears to be the same as the current conflict.

3. *Relation Between Current and Nuclear Conflicts.* See 2.

4. *Transference So Far Observed.* This consisted of initial inability to trust (defense), which was relatively easily penetrated by an interpretation implying understanding of his need to express his love. He then formed an intense and trusting relation. With the psychologist, mistrust returned but the trust for the interviewer so far has remained.

5. *Response to Interpretation.* This appears to have been dramatic (see 4. above).

6. *Motivation and Its Fluctuations.* His motivation to *come* was always high (he said he had been depressed when he learned that there would be a delay before he could be seen). His motivation *for insight* could not really be assessed at initial interview, although it appears to have been momentarily high when he responded to interpretation. His motivation during the projection test was apparently low; but his motivation both for insight and for being treated *by the interviewer* appeared, in view of his letter, to be very high indeed.

The Zoologist: Prediction Form

1. *Conflict to be Taken as Focus, Expressed if Possible in Terms of Impulse, Defense, and Anxiety.* (a) Inability to trust (*defense*) because of fear (*anxiety*) that his love (*impulse*) will be spoiled by others' lack of understanding and his own consequent anger (*second impulse*); (b) withdrawal (*defense*) because of fear of spoiling his love (*anxiety*) by his own anger (*impulse*), which is expressed in a spoiling and self-destructive way.

2. *Relation Between Focal Conflict and Nuclear Conflict.* The same.

3. *Formulation of the Triangle of Insight.* The *impulse* component of his nuclear conflict is currently being expressed in the form of self-destructive anger against his *parents* and his *university teachers.*

The *defense* component of his nuclear conflict is currently being expressed in the form of withdrawal from potential girl friends.

The *defense* component was also initially present in his relation with his therapist, but has now been penetrated. However, the whole conflict is likely to be reactivated *by termination,* in the form of self-destructive anger against the therapist.

4. *Forecast of the Course of Therapy in Terms of the Two Triads of Interpretation.* (a) The original defense of *inability to trust* has already

been penetrated in the transference and has resulted in a warm and trusting relationship. (b) Initial stages of therapy will therefore be concerned with enabling the patient to experience his trust and love in the transference, while interpreting his former defense against this, and linking this with the way in which his relation with his parents has become spoiled. (c) In the later stages of therapy, the patient will experience *disappointment in his relation with the therapist* caused by the prospect of termination. This is likely to manifest itself by *withdrawal* and possibly *self-destructive anger*. This will be the crucial part of therapy. The mechanisms involved will have to be interpreted and it is here that the transference/parent link will be most important.

5. *How Will Termination Become an Issue and What Will Be the Relation Between This and the Nuclear Conflict?* This has already been covered in (4c) above.

So, what happened in fact? First of all, an unexpected complicating factor was introduced at the beginning: The therapist went on a long holiday, and the start of therapy was delayed until three months after the original interview. Thus, the element of letdown and disappointment did not wait for the issue of termination but entered as soon as therapy started (session 2). The patient was once more in resistance, trying very hard, but tense and unable to speak spontaneously. He thus presented at once in the transference the *defense* element (withdrawal) of the second impulse–defense triad. It was interpreted that he felt tense (*anxiety*) because he *resented* the delay (*impulse*). He agreed that he had been disappointed, but this didn't help.

In session 3 he was set a time limit of a total of sixteen therapeutic sessions (i.e., session 17 would be the last), though with the possibility of keeping in touch with the therapist for occasional sessions after that. This had no effect on the tension, either one way or the other.

The patient opened session 4 by saying that he had been thinking about "this barrier" between him and the therapist, thus introducing his own word for the *defense* component of his conflict, and illustrating the kind of work that highly motivated patients do in a good therapeutic alliance. Later, talking about the future as far as jobs were concerned, he said he had been wondering whether he wanted to stay where he was or "go wandering." This gave an opportunity for, first, another *defense* interpretation, a hint at an *impulse* interpretation, then a complete *impulse* interpretation, and finally an interpretation *completing the triangle of insight* (in our notation, O/P/T). This all happened as follows:

In response to the word "wandering," the therapist said that it seemed that things were all right between him and other people for a short time (the flexible phrase "other people" was deliberately used because it could lead to any component of the triad of person and, in the context, because it had clear transference implications) and that then "something went wrong" (leaving the options open about the nature of the impulse and anxiety) and he wanted to "go wandering," i.e., to start another relation somewhere else "in order to avoid whatever it was that went wrong" (i.e., essentially a general *defense* interpretation).

This obviously meant a lot to him, and he responded by telling of a family in which there was a delightfully informal and accepting atmosphere where this had never happened.

This gave the opportunity for the following major composite interpretation, here quoted only with slight editing from the therapist's account of the session. The components of the two triads are added in brackets:

> It was obvious that this *family* (*"others"*) had provided him with the sort of *parents* that he had not had himself (*others* linked with *parents*). I suspected that what went wrong between him and other people was his coming up against his *anger* (*impulse*) with his *parents* about the things that he had not had, which got directed toward *anybody who did not behave to him exactly as he wanted* (*parents* linked with *others*). So far this family had managed to avoid this problem (*others* again linked with *parents*). In his relation with me (*transference*) he had spoken about the feeling that I was a bit impersonal, and perhaps what had happened was that I had come up against this anger (*impulse* in *transference*), and that what he wanted from me was that I should actively show him that I loved him. What seemed to have happened between him and me (*transference*) was *just what happened between him and other people* (*transference* linked with *others* and *parents*), namely, that we had started off with a very good relation in which we obviously talked the same language and he wanted to talk to me—as was shown by his letter to me after seeing the psychologist—but that after my holiday something had gone wrong. Now he wanted to go wandering. Perhaps he was feeling that he wanted to escape from the relation that had gone wrong with me (*defense, transference*).

Again, this obviously meant a lot to him, and he said with feeling that he could see this pattern occurring in his life "again and again and again." Yet, the tension was not resolved.

From now on, therapy dealt with nothing else but the problem of understanding the barrier and bringing home this understanding to the patient. The way in which this understanding finally emerged is an instructive example of two general phenomena in psychotherapy: (1) that the understanding may be already there, but it cannot be used in a meaningful way until the patient himself is ready; and (2) that the really therapeutic moments often occur not when the relation with the therapist *goes right* (as it had in the initial interview), but when it *goes wrong and this can be understood and resolved.*

Therapy continued tense and unproductive till session 9. The patient then said that since he started treatment not only had his relations with human beings become worse, but now even his relation with animals had become spoilt. This gave an opportunity for a *major impulse interpretation in the transference,* together with the possibility of the *transference/parent link*: The therapist said that whenever the patient was angry with people, he wanted to *spoil everything that they had given him (impulse)*. With his *parents,* he had thrown up college; with the *therapist* he probably himself spoiled his relations outside and then said it was all the therapist's fault *(parents* linked with *transference)*. This was the first time since session 1 that an interpretation broke the tension. The patient became animated and *admitted openly for the first time that he had thrown up college to spite his father.* In the next session he said that his relation with animals had improved again.

The climax of this stage of therapy came in an important sequence in sessions 16 and 17. This started with a complex dream. The most important of the associations to this dream was that when doing his National Service in the Army, he had been *transferred* from a station that he liked to one that he didn't, and had deliberately done his work badly so that he had failed to get a commission. This once more gave the opportunity for the *impulse interpretation* and the *transference/parent link*, this time introducing the *termination* issue as well: that he was dissatisfied with what the therapist had given him, as he was dissatisfied with what his parents had given him *(transference* linked with *parents)*, that he was now being "transferred" from *therapy* to *life,* and that it looked as if he would deliberately sabotage his life in order to get his own back on the therapist *(impulse, transference)*. The patient smiled and said it was probably right, but made no other response.

Yet, in session 17 there was, quite unexpectedly, a complete transformation. Interpretation of the self-destructive hate in the previous session now *led to an upsurge of warmth and love.* The atmosphere was one of hope, of sadness at parting, and a wish to keep a relation with the therapist to take away with him. He told a dream in which there seemed some possibility of meeting again a *girl* whom he had known previously, but with whom the "barrier" had prevented any progress (girls are mentioned for the first time for many sessions), and his associations led to his interest in romantic music, and to how he used to be taken as a small boy by his *father* to visit the crib in the crypt of a church at Christmas (the first inkling that there had ever been a good relation with his father). The therapist interpreted that he now seemed to be concerned with the possibility of expressing warm, tender, and romantic feelings as opposed to anger and hate; in parting from the *therapist* he must feel that he was parting from something that meant a lot to him (*transference over termination*). The patient agreed and went on to speak of how he had wanted to write a story about a *very motherly woman* whom he knew. Some time ago his writing had come to a full stop, but last week he had suddenly felt able to take it up again and had almost finished it. Finally, he asked if he could write a sort of "diary plus" and send it to the therapist (preserving the relation after termination), to which the latter readily agreed.

Therapeutic effects that were noticeable soon after this first phase of therapy were (1) that the patient went back to college for the next term and eventually completed his studies; and (2) that for the first time he began to make sustained attempts to make contact with girls— previously the "barrier" had always made this impossible. There was thus introduced a new class of person in the category "other" with whom the nuclear conflict was likely to arise, which assumed greater and greater importance as time went on.

Mainly because of vicissitudes in the patient's relation with girls, this first attempt at termination was by no means the end of the story. The nuclear problem was weakened but not resolved. A summary of subsequent events for the next two years can be put very simply as an alternation between hope and depression, with visits to the therapist during the depressions. In these sessions the theme of the therapist's interpretations was always the nuclear conflict: that the patient formed intense relations, got disappointed, and his hatred and desire to spoil everything interfered with the possibility of experiencing and fulfilling his love.

The degree to which the nuclear problem had been weakened, however, is illustrated by the fact that the patient attempted to form a relation with one girl; and when this failed, with a second; and when this in turn failed, with a third. Her name was Barbara, and he eventually proposed marriage to her and was accepted. In a letter to the therapist he wrote, "We are in love and can trust each other. But on occasions I get slight fits of depression in case our love fails."

Nearly two years after session 17 he asked for another session. He said that he had had an attack of depression and inner confusion that was worse than he had ever known before. He did not know the cause of this, but it was eventually traced to the fact that he had discovered an old diary of Barbara's and had been unable to resist the temptation to read it. In this he had found out that during a period in the previous year, before they were engaged, Barbara had been going out with someone else as well as him. This called for an interpretation of the nuclear conflict in relation to Barbara. The result was that he succeeded in talking over his feelings with her and their relation improved again.

Nothing was now heard for over a year. Eventually the therapist received another, rather surprising, letter, the theme of which was that *Barbara* seemed to have changed: From being full of life, she had changed into a state of apathy.

We may now try to condense the sequence of two sessions (nos. 31 and 32):

1. The patient started by trying to present Barbara's story like a case history, which the therapist brushed aside, suggesting that she was really reacting to something in *him*: Perhaps he had been less able to be affectionate since the diary incident (*defense* interpretation, *other*).

2. The therapist restated the nuclear problem of *spoiling a* relationship with *someone who disappointed him*, reminded him of *how this had happened in therapy*, and suggested that he still hadn't forgiven Barbara for the diary incident (*impulse* interpretation, *other* linked with *transference*).

3. Then, noticing something rather nasty about the patient's smile, the therapist suggested that the patient took some satisfaction in reporting to him that things had gone wrong (further *impulse* interpretation, *transference*).

4. The patient, surprisingly, immediately responded by telling how he had experienced a similar feeling when his *father* had had a breakdown after failing to get promotion at work (the patient makes his own *transference/parent* linking interpretation).

5. The therapist then took the bit between his teeth and suggested that since he seemed to have been glad about his *father's failure*, perhaps he wanted to make the *therapist fail*, too, by making a mess of his life (further *impulse* interpretation, *parent* linked with *transference*).

6. Shortly after this the patient, near to tears, began to admit how cold he had been to Barbara over the past year (clear response—again the warmer and softer feelings come to the surface).

These final two sessions of therapy illustrate very clearly the step-by-step progress from the *defense* to the *impulse* in the *current* situation (*other*), and then the *link with the transference* (*other/transference*), followed by a new *impulse interpretation* in the *transference*, and then by the *transference/parent link* given first by the patient himself and then by the therapist.

The only way in which this therapy fails to fit exactly the formulation in terms of the two triads is that the *anxiety* was never clearly formulated, and its interpretation appears to have been unnecessary.

A comparison of the *predictions actually made at the time* (not the predictions made with hindsight) with *actual events* will reveal the following:

1. The implied formulation of the patient's nuclear problem was almost exactly correct, except perhaps that one could disagree with the word "rebel" and want it replaced by the word "spoil."

2. The prediction that the patient would form a very intense relation at first was incorrect because of the unforeseen consequences of the delay before starting treatment.

3. The prediction that the patient would have to experience his hate after his love was, of course, the main theme of therapy.

4. The prediction that the hate would arise over termination was also correct, but the hate had already arisen before this over the delay in starting.

In sum, the predictions were inaccurate in some details, but accurate in all essentials.

It should perhaps be added that during the course of therapy there was at no time any useful response to a number of interpretations given about Oedipal problems.

The reader may well expect that, with such a degree of clarity and focality, this was a highly successful therapy. Well, this probably was not so. The patient made enormous progress: moving (1) from throwing up his studies to completing his degree and becoming very successful in his work; and (2) from being hardly able to make any contact with girls at all, to falling deeply in love and marrying the girl of his choice. However, at follow-up it appeared that there was a good deal missing in his relation with his wife and that the nuclear conflict was still being expressed; he had never really been able to forgive her for what he felt, seemingly quite unjustifiably, to be her betrayal.

THE MAGISTRATE'S DAUGHTER

The best recent example from the Tavistock brief therapy unit is as follows:

The patient was a girl of twenty-one complaining of inability to respond sexually, beyond a certain point, to her boyfriend.

The chief factor in her upbringing seems to have been the ambiguous messages about sexuality conveyed by her magistrate father—a man on the one hand extremely puritanical in his stated principles, who had criticized his daughter for wearing short skirts, but who yet would speak openly and somewhat lasciviously about the charms of women. The result had been an "all or nothing" or otherwise ambiguous reaction to sexuality in three of his four children. Of these, one older brother had married a girl because he had got her pregnant; while a second older brother had married a girl who turned out to be frigid, and had then turned for sexual relief to the patient herself (at the age of eighteen), who had allowed sexual contact with him short of intercourse over a fairly long period "in order to help him," although she also got no pleasure from it. The third older brother did not have obvious sexual difficulties. (This story illustrates, incidentally, the importance of the family history in making a full initial assessment).

The patient's own ambiguous attitude to sexuality was demonstrated in many ways: (1) she arrived "looking like a sexy schoolgirl with a very short skirt and a gym-slip type dress," yet somehow contrived to be demure at the same time. (2) She said she got upset when the other girls in her apartment had sexual relations with boys, but added "I sometimes wonder whether it's jealousy." (3) She obviously dressed and behaved in a provocative way at work and was continually being asked out by the men there, but she refused them and then got depressed. (4) She said that after the relation with her brother she had become "hard," and that although she had had intercourse with several men she got no pleasure from it. (5) She now had a boyfriend with whom she had had intercourse and whom she intended to marry, but she said that she just shut off her feelings when she began to get aroused beyond a certain point. She also said that she got no vaginal secretions, though this had improved recently.

In her previous history, she had always been "Daddy's girl" until she had a late puberty at the age of seventeen. She remembered being shocked from the age of twelve by her father's crude language when talking about sex, and she had actively tried to stop him. She said she had always admired him very much, but at the same time she was clearly more angry with him than she was able to admit, and she spoke of him with some contempt.

She and her brother had in fact been able to tell their mother about their sexual relation. The mother had been extremely sympathetic about this, perhaps too much so.

The (male) interviewer made a number of interpretations: e.g., underlining her own admission of jealousy of her roommates' sexual relations (impulse interpretation), which the patient now denied; pointing out that during the interview she shut off her feelings about sex in the same way as she did with her boyfriend (defense interpretation); and saying that perhaps she was afraid of getting out of control and becoming like a whore, a word probably derived from her father (anxiety interpretation). To none of these interpretations did she respond, and she ended—as she had started—by wondering whether she really had a problem and needed to be treated at all.

Psychological tests confirmed and elaborated the above picture. Her Word Association Test showed: (1) a strong and rather moralizing conscience, (2) an inability to respond to either sexual or aggressive stimulus words, (3) an idealization of members of her family, and (4) a perception of men as sexual and dirty (projection?). After projective testing the (woman) psychologist wrote: (1) that there was clearly a *focus* in her *denial of her sexual impulses* and her *anger against the sexual man*; but that there were contraindications to brief therapy in (2) her lack of conviction about actually having a problem, (3) her tendency to brush interpretations aside, (4) her rather rigid projection of all "dirty" sexuality onto the man, (5) her dependent manner of relating, which might be largely defensive or might have some primitive basis, and might make termination difficult if she ever committed herself to therapy, and (6) her difficulty in owning any of her impulses and feelings. On the other hand, it also emerged that in five months time she intended joining her boyfriend in the States in order to marry him, which would provide both a natural termination point and a further issue around which therapy could be focused.

This was a case in which the contraindications were swept aside by the intuitive feeling that with a male therapist these issues would rapidly manifest themselves in the transference, and that if the therapist possessed a considerable degree of therapeutic tact, he would be able to keep the patient in therapy and working on these problems. There was such a therapist available, and he also was a fatherly man considerably older than the patient, which would be likely to focus the issues still further. The plan was made that the date of projected departure to join her fiancé in five months time would be made the termination date *irrespective of whether the patient actually went or not.*

The reader who has followed this story will see that, provided the patient stayed in therapy, there was the material here for very detailed assessment and predictions:

The Magistrate's Daughter: Initial Assessment Form

1. The Current and Recent Conflicts.   All her conflicts seem to be concerned with her very confused feelings about sexuality. In the *current* conflict these feelings are directed toward *boyfriends* (especially her fiancé) and consist of the following: (a) the conflict between expressing her own sexuality (impulse) and rejecting it (defense), apparently because she feels it to be wrong and dirty (anxiety); an additional defense is putting all the blame for sexual impulses onto the man, a mixture of *denial* and *projection* or *externalization*; (b) the conflict between wishing to *attract* men (impulse) and to *reject* them, probably both out of *guilt* (anxiety) and *anger* (conflicting impulse).

Conflicts (a) and (b) are expressed together in various ways, e.g., by dressing provocatively but rejecting men when they ask her out, by becoming "hard" toward men, and by her inability to respond sexually. All these can be formulated as mixed expressions of *defense* and *impulse*.

In the *recent* conflict these feelings were directed toward her *brother*. She allowed sexual contact with him (impulse) but "only in order to help him" (defense against admitting any responsibility for the impulse), again presumably because she felt guilty (anxiety), and then was unable to respond (defense). Since he was presumably the prime mover in their sexual relation, this can be used to reinforce her defense of blaming the man (denial and projection).

2. The Nuclear Conflict.   In the *nuclear* conflict these feelings are presumably directed toward her father, and have been aroused in her by (a) the close relation with him, (b) his own overt sexuality, and (c) his moralistic attitude toward it. The *anxiety* is presumably the incest barrier (there is little tangible evidence for problems concerned with rivalry with her mother). She has *identified* with her father's moralistic attitude toward sexuality, which may well be the result of a kind of conditioning, but which now both reinforces her *anxiety* and can be used as a *defense*. Since her father has in reality expressed sexuality in a rather crude way, this also can be used to reinforce her defense of blaming the man (denial and projection).

3. Relation Between Current, Recent, and Nuclear Conflicts.   They are all essentially the same. Her brother acts as a kind of intermediate between her fiancé and her father.

4. *Transference So Far Observed.*   None definite.

5. *Response to Interpretation.*   Although interpretations of defense, anxiety, and impulse have been given, the response has been minimal.

6. *Motivation.*   She tends to fall back on the defense of questioning whether she really has a problem at all, and her motivation also appears to be minimal.

The Magistrate's Daughter: Prediction Form

1. *Conflict To Be Taken as Focus, Expressed if Possible in Terms of Impulse, Defense, and Anxiety.*   There will be two conflicts: (a) In the first the impulse is *sexuality,* and (b) in the second, *anger toward the man.* The *anxieties* are (a) becoming aware of and perhaps losing control of sexual feelings that she believes to be wrong and dirty (ultimately incestuous), and (b) fear of expressing direct anger toward the man. Defenses are *denial* of responsibility for her own sexual impulses, blaming the man for sexual impulses (*externalization*), sexual *inhibition,* and *identification* with her father's moralistic attitude.

In addition, *defense* and one of the *impulses* (anger) are expressed together by becoming "hard" toward men and rejecting them.

2. *Relation Between Focal Conflict and Nuclear Conflict.*   The same.

3. *Formulation of the Triangle of Insight.*   There are really *five* categories of person toward whom these conflicts have been or are likely to be expressed: (a) men in general, (b) her fiancé, (c) her brother, (d) her father, and (e) the male therapist.

The focal conflict will need to be clarified and demonstrated to be essentially the same in all these areas. Most important will be all the links to her father.

4. *Forecast of the Course of Therapy in Terms of the Two Triads of Interpretation.*   (a) A major problem will be to get her to admit that she needs help, to recognize any of the impulse components of the impulse–defense triad, and to keep her in therapy. For this purpose the therapist will need therapeutic tact of a high order. (b) It seems likely that the way into her problems will be the *transference.* The therapist will need to interpret the impulse–defense triad in the relation to himself, and then make the link with other areas, probably first the patient's fiancé, then her brother, and ultimately her father.

5. How Will Termination Become an Issue and What Will Be the Relation Between This and the Nuclear Conflict? Since the patient has shown evidence of some degree of regression, termination may well become a difficult issue once contact has been made. It will probably be best to interpret the regression as a flight from (*defense* against) mature sexuality. Provided this can be weathered, the basic interpretation will become an aspect of the nuclear conflict: feelings of grief and anger against the therapist for first arousing her expectations and then disappointing them.

What I have tried to do here—as with the Zoologist—is to make the detailed assessment and predictions solely on the basis of the information available before therapy started. This inevitably is contaminated by hindsight, but I firmly believe that essentially the same formulation could have been made, with careful thought, at the time.

What was actually written was much less detailed but contained many of the same essential elements:

> The focus will obviously be her extreme conflict over sexuality [impulse], her unwillingness to admit her own sexual impulses [defense, denial], and her tendency to put all the blame for sexuality onto the man [defense, externalization]. This is likely to manifest itself in the transference very early and it looks as if most of the work will have to be done through the transference. These feelings will need to be linked with her relation to her father. It will be necessary to keep interpretations at the right level so as not to frighten her away.

The main omissions from this formulation were (1) the other main impulse, namely *anger* against the man (which nevertheless was clearly seen by the psychologist); and (2) any prediction about the termination issue. A more detailed account of the defenses, anxieties, and the triangle (here, pentagon!) of insight could certainly have been formulated, but were not because the headings of the form had not been thought out at the time.

So, once more, what happened in fact?

This patient offers a very instructive contrast from the Zoologist. The latter was a high-motivation patient struggling against his own resistance, with whom as soon as opportunity arose the most complete interpretation could be given at once. This girl, on the other hand, was a patient with highly ambivalent motivation, who required a high degree of therapeutic tact if she was not to be frightened away, and yet who did her own therapeutic work if she was allowed to go at her own pace. Some of the issues in handling such a patient appear very clearly in the first few therapeutic sessions, which are therefore given in some detail:

She arrived for the first therapeutic session (session 2) in a trouser suit that seemed to make the best of her attractiveness without being extreme in any way. The opening was of *defensive passivity*: The clinic had requested her presence here, her G.P. wanted her to come, she felt she had nothing to lose but was afraid she could only use the time ineffectively.

Yet, she then went on to talk in detail of her central problem: that she had mixed-up ideas about sex, her upbringing was very strict, she was shocked when her brother had a sexual relation with her, she felt that men were animals and she *resented* them (here spontaneously bringing in the second *impulse* at once). The theme then developed of her *lack of trust* in men (*anxiety*) with the possible exception of her fiancé. Associations went on to include a man who had asked her out and whom she had refused, a description of her unsatisfactory sexual relation with her fiancé, her mother who didn't mention sex, her father who talked of sex extensively, which *embarrassed* her, and her second brother who had had to get married because he got a girl pregnant.

It seems almost certain that in all this there is considerable *transference* communication here about her *anxieties* in relation to men. I think a less experienced and overinterpretative therapist might well have been too explicit in terms of sexual anxieties in the transference and have frightened the patient into withdrawing; but this therapist simply asked, did she perhaps feel *"embarrassed"* at talking of *sex* with an *older man* in this room? It is worth noting here the following points about this wonderfully tactful interpretation: (1) It is essentially what is required, namely an *anxiety* interpretation in the *transference*: (2) it uses the mildest word possible ("embarrassed") about the anxiety; (3) this is the same word as the patient had already used about her father; (4) thus, this word, and also the phrase, "an older man," lead in the direction of the T/P link at once, but in the most tactful way possible; and (5) since the interpretation explicitly mentions sex, it leads toward the *impulse* as well.

She responded by laughing and exclaiming, "You?" and went on to imply that the therapist couldn't possibly have sexual feelings for her in this setting (thus she remained defensive but she was not frightened into immediate withdrawal, and she picked up part of the sexual implications of the interpretation at once). However, she ended up by intensifying her defenses, saying, "I don't need to have treatment, do I?"

What does the therapist do now? He has already made an anxiety interpretation in the transference; what is there left? He chose to deal with this on the basis of reality, saying that she had conveyed to him that she did want to become more comfortable over her thoughts and feelings about sex. To this she answered, "Not really," leaving him in a state of utter doubt as to what she did want, which he pointed out to her. She then spoke of how she was always indecisive, and this had applied to her vacillation over whether or not to accept her fiancé's proposal of marriage. The subtle transference implications of this were reached as follows: The therapist pointed out to her that this indecisiveness might well convey feelings that confused other people, and this led directly into a discussion of how she *encouraged men and discouraged them at the same time.* Thus, again the sexual transference and the link to men in general was touched on but never explicitly interpreted. (I think it is true to say that it doesn't matter whether or not the therapist saw all this at the time; there is such a thing as "intuitively not seeing something" when the patient is not ready to hear it.) The effects of this were almost immediately apparent, for the next sequence went as follows: (1) She spoke of handling her sexual feelings by thinking of unromantic things while the man was petting her (this was an admission of her direct and conscious involvement in *defense* against her sexual feelings, and a new piece of information). (2) She spoke of the brother who had seduced her, how he had a bad marriage, how he wanted sex with her, how shocked she was, and how he had cried. (3) At this point she blocked, tears came into her eyes, and she appeared to become *choked* (it is worth noting the partial breakdown of defenses and the first appearance of strong feeling). (4) She then *spontaneously associated to her father*: "My father *chokes* me. He hurts me. He has no feelings . . . He has feelings deep down but he never smiles at me . . . You can't be his friend if you don't share his moral convictions." (Again, the immediate emergence of disappointed love for her father, not explicitly foreseen in the predictions— though it should have been—is very striking.) "After what happened with my brother I didn't show any feeling and I didn't care." But the next association was to her fiancé, Mark, and how toward him she has changed and cares very much. Then, that before the incident with her brother she had been unaware of sexual feelings, "they were bottled up," and at the present time she can have about two minutes of petting and "then her bottled-up feelings [*impulse*] can't be liberated" (but thus admitting that they exist).

The therapist wrote here that "there seemed so much dynamic material at this point that it was very tempting to tie together her choking and her feelings about her father, brother, fiancé, and me [i.e., four of the sides of the pentagon of insight]. The patient was under considerable anxiety, looking frequently at the wall and sitting rather rigidly in her chair, except when at times we could laugh together about something that she had said. It seemed that we had established very meaningful communication through being able to share the sexual topic, and being able to look at her ambivalence and fence-sitting with a smile or a laugh. An interpretation would have disrupted this feeling, so I elected not to say anything other than that the bottled-up sexual feelings were indeed the things that she was concerned about, and that was why she was here to enter treatment. This was a direct answer to the patient's previous question about her need for treatment and an invitation to establish a therapeutic alliance. Again the gentle approach paid off, as the patient said first that she didn't really feel like talking about it, and then "if these feelings were unleashed it's as though my mind would be out of control" (thus spontaneously mentioning another *anxiety*). To this the therapist said that liberating these feelings was similar in her own mind to going mad, which in reality was not so (thus responding with *reassurance*).

As it was near the end of the session, he now asked the patient if she wanted to come once a week until the month in which she was due to leave for the United States. She accepted this readily but was worried about the possibility of running out of things to talk about. He said that she was free to leave therapy at any time, thus reassuring her that her therapy was basically under her own control.

This was the fourth contact with the clinic (she had been interviewed twice by the psychologist), and it can be seen (1) how many times the patient herself spontaneously leads the therapist toward *anxiety, defense*, and *impulse*, often making direct interpretation unnecessary; (2) how she has herself also begun the process of making *links* among the various people in her life; (3) how the therapist keeps communication going by deliberately going less fast and less deep than the patient; (4) that her motivation has definitely increased, though of course it remains markedly ambivalent; and (5) that therapy is highly focal, every communication of both patient and therapist being relevant to the focus.

In the second therapeutic session (session 3), she arrived dressed very provocatively in a tight-fitting blouse and a very short skirt. The session was notable for the following:

1. She told about the relation with her brother in detail. He had told her about his sexual predicament with his wife, had made some sexual advances to her which she had accepted, and had then asked if

he could use some of her friends for sex. She had said, "Use me, not them." She thus came much nearer to taking some responsibility for this relation and for her own *sexual impulses*.

2. After this she had had sexual relations with other boys, had been disgusted at herself, and said, "The more they liked me, the more I wanted to hurt them." She thus even more openly admitted *aggressive impulses* toward men.

3. The therapist then *linked* the anger toward *men* first with her *brother*, to which she agreed; and then, since she had earlier mentioned her *father* and his rigid views, suggested that she might also be angry with him (an impulse interpretation making the link between men, brother, father). This she half-denied, but she quickly associated to (a) her father making crude remarks when he saw a picture of a nude woman, (b) her boss looking at pictures of nudes, and (c) her Rorschach, which had been a dreadful experience because of her fear of seeing sexual percepts (admission of *anxiety* and partial admission of *impulse*). The therapist was then able to suggest (a) that her attitude toward sex now could have something to do with her father's attitude, and (b) that perhaps she was afraid that he, the therapist, would "bring out pictures" for her to see (a phrase that clearly had symbolic as well as literal meaning) like the psychologist and like her father (thus making the first T/P interpretation, of the *anxiety*).

One of the characteristics of this patient was that she clearly *frightened herself* by her own revelations. This was shown later on by a number of canceled sessions, each clearly following a session containing important communication. In the next session (session 4—in trousers again!) she showed this with a clear attempt at flight into health, saying that she felt much better after talking about her brother and she thought she should stop coming—"I don't have any great problems, do I?" The therapist responded to this with *direct explanation*, saying that (1) sometimes when one is discussing very sensitive things there is a feeling of being quite healthy and intensely wishing that things were all right when in reality that might not be so; and (2) that it was his experience that, though he respected how she felt today, it usually took months of work to attain a stable position. She again brought out her anxiety about being shown pictures, which the therapist again linked with her father (*T/P link, anxiety*). Then she said, "Mother said father was oversexed. He sees young women walking around in short skirts, so he never liked to see me in a short skirt." The therapist then asked her if she felt *her father might have had some sexual feelings toward her* in her teens. She said, "This wouldn't be natural," and she wears trousers at home to make it easier for her father (i.e., denial followed by unconscious confirmation). The therapist at once reminded her that in the first session she had worn trousers, in the second a short skirt, and now trousers again, then asked, "Was this to make *both of us* more comfortable?" (the *T/P link* of the *anxiety*, also leading very subtly in the direction of undoing the *defense* of externalization). Her response was, "I feel like laughing. It's a revolting kind of upsetting feeling that causes me to laugh and giggle" (again strong and conflicting feeling had been touched off in her). Though she then reiterated her denials, toward the end of the session she returned to this feeling and got as far as saying, "It seems to be *against me inside* when I talk about sex, it's not really against you," thus coming very near to admitting both her own *impulses* and her disgust at them.

The next session was a fascinating example of the translation of the *obsessional defense* (a new example of her defenses not previously seen). She spoke of "hating untidiness" and "having to get everything done." The therapist interpreted her need to *have everything under control* (a general interpretation of the obsessional defense). He had inadvertently left the phone switched on in his room, and when it rang he moved quickly to switch it off. She immediately said, *"You're jumpy, too,"* and the therapist spoke of her need to keep *emotions between them* tidy and controlled (an interpretation of the obsessional defense now in the transference, at the same time hinting at the undoing of *externalization,* since "between them" implies that the emotions are *in her,* too).

This led, later in the session, to her saying that when she was small she was always on Daddy's knee, but that he hasn't liked her since she grew up. The therapist said, "Perhaps he liked you too much," thus both clarifying what was probably the external reality, and preparing the way for the *impulse,* but for the time being accepting the *externalization.*

At the end she said that if her sexual feelings were liberated she'd be afraid that as she went out from the session *she'd go to bed with any man she sees,* thus admitting the *impulse,* and entirely confirming the interpretation of the obsessional defense as a need to keep control.

By this time it seems she had really frightened herself, and she managed to miss the next two sessions on the grounds first of illness and then of fog. It would be tempting to go over each session in detail to illustrate the step-by-step approach to the patient's central problems, but these first four sessions will have to suffice.

The climax of therapy came in session 9, when she spoke of an important incident that had happened in her apartment. One of her roommates had seduced a sixteen-year old boy, who hadn't been able to satisfy her (the roommate) sexually, and he had come to the patient crying. However, the couple had continued their sexual relation, and she could often hear it all going on. This was a year ago, and it was *about then that many of her present difficulties had started,* thus illustrating one of the fascinating phenomena of psychotherapy, the late discovery of a hitherto unknown precipitating factor. Her essential feeling was that the boy had been *humiliated,* and she spoke of "anger boiling up inside." Here the therapist made a major and virtually complete interpretation of *sexual* and *aggressive impulses toward men* and *defenses* against them, making every one of the links in the pentagon of insight:

> I interpreted to her how she feels sexually stimulated by *men,* her *brother, father, Mark,* and *myself* [five categories of men]; that at the same time she views herself as this sixteen-year old boy who has been taken advantage of, and her anger boils up inside and comes out as nausea, back pain, and passive aggressive behavior; and I further expanded on examples using incidents with her *father, brother, Mark,* and *myself.* This seemed to be a very intense interaction and the patient responded in a very dramatic and positive manner. She participated by giving additional examples and seemed to accept the entire interpretation. At the end she said, "I feel better. I didn't have any stomach rumbles this time, only my hair did stand on end five times. This understanding has helped me a great deal."

Of course, she canceled the next session, eventually admitting that she went for a drive in her car rather than come!

The termination issue was in fact never a problem, and there was no sign of the regressive element that had been seen by the psychologist and was included in my retrospectively made predictions. She denied most of her feeling toward the therapist over this issue, but came out with intense feeling about her father. She said that her father didn't want her to go to the United States—"I've got to go against his wishes. I don't know how to talk to him. He means so much. It upsets me to think of leaving . . . father may die . . . he often talks about death." The therapist asked her if she felt that leaving would be letting her father down as she felt Mark and other men had let her down; and further, if her father died, would she in some way feel responsible? (This was an *impulse* interpretation, with implications to do with *termination.*) This *led to more profuse tears than at any other time;* and, later, "I wouldn't want anyone to replace him," and remarks that he needs psychiatric help (thus, the hidden love comes to the surface quite undisguised, together with reparative feelings).

Again she left work to come to the next session but drove home instead. When she did come (the penultimate session, no. 16), she spoke of how destructive children can be, and the therapist questioned whether she had *destructive feelings* toward her parents and her fiancé, and perhaps toward him (the therapist) because of the end of therapy, and it was *safer not to come* (linking three corners of the pentagon, including the T/P link, and interpreting *impulse, defense,* and *anxiety* in connection with *termination*). Later he was able to give a similar interpretation of the reparative feelings as a *defense* against her anger (*impulse*), and this led to her admitting that last week she had "had a good cry," and that she had cried with Mark several times before he went to the United States; thus the interpretation of *negative* feelings leads to *positive* feelings, and she comes near to admitting her sadness about termination, which the therapist interpreted, linking himself, Mark, and her father. She attempted to go back to her defenses: "I'm fed up with feeling, I'd rather be a vegetable. No, I wouldn't, but it's all so complicated." Finally, she went on to admit how she bottles up all her feelings, like sex, anger, and sadness. In other words, the main message of therapy had got through to her.

In the final session (session 17) she spoke of a number of therapeutic effects:

She feels more confident, is less sensitive to other people's opinions, feels more physically than at any previous time, still gets "funny feelings" with men but now can handle them, has got back her vaginal secretions, feels more like a woman, and can admit to things about her father that she doesn't like.

She still denied any feeling for the therapist: "No, you are my robot. No feeling, no hate or love." Yet, she ended on a note of great warmth: "I *am* grateful and I am so pleased to have known you. The hurt was for my good. I hope to see you again."

We have as yet no follow-up on this patient, but even if she turns out to be no better, I have the feeling that therapy could hardly have been conducted with greater tact and skill, and she illustrates the principles of such a therapy to a remarkable degree.

Apart from the omissions already noted, the predictions actually made seem to have been fulfilled to the letter.

PART V

Extending the Limits of Brief Psychotherapy

CHAPTER 13

The Use of More Than One Focus

Although ideal patients like those described in the last chapter do occur, they are rare; and if intensive brief therapy is to make any impact on the practice of psychotherapeutic clinics, its use obviously needs to be extended to other types of situation. In fact we have very considerable evidence that this is possible, and I am quite sure that the limits have not yet been properly explored.

There are three main ways in which this extension of the limits might occur: (1) the use of more than one distinct focus; (2) limited foci in more disturbed patients; and (3) deeper types of interpretation.

Clinical examples of each of these will be given in the following pages.

MORE THAN ONE FOCUS

In much of what I have written I have emphasized the importance of therapeutic planning around a single circumscribed focus, and the question now arises of how necessary this is, and whether more than one focus can be used successfully. Where therapy is really brief—say, up to twelve sessions—I doubt very much that there is time for this; but where therapy is as long as thirty sessions it would seem *a priori* that there should be scope for more. Thirty sessions are now the standard limit set in my brief therapy unit. It is useful especially with trainees, as it gives therapists a good deal of latitude; e.g., if half a dozen sessions are wasted because some crucial interpretation has been missed, there is time to make up the loss when the mistake is discovered later. The question is whether this *a priori* impression is borne out in practice.

The evidence seems to be equivocal. When I came to consider this question, my *impression* was that there had been a number of successful therapies in which more than one distinct focus had been used; but when I came to look through our clinical material, I found I could quote a number of such therapies that had either been *unsuccessful* or had ended up as *long-term*, and hardly any that had been both brief and successful. Examples are as follows:

1. The Storm Lady (first series, see *SBP*), which had started with sexual anxieties and had quickly gone over into depressive problems, and had ended with a limited therapeutic result in a total of fifty-three sessions.

2. The Articled Accountant (first series), which had started with Oedipal problems and had also ended with depressive problems, where therapy seemed to have been entirely unsuccessful in twenty-seven sessions.

3. The Factory Inspector (second series, see *Toward the Validation of Dynamic Psychotherapy*, Malan, 1976), where the first focus had been Oedipal problems, with special reference to competition, but where the later theme was resentment at having to take too much responsibility in his childhood. Here there was a very limited therapeutic result in eighteen sessions.

4. The Interior Decorator (second series, failed follow-up), where the first focus was Oedipal, but in the later stages of therapy emphasis seemed to shift more and more toward hostility against women. Here there was a disastrous termination after an attempt to give therapy to the wife (seventeen sessions).

5. The Personnel Manager (see Assessment and Therapy Form), where the initial Oedipal focus passed quickly over into the working through of deeply depressive problems. This was a highly successful therapy but took sixty-two sessions.

This inability to find successful examples of course entirely confirms the statistical evidence discussed in chap. 5, where it was mentioned that during the first eight contacts with the clinic low focality combined with low motivation tended to lead to poor outcome, and low focality with high motivation to successful outcome but inability to terminate within the limits of brief therapy.

Despite this, I am convinced that with a limit of twenty to thirty sessions the successful use of at least two quite separate foci is perfectly possible. The clearest type of situation in which two foci are likely to be used, both of which can easily be incorporated into the therapeutic plan, is when a patient of either sex has both (1) an Oedipal problem involving the triangular relation with the parents, and also (2) a two-person problem—often of dependence—with the mother. A plan can then be formulated in the following terms: that therapy will start with the three-person problem; but that as it progresses, dependence will become more marked and will manifest itself particularly over holidays and other absences, and finally will become a crucial issue as termination approaches. It will then be necessary to deal with anger against someone the patient needs and loves, especially in the transference, which may lead quite deeply into depressive problems.

An example of this from my brief therapy unit, in an incorrectly planned therapy but one in which interpretations were made at a very deep level indeed, will be given in chap. 15. The clearest example from Balint's workshop is the Falling Social Worker, from the first series, a summary of whose therapy is given below. Even here it will be noted that the length of therapy—forty sessions in all—is at the upper limit at which it is still legitimate to use the word "brief."

THE FALLING SOCIAL WORKER, AN EXAMPLE OF A COMPLEX THERAPY

This twenty-seven-year old single woman was admitted to the Cassel Hospital with four main areas of disturbance: (1) a long-standing phobia of falling; (2) a split in her sexual feelings, which caused her to be able only to make sexual relations (short of intercourse) with "disreputable" men; (3) an inability to free herself from her seventy-year-old father, who was possessive of her and jealous of her boyfriends; and (4) a compulsive need to pile responsibility on herself at work. She had had previous eclectic psychotherapy from a psychiatrist on and off for four years.

The main focus in the initial stages of therapy was her guilt and shame about "bad" feelings, which led in the initial interview to her confession of her sexual problems—something that she had been unable, during four years, to confide to her previous therapist. This led to many interpretations linking these sexual problems to her relation with her father, with particular reference to her longing for a "pure" relation with a man who was unattainable, and her inability to integrate this with overt sexual feelings. The transference rapidly became sexualized and the therapist made a number of interpretations about this, linking it with the relation to her father. The patient at first found this difficult to accept, but she was forced to do so when, in session 10, she had to admit that over the weekend she had had a vivid sexual fantasy about the therapist. The latter used this to explore the sexual transference to the previous therapist, and it then emerged that this had been both unacknowledged and very intense, and had clearly been responsible for a severe exacerbation of her symptoms after he had given her a pentothal injection.

Side by side with this sexual and Oedipal focus another theme arose: that she felt she had to be what others required her to be, whether this was her parents, her colleagues in a superior position at work, or the present therapist, and consequently she felt unreal.

There was in addition a conflict between being what her *father* wanted her to be and what her *mother* wanted her to be. All this was interpreted as being partly a response to her father's possessive pressure on her, and partly a fulfillment of Oedipal wishes, and the identification with her *mother* was also a defense against Oedipal wishes.

Another theme that then arose was her inability to be feminine because of her mother's own lack of femininity, and the patient's contempt for her.

Finally, in the later stages of therapy, problems of termination and dependence became paramount. This occurred first because the patient had to be admitted to a medical hospital during a brief illness, and when she returned she felt that the therapist had behaved indifferently to her. This was very quickly linked with her mother's indifference, something that had always caused her to be infuriated. There was also some discussion of dependence in quite primitive terms, concerned with projection—seeing in others the greedy, demanding parts of herself.

Thus, this forty-session therapy really contained almost all the themes that one would expect to arise if this patient had had a full-scale analysis.

It is important to note that this was one of only three therapies in the first series that were shown by very long follow-up to have been strikingly successful.

The final conclusion can only be that the use of complex foci requires a great deal of further exploration.

CHAPTER 14

Partial Foci in More Disturbed Patients

The previous chapters have been concerned with patients in whom the nuclear conflict could be taken as the focus, and could be to a large extent fearlessly interpreted and worked through. In the present chapter we shall be concerned with patients in whom the pathology is far too deep or complex for any such approach, but yet in whom some carefully circumscribed conflict may be taken as focus and worked through to a much more limited extent. In colloquial terms, the last chapter was concerned with "doing a lot with a good patient," while the present chapter is concerned with "doing a little with a bad patient." As always, of course, this is not a sharp distinction and there is a continuum between the two.

It must be said at once that we have far less experience of this latter type of therapy, and that it represents a largely unexplored area of great practical importance; "bad" patients considerably outnumber "good" patients, and the systematic extension of brief therapeutic methods to them would have a profound effect on the efficiency of therapeutic clinics. Moreover, just as we found with the good patients, all the signs indicate that in terms of depth of interpretation and severity of pathology this kind of work can be much more radical than most preconceptions would suggest.

It is now necessary to introduce a diversion on the subject of the focal technique. When we started this work we were all mainly experienced in analysis or at least long-term therapy, in which the

297

transference neurosis develops, the patient may become very dependent, and therapy is inevitably drawn toward ever deeper and more complex issues. We were therefore much preoccupied with ways of counteracting these tendencies, and among the ideas put forward was the need to concentrate on a single theme and to refuse to be diverted from it; in the words of other authors, the technique must involve "selective attention" and "selective neglect," in the terminology later used by Balint, the technique must be focal. What was not foreseen, however, was that to an experienced therapist the technique might often be much easier than expected. On the one hand, there were many patients who *brought* a single theme, so that a focus "crystallized" very quickly; on the other hand, therapy could be much deeper and much longer than anticipated, so that the therapist could make exactly the same kinds of interpretation as he would make in long-term therapy, and moreover, there might well be time to deal with two or more quite separate issues. Thus, there were very few clear examples in our first series of therapies in which the patient gave material that led away from the focus and the therapist actively brought him back to it. The result was that these first cases offered very little scope for illustrating the special characteristics of the focal technique.

Another way of expressing this is to say, in the terminology introduced above, that where the aim is to "do a lot with a good patient" there will be little difference between a focal technique and that employed by any well-trained therapist. It is when the aim is to "do a little with a bad patient" that the main difference arises. It is here that the therapist has to plan a circumscribed focus from the beginning; it is here that he is most likely to need to refuse to be diverted; and it is here that the focal technique begins to have obvious special characteristics. It is with this type of therapy that the present chapter is concerned.

In these more disturbed patients, the concept of nuclear conflict is often much less useful; there may be more than one conflict that can be described as nuclear, or the pathology may be so complex that it is almost impossible to disentangle one conflict from another. The two examples that follow represent quite different situations. In the first the focus chosen was clearly fairly central to the pathology, but the aim was to work it through with reference to a single issue only, namely termination. In the second the pathology contained several major areas, only one of which was taken as focus, and at a carefully chosen and deliberately superficial level.

MISS PERSISTENCE

This was a single girl of twenty-four complaining of depression, apathy, emotional confusion, and inability to make good relationships. Her story was as follows:

Before the age of ten she seems to have had a good relationship at least with her father; but from that time he became seriously alcoholic, would come home and do nothing but shout at everyone, and the relation distintegrated. He eventually died one year ago. Her mother managed to keep the home together by going out to work but had little to give in the evenings. The patient's memory is of spending her childhood alone, waiting for her parents to come home. Her only sibling, a brother three years older, seems to have got most of the attention that was available.

At fifteen she met a boy called Norman at school and from eighteen she developed a close and sexual relation with him. The relation was unsatisfactory: He began to drink quite heavily and physically to maltreat her, and he also seems to have been partially impotent, while she is partially frigid. She began to take cannabis. At nineteen she sought treatment from the Adolescent Department of the Tavistock in order to help her break free from Norman, and although she succeeded in this for a time, she is now back with him. She was treated over a period of about three years, first in a group and then with once-a-month supportive treatment, and is now referred to the Adult Department for further help.

After her consultation in the Adult Department, she was seen for two interviews by the woman psychologist who eventually took her on for treatment. She was given the Rorschach, which she had also been given at her first contact with the Adolescent Department, and gave almost exactly the same responses as she had some five years before. The psychologist felt that this expressed a great deal of anger about coming to the clinic over so long a period and getting nowhere, which she interpreted to the patient. The result seems to have been a considerable freeing. She admitted to being angry with her former therapist, and her percepts changed in the direction of expressing greater dependence and need for affection.

The psychologist wrote that her record was that of "a deprived, empty child seeking warmth and comfort . . . unable to manage relationships except by denying and projecting her anger and responding in an impoverished, dependent way."

We may note therefore that this patient seemed to have shown a satisfactory response to interpretation, and that she may possibly have some basis for early good experience (though this was not evident in projective testing); but that apart from this the signals were at "danger": the deprived childhood, the inability to break free from a sado-masochistic relation (resembling that with her father) in which there seemed little satisfaction, and the small progress from previous therapeutic attempts. We felt that long-term therapy might well end up in an interminable attempt to work through her deprivation, even if such therapy were available, which it was not. What then could be done?

After a long and despairing discussion, we remembered a paper once read (though never published) by Dr. T. F. Main, in which he described a form of treatment offered to a series of very severely hysterical women, referred to the Cassel as just one more passing of the buck. He had adopted the policy of telling the patient that *she could not be helped,* and then of working through with her over a few months all her feelings about this, including all the acting out, suicidal threats, etc. One of the great advantages of this form of treatment was the fact that it was the first *honest* approach to the patient; all previous attempts at treatment had contained the implied promise that something would be done to make up to her for the past. Main said that he had applied this form of treatment to several women, and that when he followed them up he had found that all of them were at work and functioning reasonably well.

This girl was not hysterical or as severely disturbed as these Cassel patients, but we felt that a similar approach offered the only hope of dealing realistically with the situation. Accordingly, she was referred to the Psychologists' Workshop, a unit specializing in brief interventions making particular use of projective material. The psychologist who had tested her offered her ten sessions, stating to her at the outset that this was all we could give, that it was limited and inadequate, and that we made no promises of dealing with her needs. The aim was then to work through her feelings about this, ending if possible with a proper termination with the clinic. The account of therapy is told mostly in the psychologist's own words (whether quotation marks are used or not), which reveal something of the quality of her own feeling about this patient:

The patient responded to this offer with an "amen" statement, that she would just have to accept that she clings to people. She was at a loss as to how to use the time and was near to tears. Eventually, she said that people say she is aggressive; she doesn't feel she is, they don't give, don't respond to her. The therapist suggested that this was what she felt about her and her offer but the patient denied this, saying that she was grateful for anything. The therapist then tried making the *link with the patient's childhood,* that she was glad when her parents were around, but angry and disappointed that they weren't around enough. To this the patient responded by describing waiting around for her *boyfriend* (Norman) to show up, pleased but apprehensive when he does come. The therapist interpreted "her anger that others and myself are not there for her"; but that she feels her angry, needy feelings (*impulse*) are *unacceptable* (*anxiety*), so she *denies* them (*defense*), feels empty and depressed—she has to preserve what little she gets with gratitude. Even this comprehensive interpretation, by implication making all the possible links, and including all three elements of the impulse–defense triad, was denied; the patient restated her gratitude.

The therapist had to keep her waiting for a short time before the beginning of session 2. She fumed silently over a cigarette and gave a depressed report of her week: She had been upset by the first session because she had been made aware of her misery and she had to go home to a cold, empty flat, so she went and appealed to her mother to comfort her, which the latter refused. Norman had then come to her, himself needing comfort, but she had to accept that he wouldn't live with her. She was tired, empty, depressed. The therapist again took up the obvious transference implications: "I interpreted her wish to find a *mother* in *me,* and her disappointment" (an *impulse* interpretation making the *T/P link*). At last the patient made a response other than denial, saying that the therapist "was too gentle with her and should be tearing her feelings out of her." The therapist then interpreted the projection (*defense*) of aggressive *impulses* in the *transference*: "I put this back as her wish to tear at me for giving so little and being late, but she was afraid that I wouldn't be interested or *couldn't take it*" (this is the interpretation of a new *anxiety,* her fear of the consequences of her anger for people close to her). The patient responded at first by admitting her anger, but then "gradually the argument turned so that it was as if *she* were late and *I* the angry one (the *defense* of projection reasserted itself). The therapist interpreted the whole of the impulse–defense triad: "She seemed to feel that it is bad and unjustified to be angry with me, so she ditched the feelings and felt empty and confused." The patient responded, this time even more clearly: "She smiled as if she had been caught out and said, 'So you knew I was angry when I came in.' " She ended by admitting the *impulse* and the *anxiety*: "that she could be angry only if she knew her opponent to be strong enough to resist and calm her."

Sessions 3 and 4 consisted mainly of making the *link* between the patient's feelings about *Norman* and her *father*. She began by admitting her anger with people more openly, and went on to speak first of having to *ask* Norman to come and sit beside her, and then of being quite unable to respond sexually to him. The therapist interpreted that she needed to *control* her sexual feelings lest her *anger* with him should emerge too (*defense, impulse,* and *anxiety*). Shortly after this the therapist asked her about masturbation, and she said that she masturbated a lot and had done so from an early age. This mention of childhood enabled the therapist to make the *link with her father,* saying that her masturbation must have contained her loneliness, her longing for him, and her angry disappointment in him, but she couldn't express her anger because he was weak and ill. She said sadly, "But I did love him," and this led to interpretations about her keeping alive a good image of him, and her doing much the same with her feelings about Norman.

In session 4 she related how Norman had had a severe attack of food poisoning, had been admitted to the hospital, and she had stayed with him. This led to interpretations about having to assuage her guilt (*defense*) because she imagined she had hurt him (*anxiety*), and then again to the parallel with her father. She admitted feeling guilty about having stayed away from her father during his last years, and not having visited him on the day he died.

We may sum up the work in these first four sessions as concerned with the patient's hidden *disappointed anger* (impulse); with *defenses* of denial, projection, idealization, and unconscious control; and *anxieties* that her feelings were unacceptable, that the other person couldn't stand up to them, and guilt about hurting. Moreover, the links had been made between (1) the *transference* and the patient's *mother,* and (2) *Norman* and the patient's *father*. Thus, even in these four sessions the work had been fairly comprehensive.

The consequences were seen in sessions 5 and 6, which are reproduced here in the therapist's slightly edited words:

> These were markedly different hours—she was animated and excited and the pace was dizzying. She had been ill in bed and had been thinking. She thought she was angry because her father hadn't loved her enough, but maybe she had expected too much, so her anger was unjustified. Surely his drinking had nothing to do with her, but had she done something wrong? When I interpreted her guilt about not being able to care for him because she was so angry that he didn't love her, and her anxiety that she had contributed to his death, she broke into vehement confused criticism of her mother, father, and Norman. When I clarified that she wanted maternal, paternal, and sexual love from Norman, love she felt

she hadn't had from her parents, she responded with feelings of being selfish and overdemanding. She acknowledged that she withdrew from her father, but what had *she* done wrong? On a hunch, I introduced her brother, and it emerged that he was just then enjoying his usual prodigal son reception with her mother. She felt left out, and she poured out her resentment against this favored brother. I commented on her hurt that her father could love—but not her—and with the hurt came anger, withdrawal, and guilt. The theme of wanting too much, asking the impossible, continued.

Thus, the emergence of strongly expressed anger against the members of her family was accompanied by the expression of a new *anxiety*, that she had demanded too much.

After this central, crucial, and essentially nontransference pair of sessions, the last four sessions were, of course, mainly concerned with termination. It is worthwhile quoting Mann (1973) here, whom none of us had read when this therapy was carried out: "The last three or four of the twelve meetings must deal insistently with the patient's reaction to termination. It is in this end phase that the definitive work of resolution will be done."

I continue in the therapist's words:

> Anger gave way to sadness and depression. She irritably described many people who angered, frustrated, or upset her, which I interpreted as her feeling about me and the limited therapy. She protested furiously that it had been good therapy, but she hated being put in the position of having to ask for more. . . .
>
> Suddenly she felt exhausted, with the desperation she felt to get all she could from treatment, and very depressed—why was she feeling depressed now? [At this point the therapist brought in her own need for follow-up, thus both softening termination—and why not?, though Mann wouldn't agree—and making an important point about the patient's inability to ask for things.] I said it was the end of the hour, we have only three hours left, and she feels she is about to lose me. I finally said that she felt so needy and hungry for love that she couldn't tolerate waiting for people to offer it, so she ended up feeling greedy and demanding and guilty. It was true that our regular sessions would end at Christmas, but I would want to see her again, perhaps in three months time, to know how she was getting on. She smiled and said she had wanted to ask for that but hadn't been able to.

In session 8 she reported having gone to her mother, crying for two hours, and having to defend her therapist against her mother, because she felt what was happening in therapy was right. She said that last session she had been beyond crying. This caused the therapist to make a link with the *father* she had never mourned, saying "she felt she had had something good with us and wanted more, felt angry about not getting more, felt sad about losing a good relationship, and felt guilty about wanting to ask for more and about being angry with someone who had been good to her."

In group supervision it was emphasized that the therapist should now not only work with the feelings about termination, but also emphasize the patient's resources that she could now use on her own.

> Session 9, the penultimate session, had the quality of a final session. She looked and felt happy and alive. She had made love with a man to whom she feels very close as her confidant, but with whom hitherto she had kept sex out of the relationship. It had been very good but she felt frightened. She wanted to give Norman up, but didn't want to hurt him; besides, what if this new relation didn't last? I interpreted her anxiety about being loved and left, about driving him away by wanting too much, linking her anxious expectations with her experience with her father and her feelings about the termination with me.
>
> She now wants to be dependent and independent—grateful for what she had from me, wanting more, but also wanting a rest from me. It emerged that she regarded the time until the follow-up as a kind of homework assignment, and she reserved the option of contacting me if she wanted to. My uneasiness about having softened the termination prompted me to emphasize that we had *one* more session, and that she was leaving with her reclaimed resources and feelings that she could use independently of me.

In the final session she appeared to have withdrawn and there were a number of issues that she didn't want to go into. These included the fact that her period was late and she might be pregnant (in fact, as discovered later, this was a false alarm) and also that she had woken up one morning with no further interest in this new man. It eventually emerged that he had asked her about her treatment and she had mentioned that it concerned "negative" feelings about him, which had upset him. The therapist interpreted that she had withdrawn from him because she felt he couldn't handle her angry feelings and had to protect him from them, like her father.

At the end she reported some improvements: She feels more content, now likes to be alone, is not so worried about feeling depressed, is more confident, and worries less about what other people think of her. People were commenting on how well she looked. The therapist said that the next three months were *not* a homework assignment but were for the patient to live her own life. The patient thanked her with some tears, and treatment ended on this positive note.

It will be remembered that the original aim of therapy was no more than to achieve a satisfactory termination with the clinic. As far as this question of termination is concerned, more has been achieved, because she has continued to visit her therapist from time to time in crises, a realistic and efficient way of using therapeutic time. She has come eight times in all in the subsequent two and a half years.

It will also be clear from the last session that our ultimate hopes were much more ambitious than simply to achieve termination, and the question therefore arises whether there have been any permanent major improvements. The answer is that it is not really clear; certainly the dramatic improvements seen during therapy did not last more than a few months. The relation with Norman has ended but she continues to pick her men badly and to have unsatisfactory relations with them. However, she appears to be in touch with her anger and to be able to express it; and as a result, although she still gets depressed, there seems to have been a change in the quality of her depressions— formerly she felt that she was empty and had nothing, whereas now she feels more guilty and that what she does have isn't what others want. She can also sometimes use the insight that she achieved in therapy to help her out of emotional crises.

The main result therefore seems to be that she is still working on her life and making use of the therapist's help in a realistic and undemanding way; and that the cards-on-the-table approach has left her with a good relation with us, in contrast to the hidden resentment that she showed after her previous course of treatment.

THE STATIONERY MANUFACTURER

This is the patient who scored highest for outcome in the second series. The therapist was Michael Balint, and he devoted his last and posthumous book to a complete presentation and discussion of this therapy, with the aim of illustrating the special characteristics of the focal technique (Balint, Ornstein, and Balint, 1972). For this purpose, and particularly for illustrating the use of selective neglect in the interests of sticking to a chosen focus, and refusing to be drawn into major psychoanalytic interpretations, this therapy cannot be bettered. As the reader will see, it differs very markedly from the type of therapy presented in the previous chapter, or that presented in the next.

The patient was a married man of forty-three, joint owner with his two brothers of a printing and stationery business, suffering from a severe state of "jealousy paranoia." The story was as follows: Twenty years before, while he was in the Army, he had courted his future wife, a Turkish girl named Farah whom he had met in Cyprus. He had then been posted to India, and while he was there his wife had had a passing relation with another officer, whose name was James. For some time she had hesitated which of the two men to choose, but in the end had chosen the patient.

Since then, he had often pondered on the relation between his wife and another man, but this did not make him ill. However, about six years ago, and again eighteen months ago, he had become so preoccupied with this relation and with questioning his wife about it, that both he and his wife were near breakdown:

> He could not understand how his wife could have affectionate feelings for another man, although he could understand that she might have been sexually stirred up; so he had to go on and on and on grinding her down until he extracted from her the minutest detail about what happened between the two young people; when and how they kissed, which part of her body was touched, what she felt in response, and so on.

Here it should be added that this very severe illness occurred within a personality that was in other ways unimpaired and indeed functioning excellently; otherwise, of course, the kind of brief therapy used would not have been considered. For instance, it was largely the patient himself among the three brothers who had been responsible for building up the business to its present state of success; and, more important than this, there seemed no question that he and his wife genuinely loved each other, and despite the strains that his illness imposed on her, she would sincerely do everything in her power to help.

I wish now to discuss the patient's psychopathology in depth, and in doing so I shall, where necessary, introduce information revealed during therapy. My reason for this will appear later. In chap. 11 I emphasized the importance of identifying *precipitating factors* in order both to understand the pathology and to formulate a therapeutic plan. Here, when the patient was asked for events in his life at about the time of his two breakdowns, he said (1) that six years ago he had just moved into a new house which he had had specially built, and that his father-in-law, of whom he was very fond, had died; and (2) that eighteen months ago he and his two brothers had finally bought their majority interest in the business from their father.

These three events: success (the new house), death of a father-figure, and superseding a father, have obvious Oedipal implications. So has a man's preoccupation with his wife's relation to another man. This latter kind of symptom is also often found to be a disguise for homosexuality; the patient is found to be at least in part identifying with the woman. If this is true, then it is likely that the origin of the presenting symptom lies in the relation to the patient's father.

Now, at this stage of the assessment little was known about the patient's early relations with his family. During therapy, however, it was discovered that the father was a crude and dominating personality, who had not only squashed the patient's mother, but had lost no opportunity for squashing the patient also, though the impression is also created that, side by side with this, he had his own special kind of warmth.

With the aid of this information, one can speculate along psychoanalytic lines that the patient's presenting problem involved latent homosexuality, and that a full interpretation of this might well include (1) the unsatisfied longing for closeness with his father (one *impulse*), and (2) a *defense* against his Oedipal hatred of his father and against the second *impulse* to humiliate him, cut him down to size, displace him, castrate him, or whatever terms one likes to use; together with (3) the *anxieties* commonly associated with such an impulse, namely guilt and fear of retaliation.

But can this rightly be described as the patient's "nuclear" problem? This formulation has many deficiencies. First of all, it entirely leaves out of account the patient's direct relation with women; after all, his main symptom not only involves a preoccupation with another man's relation to his wife, it also involves an active persecution of his wife to the point that she is near breakdown. Moreover, it in no way accounts for either the severely *obsessional* or the *paranoid* (i.e., potentially psychotic) features of the patient's illness. If with the aid of both classical Freudian and Kleinian theory, we speculate on what might be revealed by a full analysis, we are likely to think of intense *anal* impulses, and severe early *oral* conflicts, lying behind the manifestly genital nature of the presenting symptom. Let it be said at once that I do not indulge in such speculations lightly, and in therapy there was indeed abundant evidence for anal impulses, and in the Rorschach for primitive attacks upon women. The Rorschach was in fact given by a woman psychologist, and quotations from her report read as follows:

> He feels challenged and threatened by the woman, who unconsciously is felt as a powerful, phallic, dangerous person. There is a recurring phantasy of the combined male/female object—the vagina that contains a penis . . . He cannot maintain for long the illusion that the woman is harmless, and so he resorts to violent, sadistic, ruthless attacks against her. At some moments in the test he is quite literally tearing the woman to pieces, a particular concern being to divest her of her phallic properties. . . He seeks

for genital contact with the woman, though he is plagued by anxiety lest she should turn out to be dangerous and castrating—thus he must turn his attack against her. This situation is mirrored by an identical fantasy at the oral level, where the feeding mother, whom he seeks, is represented as the wolf who fed Romulus and Remus, but the same area of the blot is also seen as an animal crouching, about to leap.

It should be added, that, in complete accord with the psychiatric appraisal, the Rorschach also gave evidence of *concern* for the woman and of considerable strength, though he was described as "threatened by breakthroughs of irrationality" and his control was described as "precarious."

The purpose of this prolonged discussion is to point the contrast between this patient and the two described in chap. 12, where—even with the additional information derived from therapy—the observed pathology could in each case be described in a few sentences. Where on earth does one start if one wishes to find a focus in such a patient?

Perhaps it is best to start by saying what one does *not* want to get involved in. This will certainly include (1) oral attacks on the persecuting mother, (2) dangerous, castrating women, (3) the vagina that contains a penis, (4) obsessional defenses against anal impulses, linked with toilet training—to name but a few. It seems certain that if a focus is to be found it must be *Oedipal* in nature, but: (1) Should homosexuality be mentioned, and if so in what terms? (2) Should the problem be related to his father? (3) At what depth should the Oedipus complex be interpreted? (4) Should castration be mentioned? (5) If so, should one deal with *fear* of castration (the anxiety) only, or bring in the *impulse* to castrate as well? (6) In what terms should one interpret the patient's persecution of his wife? (7) How much should projection be dealt with? (8) What about the transference? And so on and so on; there are endless possibilities.

It is interesting to note that there was a patient in the first series, the Paranoid Engineer, who presented similar problems, in the sense that he was near to a paranoid psychotic breakdown and his presenting symptom was genital in content (fear that he would involuntarily shout out that he was homosexual). There, homosexuality and the wish to kill his father, together with the transference/parent link, were all interpreted in the most literal terms, and the result—though in the end uncertain—was that the patient seemed to be afforded considerable relief. This was an example of taking a purely Oedipal focus in a basically psychotic patient.

Anyhow, there is little point in further speculation. What Balint did was to cut through all the complexities, to make use of his own vast clinical and psychoanalytical experience, and to formulate a basic hypothesis, which as later elaborated by his two co-authors (see Balint, Ornstein, and Balint, 1972, p. 29) ran as follows:

> . . . the most important factor was the patient's homosexuality, which could not tolerate that there were men who would not love him . . . [what] he could not accept was that in the case of his wife he defeated his rival, which was the final proof that his rival will forever remain his enemy and could never love him.

Balint's main focal aim was therefore to enable the patient "to accept his ultimate victory, that is, the fact that he will never be able to enjoy the love of his rival."

Balint formulated this as his more ambitious aim. If this failed, he had a secondary aim: to enable the patient to share his wife symbolically with him, the therapist, as another man; then "he dispenses with the victory, nobody is the conqueror, so perhaps the men need not hate each other."

It will be seen at once that this second aim has nothing whatsoever to do with *interpretation,* but that it uses psychodynamic understanding to collude with the patient's pathology in a way that it is hoped may help him. This introduces an entirely new element into the form of therapy to be used, and once again points the contrast with the types of patient presented hitherto.

It would be impossible to go through every detail of this complicated therapy (for which the reader is referred to Balint's book), but instead I shall consider five main aspects: (1) the way in which Balint employed selective neglect in the early stages of therapy, in order to keep to his focus and avoid getting involved in the very deep pathology that the patient offered; (2) the degree to which the patient's direct relation with his wife was interpreted; (3) the depth of interpretation employed in the interests of the first focal aim; (4) the part played by the second focal aim; and (5) the use that Balint made of directly confronting the patient with reality.

Balint offered his first focus to the patient in session 2, saying that "something must have happened to him about six years and again about eighteen months ago that brought things to a head; perhaps if we could find out what these things meant to him he might be in a better position to prevent another breakdown." It is interesting that the patient firmly rejected this offer, and proposed instead that he should have five or six sessions in which he used the therapist as a sort of sounding board, in order to work through what he had recently learned from his wife about her relation to the other man. At the end of the session he promised to let Balint know his decision about coming, and wasn't heard from until fifteen weeks later, when he was driven back to therapy by a severe relapse.

This was a fascinating example of a sudden drop in motivation, presumably due to the therapist's trying to go too fast, which was followed by a rapid rise, since in sessions 3–5 there was a precipitate deepening of material to the point at which it threatened to get out of hand.

Session 3 started with an account of recent questioning of his wife, and Balint immediately said that the patient "had obviously felt very badly hurt by her and ruthlessly took revenge for it." This was as deep as he ever went in interpreting *aggressive feelings toward women*, which—with much more primitive implications—had been such a feature of the Rorschach. There was at no time during therapy any suggestion that women were dangerous or castrating or had phallic properties, which clearly would have led into much too deep water. Instead, the interpretation was essentially focal, in the sense that the patient clearly understood that his aggressive feelings were concerned with a three-person situation, and were caused by his wife's relation to the other man. Moreover, it was put in everyday terms, implying the kind of revengeful feelings that any man might direct against a wife whom he suspected of infidelity.

This interpretation, which was repeated, seems to have had a considerable freeing effect, because the patient then made what in the book is referred to as an "independent discovery," namely that there must be some special significance to this particular hurt, since he had been hurt before but it had not had this kind of effect on him. Balint immediately took the opportunity to begin to *make the link with the past*, saying that the hurt must have had a long prehistory and have started long before Farah had appeared on the scene. This again produced a response, the patient beginning to admit that he had *always felt inferior to other men*.

It is again very interesting that whereas in session 2 the patient had firmly rejected examining the *recent* past, he now quite spontaneously entered on an examination of the *distant* past, taking up from where he had left off and saying that the reason why he could not now accept the facts and have done with them "must go back to his experiences in childhood and adolescence, especially in relation to his father." He said that his father constantly humiliated every member of the family; and then, suddenly plunging into the depths, spoke of one of his earliest memories, of a dream or fantasy that his father comes into his bedroom at night with his false teeth sticking out and a red-hot poker in his hand, looking like a monster; and from this, straight into an account of (1) homosexual experiences at school, (2) being caught, (3) his father hearing of it and missing no opportunity to humiliate him, (4) an occasion on which he had been so frightened of his father that he had run to his mother, saying that "he could not stand that man," and finally (5) to his being lonely in the holidays and being seduced by an older man, an engineer, with whom he continued to have a homosexual relation until the age of about twenty.

It is worthwhile observing here the complete confirmation of what may have appeared to be rather speculative psychoanalytic theorizing both about the patient's homosexuality and about the possible connection between this and the relation with his father. But what does the therapist do about this material? There are endless opportunities for interpretations about his father's terrifying penis (the red-hot poker), his fantasy of his father's oral attacks on him (the false teeth), the projection of his own castrating attacks on his father (*defense* and *impulse*), and homosexuality as another *defense* against his father's retaliation (the *anxiety*), together with homosexuality as an expression of his need for love from his father (another *impulse*).

No one can tell what would have happened if any of this had been interpreted, but suffice it to say that what Balint did was to pick the aspect of all this that fitted in with his main focus, saying that "the experiences in his childhood and adolescence created in him a feeling that he was not a proper man, that other men were superior to him, and that he had to lose whenever he competed against anyone else, like father or the other officer."

This interpretation was clearly very carefully formulated in such a way that it could lead toward the anxieties or not, as the patient chose. It makes the link between the *father* and the *other man*, it mentions the word *"compete,"* which can lead toward problems of competition with the father; but, on the other hand, it also implies that the patient is the helpless victim of circumstance, and in that sense can be regarded (in Sifneos's terms) as anxiety-suppressive rather than anxiety-provoking.

However, in the next session (no. 5), Balint led toward more anxiety-laden feelings by saying that the patient apparently could not *rebel* against his father, and expected and perhaps *desired to be dominated* (which has implications of homosexual submission as a *defense* against aggressive *impulses*). This again seems to have had a freeing effect, for shortly afterward it led into what can be seen both as a confirmation, since it dealt with passive homosexuality, and also into the most disturbing material of the whole therapy: (1) how when he was a boy his father had caught him putting on a towel as a sort of diaper round himself, something that had fascinated him for as long as he could remember; (2) an account of a number of anal games (including passive anal intercourse) that he had practiced with other boys or men up to the age of twenty; (3) forcing water up his penis in various ways; and (4) running a low-voltage electric current between his penis and his anus, which he found intensely exciting.

It is an interesting and perhaps not too difficult exercise for the reader to predict what Balint did with this material. Naturally, he did not get involved in toilet training, etc., but made the interpretation closest to his focus: that apparently the patient used his penis in the way a woman would use her vagina (thus implying an *identification with the feminine role*). The patient responded by saying that he had always wondered if his penis was too small.

In session 6 the patient reported one of this father's "robust jokes." His father used to come up to the patient's bedroom when he was a child and try to grab his genitals, saying "All this is mine." Here it is noticeable that Balint totally ignored the implications of this in terms of *castration anxiety* and instead chose these in terms of *homosexuality*, asking the patient if he found it more frightening or more exciting, to which the patient replied that it was difficult to say.

The patient went on to speak of having had a suspected heart condition while at school, which had meant that he was not supposed to take part in sports. Balint again ignored any implications in terms of castration, and interpreted that all this contributed to making him into a kind of weakling or sissy, which seemed to link with his interest in the woman's role in intercourse.

This led the patient to speak of his *mother* for the first time, and how she had lost all her warmth as a result of being squashed by her husband. Balint immediately made the link between the *parents* on the one hand, and *Farah and the other man* (James) on the other: how the patient couldn't understand how a nice woman like his mother could have fallen for a crude man like his father, just as he couldn't understand how Farah could have fallen for James—an interpretation with highly Oedipal implications.

One can always judge the correctness of one's interpretations by whether or not they produce a deepening of material or of rapport. Here, the patient showed that the interpretation was correct by immediately reporting a highly exciting sexual fantasy, in which Farah is having intercourse with another man while he is present. Once more, Balint gave a carefully focal interpretation to this, suggesting that the patient was trying to realize this fantasy in his constantly pressing Farah for details of her sexual relation with James.

Toward the end of this session they went over some of the old ground again: (1) that "what the patient cannot accept is that any man might become a rival to him," and (2) that he is immensely interested in what happened (a) between his father and his mother and (b) between Farah and James "because he simply cannot imagine that in Farah's case he scored a complete victory [note that this leaves out any mention of victory over his father]. This cannot be, because his rival, father, or the other man, might upset everything at any moment." Here Balint by implication touches on the *anxiety*, namely fear of *retaliation* by the man.

The patient showed his appreciation of this interpretation by immediately saying how much he enjoyed coming to the sessions.

It is interesting to note that at the beginning of all four sessions, nos. 4, 5, 6, and 7, the patient reported *improvement*. Almost certainly the confession of all this disturbing material had been a relief to him, and Balint's interpretations must have been at just the right level. In session 7, however, nothing new was said, and the patient now responded to a repetition of a previously given interpretation ("inability to win in competition with a man, whether it was his father or the officer") by the first manifestation in the sessions since the first interview of his *paranoid preoccupations*, which soon got the therapist confused, as it did the patient's wife. Then, toward the end of this session, the patient himself proposed that *he should bring his wife along to the next session*, thus suddenly switching away from Balint's primary (interpretative) focal aim to his secondary (collusive) one. Moreover, at the beginning of session 8 (a fortnight later) the patient for the first time reported that he had been worse for three days after the last session, though he had then had the best ten days for years.

This eighth session, after some further paranoid ruminations, then involved further important work, together with the first report of what seemed to be a major alteration in one of his relationships. Balint got an opportunity to complete the interpretation given in session 6, stating that the patient "cannot accept the fact that for some time there was a struggle between [him and his *father*] and now the fight has been decided. He is the managing director of the firm, that is, he has won." This was a direct interpretation of the significance of the *precipitating event* of his recent illness, and thus one of the crucial moments of therapy. This led later to the patient's saying that in coming to therapy he was *trying to have a better marriage than his father*, and then to reporting that in the previous week he had— apparently for the first time in his life—*stood up to his father* and "simply squashed him," and moreover that this was in defense of Farah, since his father had been trying to make fun of her.

In the next session (no. 9) the patient introduced an entirely new theme, his dread of "utter loneliness," referring at first to his relation with Farah. This is a point at which the therapist needs to be careful, as the introduction of *dependence* into the therapy of a paranoid patient carries the danger of getting involved in the relation with the *mother*, and one then may be into the early feeding situation, with projection of oral attacks on the breast, etc., in no time. However, the patient himself avoided this danger by asking whether this might have a connection with his relation with his *father*, who had often behaved toward him with utter unconcern. At this point Balint brought in the first important *transference* interpretation of the whole therapy, and moreover one that dealt with *homosexuality* and made the *transference/parent link*:

> I interpreted here his marked dependence on father in the past—and on me at the present time. This dependence might explain why he so easily accepted any homosexual approach, especially if it came from a man who was his senior or superior: the engineer, the older boys at school, and me.

The patient made as beautiful a response to this interpretation as any therapist could wish for, speaking first of his "fear of snakes, which he fully recognized as having a homosexual significance," and then saying that in the last week he had in contrast had a dream in which "a big snake, a very friendly creature, snuggled up to him and put his head in his lap." "Of course, this was interpreted in the transference."

At the end of this session Balint mentioned that in a few weeks time he was to be away for six weeks, and he proposed to the patient that they continue to meet for the next four weeks, but then might consider discontinuing.

Since I am by now very used to this kind of therapeutic situation when supervising brief therapy by trainees, it gives me some pleasure to be able to supervise my former mentor. It seems to me that to propose termination at the point at which the patient had reported such an obvious manifestation of positive transference as the snake dream, may well have been quite traumatic for the patient, and that although he reacted at first with relief and satisfaction at the thought of being better, after a time lag he reacted by markedly increased disturbance. In the next session the patient *brought his wife,* which looks like a defensive move, and the first part of the session was with the two of them. They reported that the last week had been one of the most peaceful and harmonious of their whole lives. Then, in the next session (no. 11) there was a major relapse into his paranoid ruminations, and Balint writes: "Although every sentence was perfectly constructed and sensible, the whole thing got me more and more confused"—this is one of the hallmarks of paranoid thought disorder. The possible significance of this as a delayed response to the proposed termination—if it is right—was missed by Balint. The patient got involved in his endless ruminations in both of the next two sessions, the second of which was the last before the six-week break.

At this point I propose to stop going through the therapy in detail. These first thirteen sessions before the attempted termination may be regarded—to use a musical analogy—as the *exposition*. It is a characteristic of expositions in classical sonata form that they often state all the material that is going to be used, and that this is then developed ("worked through!") and recapitulated in the rest of the movement. If I am not mistaken, this is what happened in the present therapy.

First of all, let us consider what this exposition involves in terms of the patient's insight and the depth of interpretation. The precipitating factor of the recent illness had been *superseding his father*; and the presenting symptom had been paranoid and obsessional *preoccupation with his wife's relation to another man*, together with using this to *persecute her* to the point of breakdown. Balint's hypothesis had been that this symptom concealed *latent homosexuality*, and that the patient could *not tolerate victory over his rival* because it meant that *a man would not love him*. I have made my own addition to this (which Balint would certainly have made himself if he had been asked) that the homosexuality must have its origins in the patient's relation to his *father*, and that it must contain both the first *impulse* of unsatisfied love for his father, and the *defense* (submission) against the second *impulse*, which is *Oedipal rivalry and hostility*, with the *anxieties* of *guilt* and *fear of retaliation*. Moreover, Oedipal fantasies at their most literal mean *castrating* or *killing* the father and displacing him in the relation with the mother; and the consequence of this in terms of guilt and/or fear is the *patient's* being castrated, either by his father (retaliation) or by himself (guilt). Oedipal fantasies may also involve fantasies about, or experiences of, the "primal scene." Finally, the symptom must in addition contain a considerable element of *hostility toward the woman*, which can have its origins both in Oedipal jealousy and (as shown by the Rorschach) in very primitive fantasies indeed.

The question is, How much of all this has been either interpreted, or realized independently by the patient? The answer appears to be that a very great deal of it has been interpreted, but always in the gentlest, often most veiled, and least anxiety-provoking terms; one could say, with carefully calculated superficiality. The more primitive implications were always carefully ignored, and indeed the interpretations were usually less deep than the patient's material.

The essence of what has been conveyed to the patient is as follows:

1. That he cannot accept that any man should become his rival;

2. That therefore he cannot accept that he has scored a complete victory over his rival, by winning Farah;

3. That in the same way he cannot accept that he has scored a complete victory over his father, by buying him out of the business (the precipitating event);

4. That the way his father treated him (and other experiences that he has had) have made him feel that he is not a proper man, and therefore that he *has* to lose in competition with any other man, including his father;

5. That these experiences have led him to feel himself to be in some way feminine, and hence he has a preoccupation with the woman's role in intercourse, which is expressed in various anal and urethral games;

6. That he cannot *rebel* against his father, and expects and even *desires* to be dominated by him;

7. That his need for love from (or his fear of being abandoned by) his father (or the therapist) has made him easily accept homosexual advances;

8. That he is afraid that in a triangular situation the other man "might come and upset everything at any moment";

9. That there is a parallel between his preoccupation with (a) the relation between his parents and (b) that between Farah and James, (because he cannot understand how a nice woman like his mother could marry a crude man like his father);

10. That in questioning Farah he is symbolically putting into practice his fantasy of being present while she has intercourse with another man; and finally,

11. That he persecutes Farah with his questioning because he needs to have revenge on her because of her relation with the other man.

From all this the reader will also see what has been left out. Of course this includes:

1. Any implications of the anal material other than the preoccupation with a woman's role;

2. All primitive two-person problems with women. But it also includes the following aspects of the Oedipus complex:

3. Any implication of hidden *hostility* toward the father, except

what may be implied in the phrase "cannot rebel," which was in any case apparently only used once;

4. Any mention of *castration*, whether the impulse to castrate, or the fear of being castrated (although the patient had given clear material relevant to this), or the wish to castrate himself out of guilt;

5. Any attempt to lead the patient toward the primal scene;

6. Any mention of sexual feelings toward the mother, or the wish to displace the father in relation to her;

7. Perhaps surprisingly, any suggestion that *the other man* was in any way involved in the patient's homosexual feelings;

8. Moreover, the basic interpretation as originally formulated, that he cannot tolerate any man becoming his rival *because this would mean that a man did not love him*, was apparently never explicitly given, nor was it ever given in the stages of therapy not yet considered.

Thus, in the terms elaborated in chap. 10, the "positive" *impulse*, homosexuality, was considered in detail; an anxiety involving positive feelings toward the father (fear of being abandoned) was interpreted; an anxiety involving "negative" feelings *by* the father (retaliation) was touched on once in very mild terms; the positive impulse of homosexuality was *never interpreted* as a *defense* against *negative* feelings; some very mild negative feelings, inability to "rebel against" or "compete with" the father, were interpreted, but it was never stated *why* he was unable to do this, i.e., what the *anxieties* were; and the much more negative impulses such as hostility, murderous feelings, or castrating impulses, with their accompanying *really disturbing anxieties*, were never touched on at all.

All this may be contrasted with the two therapies presented in chap. 12. In the Magistrate's Daughter, there was a similar carefully calculated superficiality to the early interpretations, but the aim was to lead up to the climax: "that she feels sexually stimulated by men, her brother, *father*, fiancé, and *myself* . . . and her *anger boils up inside* . . ." in which no words were minced in any way. And *a fortiori* the Zoologist, where there was never any need to pull punches, and one of the climaxes of therapy involved saying: "that he was dissatisfied with what the therapist had given him, as he was dissatisfied with what his parents had given him . . . and it looked as if he would deliberately sabotage his life to get his own back . . ."

Thus, in these two therapies the aim was to lead toward interpretations in terms that would have the maximum impact; while in the Stationery Manufacturer the aim was to interpret only the surface layers, and often layers far less deep than those toward which the patient himself seemed to be heading.

This is the main difference from more intensive brief therapy.

We may now consider briefly from this point of view the rest of therapy, which consisted of fourteen more sessions in all. In my opinion, no deeper interpretation, and hardly any really new interpretation, was given during this phase. The two most important interpretations probably came in sessions 18 and 22, and as in intensive brief therapy they involve *links*. In the first, the link was made once more between the other man and the patient's father, but in addition the link between hostility toward Farah and toward the patient's *mother* who, like his father, had also tried to make him feel inferior. In the second, there was a major link made between the transference situation, the recent past situation, and the early situation, but (in contrast to intensive brief therapy) this was put in the most anxiety-suppressive terms:

> In the traumatic situation there was a man, James, and a woman, Farah, who were together to his . . . detriment. Here in the treatment a man, me, and a woman, Farah, are together to help him and this has a good effect on him. Perhaps the reason why the situation in Cyprus became so traumatic to him was that it repeated a long drawn-out situation in his childhood when father (a man) and mother (a woman) were together against him.

Were *paranoid mechanisms* ever interpreted? The nearest to this was when Balint said in session 24 that the patient "is convinced that Fate is hostile to him in general, and in particular if he discovers that two people have anything to do with each other to his exclusion, he feels that there is a conspiracy against him." This is a *clarification* of paranoid feelings, but not really an *interpretation* of them.

Was *projection* ever touched on? Again, only in the most veiled way, through one of the patient's independent discoveries. In session 26 he said that "he realizes now that it was an impossible task to try to understand Farah's emotional involvement on the basis of his own feelings. If Farah had exactly the same feelings as he, it would have meant that she would have been a man. . . ." The two co-authors state (p. 96) that "the recognition that this was the result of projection meant that Farah now became understandable to him as a woman."

This long discussion completes what I have to say about Balint's use of *interpretations*. There were, however, two more elements that had far greater importance than they would have had in any ordinary therapy. The first was the therapist's collusion with the patient's wish to share Farah symbolically with him. The patient tried to get Balint to see his wife alone on a number of occasions, which Balint managed to avoid, except once for a short time at the beginning of the very disturbed session 17, which will be discussed below. On all other occasions, though he did agree to see the wife, he did so in the patient's presence. In this way he both colluded with the patient's wish, and at the same time avoided the very great danger that the homosexual sharing might suddenly turn upside down and go over into paranoid suspiciousness about the two of them plotting against him. At the very end of the therapy, the patient proposed not only that he himself should be free to consult the therapist at need, but that his wife should also. This latter Balint firmly refused.

The second noninterpretative element of which Balint made extensive use was *confronting the patient with reality*. Here it needs to be said that this is a kind of intervention much despised by analysts, who believe that true help can only be given by interpretation of the deep anxieties; and I would imagine that its use on a near-psychotic patient would be despised even more, especially by anyone who has ever tried to argue with a paranoid schizophrenic about his delusions. Yet, in this particular patient—probably because his personality and sense of reality were so well preserved—these interventions seem to have been particularly effective (see Strupp, 1975, for a further discussion of this question).

The first example was in session 3, where the patient insisted that his rival, the other officer, was in every way a better and more attractive man than he was. Balint firmly pointed out to him that since he had eventually won Farah from the other man, the facts pointed to an exactly opposite conclusion. "He was greatly surprised but could not escape its impact."

There are many examples of this kind of intervention throughout the whole of therapy. Here is another, directly concerned with the patient's persecutory questioning of his wife: "I asked him whether *he* had ever found any other *woman* agreeable or exciting" This indeed turned out to be so, and Balint pointed out that although he was sincerely in love with Farah, it was possible for him to forget her for short periods and find another woman very attractive.

The most striking example comes from the very disturbed session 17. This session was the result of a serious relapse that followed the first attempt at termination. I shall quote passages that illustrate the extreme tension of the session, together with Balint's handling of it.

> He was definitely near-psychotic—peremptory, unapproachable, hardly allowing anyone to speak, and not tolerating any contradiction . . . He almost shouted at me . . . I started by admitting that I was really worried about him. I had never seen him in such a bad state . . . He then started a long tirade about his love for the truth, about his wife's game of hide-and-seek, that she has secrets that she must hide from him . . . that what he asks is only logical answers to logical questions, and so on . . . Then he

reverted again to his paranoid ruminations about what is the difference between being in love or being attracted, and so on. I could show him that all these fine and precise distinctions serve only one purpose—to trip his wife up and involve her in irresolvable contradictions . . . He then asked me what I meant when [I said] that he had to accept the fact that for some months his wife hestitated which of the two men to choose, but in the end she chose him. Did this phrase mean that she chose him but loved the other man? I showed him again that he tries to do to me what he does with his wife, namely, to trip me up. *He knew just as well as I that what I meant was that she had chosen him because she felt she loved him.* By that time the tension had largely disappeared and we were again working together, although the paranoid cloud did not disappear altogether (The italics are mine throughout.)

A less secure and less experienced therapist might well have been intimidated by the severity of the disturbance, and indeed by the patient; or might have been intimidated by his own failure to understand the situation and desperately searched for some "deep" interpretation, reached largely by guesswork, which might have been ineffective or worse. Balint simply stuck to *very limited interpretation* and *confrontation with reality*, as a result of which the situation was greatly relieved and therapy could proceed to its ultimately highly successful conclusion. I think it is probably true that this patient, who had suffered so much at the hands of an *overbearing* and *mentally brutal* father, very much appreciated having a *strong* father who both *cared* and would *stand no nonsense*.

It is worth saying that the other two therapies that Balint conducted for the workshop were singularly unsuccessful. But this therapy was a *tour de force,* and the patient and his wife may count themselves very fortunate in having found perhaps the one therapist in Britain who knew how to handle their situation within the limits of brief psycho-therapy. If we who follow are never likely to be able to emulate this, we can at least learn some partial lessons from it and perhaps apply them in the future.

CHAPTER 15

Deeper Therapy in More Disturbed Patients

The highly successful therapy of the Stationery Manufacturer, presented in the last chapter, must raise the question of what would have happened if deeper interpretations had been used. Of course, no one can say, but in my brief therapy unit we have experience of taking on some relatively disturbed patients and fearlessly interpreting some of the deeper layers of their pathology. The results seem to have been not only not harmful but definitely beneficial. Thus, the limits of brief therapy in terms of severity of pathology and depth of interpretation do not yet seem to have been fully explored.

The present chapter consists of an account of two therapies, both conducted by American trainees under supervision in my brief therapy unit, in which the interpretation of primitive mechanisms, especially (1) *paranoid projection*, and (2) the inner destruction of good experience leading to feelings of emptiness and contamination, played a major part. Emphasis will not be laid on striking therapeutic effects, which there were not, but only on the fact that this type of interpretation afforded relief at the time and did not in any way lead into uncontrollable situations. In the presentation I shall mostly describe in detail only those sessions that are relevant to this theme.

THE HOSPITAL PORTER

This was a young man of twenty-five, married, complaining of crippling anxiety in the presence of male authority, which had caused him to have over one hundred jobs since leaving school at fifteen. Despite his limited education he was extremely intelligent and was clearly working well below his potential. He also suffered from depression and excessive drinking.

At interview he started by presenting a mass of intellectual insight about the link between his hatred of authority and his feelings about his father; ending, however, with the communication that once he had asked himself the question, "What would happen if God, who was so good and reliable and protective were to suddenly become horrible and brutal?" The male interviewer interpreted that perhaps this meant that he had once had a warm relation with his father, but had lost it and had never forgiven him. This produced a complete change of atmosphere, followed by a flood of highly charged material: The patient told how he had been admitted to the hospital with tuberculosis at the age of five; how when in the hospital he had deliberately withheld his feces and had soiled his bed; how he had had to be given enemas, and had incorporated this into his sexual fantasies; how he had deliberately put soap into the water of the fish tank in the ward, and had killed the fish; and how he had had the feeling, "Why can't men marry men?" A further interpretation about disappointment with his mother met with little response.

This flood of primitive material, of course, made us need to go into his strength and weakness very carefully. His Rorschach showed much phallic preoccupation and rivalry with men, and behind this both clear paranoid elements and a wish to return to the warmth and comfort of a womblike existence. On the other hand, there was also evidence that he had the strength to face his disturbing feelings without breakdown. There was a male therapist available to treat him.

On the basis of the above information we were able to make a very detailed psychodynamic formulation, as follows: (1) a massive Oedipal problem, hiding (2) much love for his father and disappointment in him, expressed in homosexual feelings, and behind this (3) anal problems, (4) a paranoid element, and (5) a deep longing for maternal warmth.

It was, however, beyond us to say exactly what part these deeper layers might play in therapy, and we wrote only as follows: "We will try to get behind the Oedipal hostility, which he will present at first, by interpreting positive feelings toward men. We will have to play the other layers by ear."

A time limit was set by the therapist's intended departure for the United States in seven months.

The following is a summary of the course of therapy:

The first three sessions contained the theme of anger against the therapist, which was interpreted both as a testing out and as a defense against need and disappointment.

In sessions 5 and 6, spanning the Christmas break, the therapist linked the transference with the patient's father, saying essentially that if he couldn't get all he wanted from someone he refused to accept anything at all.

This led in session 7 to the patient telling of reaching a crucial piece of insight: that he was rejecting his parents just as much as they were rejecting him.

In session 8 the patient admitted that he had previously tried to fill the sessions with less meaningful talk because he was afraid he wouldn't be accepted if he was silent, and that he would often just like to sit in silence in the therapist's presence. He ended with a fantasy about what a special case he was.

These important communications leading in the direction of positive feelings were followed by two sessions, both admitting anger with the therapist and containing *paranoid projection*. He said he felt "like a robot being controlled"; that he had been angry with the therapist for a day and a half after the last session, feeling that the therapist could end the depression he was feeling if he wanted to; he spoke of the therapist's silence as being "sadistic"; and in session 10 he spoke of formerly feeling that the therapist was trying to "lead him into a corner and pounce on him." With hindsight it now seems that these communications concerned his own anger at being rejected, which he projected onto the therapist; but this was not seen at the time either by therapist or supervisor, and it was not interpreted. The main theme of interpretations was a continuation of the mechanism of expressing negative feelings as a *defense* against expressing love.

Nevertheless, in session 11 he said (1) that he had stopped taking antidepressants, (2) that he felt much better, and (3) he was now able to describe in detail his technique with bosses: driving them into a corner with his intellect, provoking them into threatening to fire him, then saying he doesn't care anything about the job, and ending by being fired in actuality. The therapist said he wondered if the patient wanted to break off treatment rather than face his feelings about *termination,* a theme thus brought in very early.

This was followed by two sessions concerned with his need to be *mothered,* together with a dream expressing very primitive Oedipal anxieties about this (the therapist disemboweling him). There was no very clear response to an apparently correct interpretation of this material.

In session 15, under the shadow of another impending holiday, it was possible to link the patient's behavior with bosses to the transference—wanting to leave to avoid pain—with which the patient vehemently agreed.

Session 17 was the last before the holiday break. A long quotation will illustrate the contrast between this therapy and that of the Stationery Manufacturer, how in this *less* disturbed but still *relatively* disturbed patient the themes of dependence and ambivalence could be handled without any need to soften them, leading to moments of great intensity:

> I pointed out how there were two parts of himself working, the one part that values the experience here and makes the effort to come, and the other part that is angry about my announcing a holiday and the end of therapy and wants to devalue the experience here in preparation for being disappointed. He agreed and pointed out that he often has feelings about not coming at all.
>
> He expressed in rather direct terms his appreciation for what he felt to be an improvement since coming here. I answered that it is very hard to express this kind of appreciation when there is a break coming up. The following comments seemed to develop very rapidly into a mood of intense feeling and silence. This included his agreeing that it was difficult to express positive feelings with the break coming up, and my pointing out that part of the difficulty had to do with the anger about the break which comes in and destroys the good experience. He commented that this was a pattern for him, and I emphasized the way in which the important aspects of a feeling relationship with me became ruined by this anger. The silence that followed was very intense and he seemed almost on the verge of tears. He said that he guessed he was testing me to see if I would now make the session end.
>
> I said that it was as if the only way the feeling experience could be valuable was if it went on forever; and that he seems to be expressing difficulty in taking this experience away with him, even to help him with other experiences which are not as positive. He agreed with this and then said that actually he was becoming ashamed that he had been angry previously. I pointed out that what he was doing now was still to say that he was unable to handle a relationship with me that involved both positive and negative aspects. Whereas previously he was expressing difficulty about appreciating the positive aspects when anger interfered, now he seemed to be saying that he could not allow a negative experience if there was a positive one. I pointed out how in reality there will always be a combination of the two and that the one cannot be seen as a negation of the other. He vehemently agreed with this and said a warm good-bye for the two weeks break.

In session 18, immediately after the break, the patient was in resistance and finally admitted that because the break had been painful he'd decided not to relate deeply to the therapist any more. He said he was glad he'd been able to speak of this despite deciding not to.

My own interpretation of the next session is that the patient came full of positive feelings, which started as genuine but became defensive because he was unable to face the negative component in them.

Then, starting with session 20, there were a number of sessions containing more paranoid projection, which this time was interpreted. He spoke of the therapist's having the power to create a good or bad week for him, and this time having (deliberately?) created a bad week; and he felt the therapist "took apart" things that he said.

The therapist wrote:

> I said that he was seeing my interpretation as an attack. Perhaps this was related to his wish to attack me because of his anger. He responded that this was true and spontaneously remembered wanting his father's love very much and seeing his father as both angry and disappointing.

Toward the end of this session (no. 21), the patient told a dream in which he had had a homosexual relation with a friend that he did not want or enjoy, but he did it to please the friend. Thus, the mechanism of projection continued to operate. This was not in fact interpreted, but two sessions later the projection became undone and he more or less openly admitted his need for the therapist's love.

The last few sessions contained much further work on the problem of whether he could take away something good from his relation with the therapist without destroying it because of his anger about termination. A crucial communication in the very last session (no. 26) occurred when he said that this was the *first time he had ever stuck out a relation to the end*.

If we compare actual events with the original therapeutic plan, we can see that the exact sequence could of course not be foreseen, but that the prediction was clearly fulfilled that therapy would start with Oedipal hostility that would be interpreted as a defense against positive feelings toward men; and that of the other layers described in advance, paranoid mechanisms, homosexuality, and longing for maternal warmth, all played their part.

This patient was followed up one year four months after termination. There seemed to be considerable symptomatic improvement and he conveyed the feeling that he could now handle his problems with bosses, though it was also true that these problems had been to some extent avoided by his becoming self-employed. He was free from defensive intellectualization and seemed much more in touch with his feelings. On the other hand, his relation with his wife seemed little improved, which was perhaps not surprising since therapy had been almost entirely concerned with his relation with men. He and his wife were taken on for a course of marital therapy, which at the time of writing still continues. It is a very interesting fact, however, that in this therapy there has been no trace of the paranoid feelings observed previously.

THE GRADUATE CLERK

The patient was a man of twenty-eight, whose disturbances seemed to consist essentially of the Oedipal syndrome (symptoms, difficulties with male authority, difficulties over achievement, and inhibition in relation to women):

1. *Symptoms*: tension, headaches, gastrointestinal symptoms;
2. Severe difficulty in getting on with male authority;
3. After getting third-class honors in engineering, he has gone from job to job (he listed twelve since the age of twenty-two) and is at present working as a clerk;
4. He falls in love with girls from a distance but feels paralyzed in their presence.

The precipitation of his symptoms had occurred when one of these girls got married.

He was the elder by two years of two boys. The chief disturbances in his childhood seemed to be (1) intense jealousy of his younger brother's relation with his mother, and (2) a severe deterioration in the relation with his father, to whom he was quite close as a child, but who he felt became a tyrant in his adolescence.

At interview he showed remarkable and genuine insight, spontaneously linking his present situation with his childhood on several occasions. He also responded dramatically to an interpretation linking his resentment against authority with his feelings about the male interviewer, first experiencing intense anxiety but then relaxing when he was able to speak about it.

He was given routine projection tests. In the preliminary interview with the (male) psychologist, he said that the interviewing psychiatrist had brought to light some aspects of his relation with his parents that he hadn't seen before. He was able to see a link, put to him by the psychologist, between his difficulty over achievement and that with women, realizing that the underlying anxieties were fear of failure and of rejection. The psychologist wrote that he seemed to be a "complex personality"; that his drives received little outward expression but were bound up in fantasy; that in the Rorschach there were a large number of responses to texture, suggesting dependence; that the main feature of the ORT seemed to be fear of retribution for sexual and aggressive drives; that there were no psychotic features; and that he seemed to have many resources.

Here the factors in favor of brief therapy were the apparently high motivation for insight, the clear response to interpretation, the fact that the overall picture and the precipitating factor fitted into an Oedipal focus, and—despite possible complicating factors such as dependence—the impression that he had the strength to face disturbing feelings. He was assigned to a male therapist with a time limit of about thirty sessions and the following therapeutic plan laid down before therapy started:

> It seems that the focus is likely to be his anger against both the other two people in a triangular situation. This needs to be brought out and linked with the situation (1) with his mother and father, and (2) with his mother and brother. Probably difficulties with authority will manifest themselves fairly early on in the transference to a male therapist. The therapist needs to be on the lookout for a third person whom the patient is jealous of. I would expect the patient to work well in therapy, but his difficulty with authority may manifest itself in lateness, as at work. He will probably need to go through feelings about termination in the form of anger with his therapist for replacing him with someone else.

As will be seen, this plan was remarkably accurate *in the letter*: Therapy did indeed concern his anger with both people in a triangular situation; this was in fact linked to his mother and father and his mother and brother; and feelings about replacing him with another patient did appear over the issue of termination; but *in spirit* it was quite wrong, for the nature and quality of the feelings involved were entirely unforeseen.

The opening theme in the first therapeutic session (session 2) seemed to be his anger at people (the interviewing psychiatrist, the psychologist, and the therapist, all of whom of course were male) who tried to thrust theories on him. Session 3 is then worth describing in some detail:

The previous session had been in July, immediately before the (American) therapist's return home for the rest of the summer, and arrangements were made to meet on his return in late September. Owing to some misunderstanding the patient failed to keep this appointment, but came the next week (session 3). He then started with a lot of intellectual (though accurate) analysis of his own pathology: how he was a "schizoid personality"; how, according to Anthony

Storr, this was based on paternal rejection, but he suspected maternal rejection as well; how he recalls at the age of two his mother coming home from the hospital with his younger brother and he "threw muck on her," etc. The therapist interpreted both the missed session and the intellectual insight as a *defense*, expressing the patient's uneasiness about looking at these sensitive areas (leading toward the *anxieties*).

The result was that the patient immediately began expressing these anxieties openly, describing (1) how he felt he bored friends and was afraid they would *laugh at him*; (2) how a Catholic chaplain had ended by saying he could not help him; (3) how the interviewing psychiatrist here had said he would *always* have difficulty in loving; and (4) how another psychiatrist "with white hair and *pretensions of wisdom*" used to show immediately by his face when things were not getting across, and had ended by merely giving him Librium.

With hindsight one may see in this (and in the previous session as well) a definite *paranoid flavor*, and the start of the emergence of the *impulse* (hostility toward male authority).

What followed is a fascinating example of how, with certain patients, the therapist need do no more than clear the way by limited interpretation—particularly of the anxieties—and the patient himself will then spontaneously lead into the next area, and sometimes indeed into the depths. This is far more satisfactory than the situation in which the therapist tries to know better than the patient and himself makes deep interpretations based partly on guesswork—which may be incorrect, or premature, or too disturbing, or may divert the patient from his central feelings.

Here the therapist confined himself merely to linking each of these expressed anxieties in turn to the *transference*. The patient then spontaneously associated to rows with his father when he was eleven, thus both unconsciously making the *transference/parent link* and bringing out the *impulse* of hostility. He told of an incident in which his mother was in the hospital, and his father, who was doing the cooking, tried to make him eat something he didn't like. There had been rage and tears on the patient's part. With some pressure of speech he went on to tell how his mother had later had a hysterectomy, how this had upset the whole family, and his father had had to see a psychiatrist. At this time the patient felt that "his whole world had fallen to pieces." The *hostility to his father* continued, however, and by the time he was thirteen it had got to the point of his singing rude songs about his father's peculiarities in his presence. Then in the session there came the real warning to us all: "He saw his father as a vampire–lover, one who wanted to possess you and literally take the blood of life from you." When he reached the age of eighteen to twenty it seemed that there was some reversal of the relation with his father, who now was seen as rather shy and an object of contempt. The patient had wanted strength from him and was unable to get it, and at one point his father said he had washed his hands of him. Here, again, the therapist did no more than make the link with the *transference*—was he afraid he might do something that would make the therapist wash his hands of him?—to which there was an extraordinary response: "When I pulled my cigarette pack out and kind of stumbled with the cigarette I felt you were disapproving of me. If I brought a cigarette out you'd ridicule me, so it seemed I couldn't do anything." To this the therapist deliberately made some neutral comment.

It is interesting to note that, as supervisor, I was so unprepared for the idea that this patient would turn out to be suffering from anything other than an ordinary Oedipal problem, that even here I failed to see the warning signs, but in the next session (no. 4) I could hardly avoid them. He opened by saying with a half-smile that he divided people into *"authority figures* and *friends"*; he went on to speak of fantasies that were all *confused*; he said that if he didn't win arguments with his father he would be *annihilated*; that his lack of concentration resulted in *chaotic* situations. He then spoke of a man who had come into his office and threatened to smash all the glass in the windows. The therapist, undoing the projection (*defense*), asked him if *he'd* like to smash things and do away with anyone who restricted him. This led to his speaking of violent and rebellious feelings against his work, and eventually to fantasies about patients rebelling against their doctors and nurses; "using tablets as missiles *to undo the evil medical team with"*; people being *planted with drugs and then arrested*; a patient who had drawn a "doodle" that had been shown to a psychiatrist, who had said he was undoubtedly *mad*; and he ended by saying that he had the feeling of being able to *tune in on people's wavelengths.*

Although there was no suggestion that this patient was in danger of becoming overtly psychotic, it will be obvious that our initial assessment was quite inadequate and we were suddenly in the midst of paranoid fantasies. The question was what we should do now. The answer was quite simple: Though we would proceed with some degree of caution, we saw no reason why we should not just go on with therapy and interpret many of the mechanisms without fear. In this we were helped by the experience that we had already gained with the Hospital Porter presented earlier in this chapter.

From this extremely rich therapy I shall pick out only some of the main themes, with some assistance from hindsight, and I shall also illustrate one extremely important observation concerned with handling confused material in focal therapy.

In session 6 he mentioned being angry when feeling *rejected* as a child, then that he once hit a friend with a rock, and shortly afterward said that "Cain didn't get a fair hearing over his aggression toward Abel," and extraordinarily enough his really excellent therapist seems to have missed the obvious reference to the patient's brother.

In session 7 he mentioned the following sequence of events: (1) He had had a conversation with a priest that had gone well; (2) he had felt well for two days; (3) he had gone out on Friday night with his friends; and (4) he had woken up on Saturday morning in a "numb" and "bored" state. It eventually emerged, apparently, that on Friday night he had been *rejected* by a girl; and when this was brought out he also mentioned having been *rejected* by a girl when at the university. He spoke of yearning for her and then said that his feelings for her were emotional and not just a "professional meeting of minds." I think that the therapist, instead of clarifying the very intense feelings produced by rejection, justifiably enough tried to link this with the transference prematurely, and getting some response, later spoke of the patient's needs for "nurturing" and "strength" from him, and how these warm feelings in turn brought uneasiness. However, the patient's responses showed that the tension was not reduced.

The next session (no. 8) started with some *paranoid* material about being *laughed at* by superior men who were *more gifted and cunning*, which the therapist related to the *transference*. Later in the session there was again the theme of *rejection by a woman*: a girl at the university had "given him the push," and a little time later he spoke of having got a knife out and "slashed at this books." Again the therapist, preoccupied with the transference, missed the connection between these two communications, and made an interpretation about attacking the source of what he wanted, including the authority whose strength he needed. The patient responded by talking about a "missionarylike categorizing friend" who tried to be too clever.

This was followed by session 9, which alternated clear communications, on the one hand, with some of the most obscure material that it is possible to imagine in this kind of therapy, on the other:

He started with a story about his feelings having gone wrong at work, which was possibly connected with a woman having been angry with him and his department; and he went on to tell a dream that first of all involved helping his brother through a hole in a fence, with associations that there were protective as well as jealous feelings toward him, but which continued: "Through the hole in the fence there was a suburban road, and there were a couple of dogs guarding coal or something. There was another substance on the ground that was reddish-orange-brownish. There was a feeling that my parents were somewhere around." This led to his discussing his mixed feelings toward his brother. The therapist did what he could with the details of the dream, suggesting that the dogs who guarded something valuable represented his parents hiding their love from him. This led to open discussion of his mother's sexual inhibition, and her affection for furry animals instead; then, to his chatting intimately with his mother, and his father trying unsuccessfully to talk to him when he was older. The therapist pointed out that he seemed to be closer to his parents than they were to each other, and he then spoke of feeling he had some "mystical power" that was needed to keep them together; and an incident in which he had slept between his parents and his father had said "now it is complete"; but, on the other hand, of moments when his father had shown intense jealousy of him.

The therapist asked for associations to the substance in the road. The patient said it was "rather like afterbirth," and went on to describe a recurring dream: "It's a sensation of being closed in, yet expanding, like in a womb. There is a bright and sharp thing like a needle being enclosed in a blanket. It is associated with losing consciousness and my whole body expanding." The therapist—operating near the limits of understanding—interpreted that side by side with a feeling of great power (feeling himself to be the mystic go-between between his parents), there must have been great anger against them, expressed by the needle. The patient said, "Yes, they overprotected me. My bedtime was half an hour earlier than any of the other kids. I couldn't have a bike until I was thirteen, but my brother got one at eleven."

Here, although the content of the dreams is extremely obscure, the material other than dreams can all be seen to hang together in terms of *triangular relations* within his family (even the afterbirth may have been some reference to his younger brother's birth); but on the other hand, the overall impression conveyed by this session at the time was one of confusion and near-psychotic disturbance. What this session taught me was that where confusion of this kind suddenly arises *the therapist should look for an important missed interpretation in the previous session.* In this case the missed interpretation was the connection between *rejection by a woman* and *very primitive aggressive feelings* represented by slashing the books. In supervising this session

I pointed out this missed interpretation, though I did not fully see its significance.

The result was that in the account of the next session (no. 10) derivatives of the verb "reject" occurred twelve times. Here one can pick out a single vital sequence, which occurred twice: (1) rejection by a girl, who goes off with another man; (2) feeling that other men (referred to as "wise guys") are sneering or laughing at him because of his failure.

My interpretation of this sequence is: (1) rejection by the girl produces very primitive rage; (2) this results in paranoid projection and he sees the world as hostile; (3) the fact that the girl goes off with another man activates his intense Oedipal rivalry; and (4) the feelings under (2) and (3) become fused into *paranoid feelings about men laughing at him*.

What was needed at this point, therefore, was a clarification of this mechanism. The therapist did not see this, but he did the next best thing, which was to link all these feelings with the patient's father and mother, leading to the expression of considerable rage against them.

The themes that I shall pick out from the next few sessions concern his paranoid feelings, and especially those concerning the situation between him, a girl, and the "wise guys." He opened the next session (no. 11) by saying that he had taken two days off work with the feeling that *everything was against him*. However, he then told a dream in which, although the men were enemies, his feelings toward the girl were positive: He wanted to protect a girl from a "wise guy" type, who had insulted her.

In the next session (no. 12) there was material first about a woman who had got angry with him in the office, and then about his father's anger at home. The therapist interpreted this as partly being concerned with the projection of the patient's own anger, and he linked this with the mixed feelings in the transference that interfered in the sessions. The patient accepted this interpretation and immediately went on to envisage the possibility that *he* might get the girl and then the wise guys would feel the rejection that he felt. Moreover, he then said that maybe the wise guys weren't that vicious. Thus, interpretation of the projection seemed to have reduced the paranoid feelings and the anxieties in the triangular situation.

Then, however, feelings about others laughing at him returned, and this now included especially his mother. Then he said that *"she was the type that likes to be with the wise guys"*; and finally the crucial communication came out, that his brother was married but that his mother had once said "no woman would ever have *you*." Thus, it was possible to interpret that his feelings about the woman and the wise guys referred originally to his mother and his brother, and to bring out both his rage and his sense of rejection and helplessness.

This was followed by an extraordinarily rich and deep session (no. 13), which included the following:

1. There was a dream about a sisterlike woman whose breasts he wanted to feel, who seemed like "someone close to him with whom he had shared his life for a long time."

2. There were other dreams that included his father and a priest and "two fighting, vicious guys."

3. In one of the dreams a brother-figure turned into a mother-figure and her nipples grew long and protruding.

4. The therapist commented that the nipples seemed to grow into an erect penis, and this led immediately to the patient's speaking about masturbation, which he had discovered at 14.

5. The therapist made an interpretation about being sexually stimulated by the mother, and fear of the father's disapproval.

6. This led to memories of a priest's denunciation of masturbation and his mother having said that if he didn't wash his penis "a dog would come and bite it off." He also asked the therapist if babies became sexually stimulated when feeding.

It seems that what we can see here is (1) a great reduction of paranoid anxiety resulting from the previous session, leading to (2) openly acknowledged warm feelings toward mother-figures that included direct references to both feeding and sexuality, which in turn aroused (3) Oedipal anxieties, but now of a *nonparanoid* kind, which (4) could be interpreted in quite literal terms.

This was followed by two sessions (nos. 14 and 15) spanning the Christmas break. The therapist was very careful to interpret negative feelings concerned with being abandoned, but it really did seem that the patient was able to preserve something valuable from his therapy that he used to good effect during the break. He had—against all expectation—got through a probation period at work, he was getting more pleasure out of playing his guitar, authority figures seemed less threatening, he had managed to get on with an uncle whom he disliked, his father had asked him if he'd be willing to help over something, and so on.

In my annotations to this session I wrote, in addition to much praise for the therapist, "I think we want it to go wrong and then be made right again several times."

At this point I shall stop giving a detailed account of the sessions and pick out only a few essential themes from the rest of therapy. My wish expressed above was fulfilled. Session 16 opened with a denial of anything good, and in session 17 paranoid feelings returned in the form of being "used" and "persecuted." What eventually emerged, in session 19, was the feeling that he had been made to fulfill some of his father's unfulfilled longings, which the therapist related to his own need to make the patient better and the patient's reaction against this. The patient's comments about his father seemed insightful and quite probably accurate, and not paranoid. Then, in session 20, he reported a dream in which his mother was pregnant again. This led to anger with his mother when she gave birth to his brother, and to interpretations that termination meant the therapist "getting pregnant with another patient." The patient eventually said "I guess there are brother-figures all around me."

During the whole of this time the therapist reiterated interpretations about the patient's need to destroy and spoil inside himself the good experience he had had from therapy; and, whenever the patient felt all was spoiled, the therapist reiterated that there *were* good things that he had received, and his dilemma was how to preserve them despite his anger at being abandoned. Something of the depth of communications on this theme can be conveyed by a single quotation, from session 24:

> He said that somehow it is more difficult to trust women than men. He commented on having known a sensual woman, but having quickly got bored with her. "If I became dependent I'd become more demanding, and then it would be hopeless." We talked about how when one has great demands there is a feeling of devouring a person and damaging that person, and then feeling a great void inside for damaging what was a very good relationship. He said that it was a very helpless feeling indeed to destroy the thing you are dependent on and want most. He went on to associate this with how it must feel to have the golden touch of King Midas. This was followed by, "I'm a masochist with sadistic desires. I am afraid of bringing these sadistic desires out, especially as they relate to mother and father. It's like I could destroy the thing that's good for me." I interpreted that he must feel like striking out at me because of his anger at the one-sidedness of our relationship, and at the same time is afraid of destroying the good and helpful part of our work together. His response was to say, "The only thing I can do at work is not to turn up. If my dentist makes a mistake, I get angry; it's harder to get angry with father, for he was absent so much of the time." I brought out the abandonment he must feel at our termination, and how this must make him feel he was destructive and could produce nothing of nurture or lasting good, like the King Midas touch.

Three aspects of this later phase of therapy seem to stand out: (1)

The patient was much more in touch with his strong feelings: "I have more awareness, I feel more pain than I've ever felt. In the last two or three years I've developed a protective obtuseness and a failure of memory. Somehow these have been got rid of" (session 23). (2) Although paranoid feelings recurred on a number of occasions, he was much less *unremittingly* paranoid than in the first half of therapy. And (3) perhaps the most hopeful sign was his ability to speak of "good" and "bad" together, and to preserve the good after having spoken of the bad. Some quotations from the final session of regular therapy (no. 33) will illustrate this:

> He opened by saying he had been depressed, his appeal against being censured at work had been quashed, and it had been brought to his attention that he had made a number of clerical mistakes that were shown to him and discussed. He did recognize that this was a fair comment on his work and he hadn't realized how many errors he was making [it is worth noting the utterly nonparanoid reaction to this]. The next association was to being bored on weekends, rather overwhelmingly so, but he did add that his relationships with other people, especially at work, seemed to be better. I commented on the good aspect that seemed to be present despite his other feelings, and he took this in his stride by speaking of his interest in looking for a new job. Within a minute or two he was back to the good aspect of his dealings with people and how in a way this had allowed him to forget his anger and depression. I commented that he must fear I would encourage him to stick to his job because it's good for him, instead of respecting his individuality and his needs. He agreed with this and said, "I do want guidance from you, but I know it can't be that way. The child part of me fears I might not be getting the guidance I'd like here because I know the feeling toward my father gets in the way." Towards the very end of the session he said that there is a little boil on his eyebrow and "I feel that it will expand and somehow I will be all filled with pus and poison." I commented on his preoccupation with his bad part, expanding in an invasive way and filling his body with pus as though he were untouchable, just as he feels his irritation might extend to total rage that would likewise make him feel untouchable and unwanted and rejected. This threatened to prevent the warmth in him from being nurtured and becoming a greater part of his life; further, that it was easier for him to talk about his angry part than it was to talk about the more soft sensitive part. He smiled at this point and some silence ensued with rather hesitant phrases. We seemed to leave the session on a very positive note. We had set up a definite date for a meeting in three months time and the understanding was firmly made that he could call me in the interim should there be any need.

In our discussions we had concluded that it would be quite wrong to leave this disturbed patient without support, and in fact the therapist has been seeing him since then at monthly or two-monthly intervals.

We thus have no definite follow-up. The material has continued to be primitive and disturbed—e.g., a dream in which he and a girl were looking at an ogre who became his mother—but there have also been hopeful signs such as his ability to admit openly his warm feelings for the therapist and his feeling of loss.

It therefore remains to be seen whether this kind of work can result in any lasting benefit; but we appear to have shown at least that a therapy based on interpretations of such depth and primitiveness—*with the right kind of patient*—does not immediately and inevitably lead into increased disturbance and insoluble problems of termination.

Whatever the final outcome of this particular therapy, therefore, we have come upon an immensely important finding: that—again, *with the right kind of patient*—there appear to be very few limits to the kind of interpretation, or the depth of interpretation, that can be used in therapy that is presented to the patient as time-limited from the beginning.

In a way we have stumbled upon this observation fortuitously, through an inaccurately assessed patient; but in a way it is not fortuitous at all and would have been reached eventually, because it represents simply the continuation of a trend toward more and more fearless interpretation, which has been present in our work from the beginning. The full exploration of the limits of this kind of therapy, and the accurate definition of selection criteria, are tasks that remain for the future.

CHAPTER 16

Some Contraindications

The main theme of the previous three chapters has been that the limits of brief therapy have not yet been fully explored, and the clinical examples have consisted of successful work with apparently very difficult patients. It is, however, very important to know that at times we have tried to exceed these limits, and that the consequences have ranged from wasted effort to catastrophe. During the course of all this work we have steadily accumulated a fund of mistakes, and some of these, of course, may often be more instructive than successes; and indeed satisfying *scientifically* (though certainly not from a clinical or humanitarian point of view), since they often result from ignoring the selection criteria so carefully built up over the years. The present chapter consists of four cautionary tales.

The first example underlines the importance of *response to interpretation* as a *sine qua non* for brief therapy.

The patient was a single man of twenty-four who was brought to the clinic by an acute attack of anxiety some five weeks before. He had been to a concert with his girl friend and a male acquaintance. His girl friend had seemed attracted by this other man and had paid him a good deal of attention, and the patient had become so anxious that they all had had to leave the concert. It had apparently taken a week before he felt calm again.

Further exploration revealed additional aspects of one of the most strikingly Oedipal stories I have ever encountered. The girl friend was married, was old enough to be the patient's mother, and in fact had a son of almost the same age. The patient lived in the same house as her and her husband, who was crippled with multiple sclerosis and seemed to connive at the patient's relation with his wife. One of the patient's additional problems was hostility toward men in authority. There had also been a previous episode of anxiety at the university at the age of twenty-one, when he had begun to feel unable to compete and had had to take time away from work to recover.

He said that he had been very close to his father, but had had the feeling that this kept him away from his mother. His father had died suddenly when the patient was eleven, the patient had been extremely upset by this, and had had to spend two or three weeks in bed under heavy sedation.

There was evidence of a sound basic personality in that he had been successful academically, had had a number of previous satisfactory relations with girls, and had no overt sexual difficulties.

In all this I was dazzled by the extraordinary clarity of the Oedipal pathology, and of course had absolutely no problem in formulating a therapeutic plan. I quite omitted to give any weight to the fact that the interviewing psychiatrist had made no attempt to explore his response to interpretations, or, therefore, his motivation for insight, and I assumed that with such clear material the response and the motivation would come as soon as interpretations were made. In view of later events, we may also note the absence of either a detailed sexual history or a routine projection test, both of which might have served as dampers to our therapeutic enthusiasm. So we took him on, assigning him to a male therapist with a time limit of twenty-five sessions.

His response to interpretation was never satisfactory and his motivation for insight was very limited. He seemed unable to face painful feelings, he defended himself against them by much intellectual and rather obsessional talk, and he shied away from them whenever they came close. Nevertheless the therapist did confront him with some of his grief about his father's death. Typical of him was that in the last third of therapy he began to speak of sexual fantasies, the exact nature of which *he felt unable to reveal*. Sessions became resistant and little further progress was made; but he revealed some details of the fantasies *in the last paragraph of the last session*, saying that "he knows it is a crucial part of his treatment, but now it is too late and it is his fault that he has been unable to bring it earlier."

He was followed up five months later. He insisted that he had benefited from therapy, and there did seem some improvement in his ability to stand up to other men. However, he was still involved with the same strange triangular setup. He became very defensive when painful feelings were touched on, but there were tears running down his cheeks when he began to speak of his father. Thus, the uncompleted mourning for his father may have been continuing, but he did his utmost to avoid this. The therapist asked him to come again, which he did. He sat down, said he felt angry with the therapist and hadn't wanted to come, and immediately got up to go. The therapist felt he had no right to stop him and the interview ended there.

Thus, there may possibly be some improvements, but neither the therapy nor the final situation can be described as satisfactory.

The second example shows the importance of (1) giving routine projection tests, (2) having the sex of the psychologist different from that of the original interviewer, and (3) gathering all the evidence before taking a decision, let alone acquainting the patient with it.

The patient was a young man of twenty-one complaining of tension, anxiety, and blushing due to lack of confidence. His history showed a pattern of breaking down into symptoms about six months after each step forward in his career—in the sixth form at school, in his first job, and in a second job at a considerably higher salary. He also said that, until the sixth form, he had been confident and a leader, but that since then he had become the opposite, feeling excluded from groups and unable to find anything to say.

He said he had had to fight his father (sometimes literally) for his freedom, and he described girl friends who seemed to bear a striking resemblance to his mother.

He treated the male interviewer in a remarkably forthright manner, but his response to interpretation was not fully explored.

At the case conference we felt that he might well make a good brief therapy case, with an Oedipal focus, although we were slightly uneasy at the way in which the Oedipus complex seemed to be already out in the open.

We told the patient that we would accept him for psychotherapy and wrote to the G.P. to the same effect; and then—as what we thought was routine—asked for projection tests. It so happened that the psychologist with a vacancy for this was a woman.

His behavior here was entirely different. He seemed to be alarmed to the point of paranoia about the prospect of a woman's seeing through his façade; e.g., he opened by speaking about people with ulterior motives who were trying to do him down, and he thought there were tricks in the tests designed to expose the aggression in him. He put on a tremendous phallic display, ending by turning the tables on the psychologist and giving her a rundown on her own character and problems. There were two bizarre responses, in one of which he used one of the ORT cards as a sort of Rorschach, turning it on its side and seeing the face of a witch, to which he returned, fascinated, several times. On Card VII of the Rorschach, in which the soft shading often evokes responses to do with maternal warmth, he saw a hideous, grotesque doll, or a wolf. There seemed little evidence that he had any basis of good experience, and he fobbed off all interpretations.

In view of the successful work with paranoid patients described in the last two chapters, it may well be asked why this patient was now regarded as unsuitable. The answer lies mainly in the feeling that he could be *taken over* by paranoid feelings and become *identified with them*, as opposed to the previous patients who gave the impression of a strong healthy part *struggling against* paranoid feelings.

We thus ended by feeling that the removal of his façade might well result in a paranoid breakdown. Having already accepted the patient as suitable, we were now faced with a most embarrassing situation. We recalled the patient and explained to him as best we could that we felt our form of treatment might well make him worse rather than better, which he seemed to accept. We have no further follow-up.

These four cases are arranged in order of increasingly dangerous consequences of clinical mistakes. The third case illustrates the consequences that may arise from taking on a patient without (1) giving projection tests, or (2) understanding anything much about the psychopathology. Hindsight also enables me to include some warning signs that were missed at the time.

The patient was a girl of twenty-six, married for six years, referred to us by her G.P. Her complaint was that about nine months ago she had started to suffer from an inability to focus her eyes. She had been investigated at an eye hospital, and part of their report reads: "Of course, this symptom of blurring, associated with ciliary muscle spasm with otherwise normal eyes, is the expression of an emotional disturbance." She was also depressed (worse in the mornings), and complained of over-reaction to emotional stimuli that left her completely exhausted. The G.P. wrote that "she often sits and daydreams at work for long periods," and the patient wrote that her eye symptom caused her to have "a surrealist, sharp view which is most upsetting" and that she feels "numb and cut off."

There were a number of significant events in her history, but it was extremely difficult to see any intelligible thread in them. She was an only child and remembers violent quarrels with her parents in which she would shout at them and hit them; there is no record of why. At eight she remembers often going and crying on her father's vegetable plot; again she didn't know why. At ten she was sent away from home for six weeks, presumably because the situation at home had become intolerable, and the night before her departure she cut the curtains in her bedroom to pieces with a pair of scissors (on her return her parents had put up new curtains and nothing more was said).

She married her husband after an affair with a much older, married man. She said that her marriage was happy, but when we saw her husband it seemed clear that there was no communication whatsoever on emotional topics. There was a significant incident in which, on learning that her husband had had an accident in which the windscreen of her car had been broken, she threw a chair across the room in a rage. Like her parents, her husband did not react, but merely repaired it.

No precipitating cause for the onset of her eye symptom was found. There was, however, an important more recent incident. Four months ago her mother told her that after a car accident in which her father had been involved, she had discovered that he had been with another woman; and she remarked gleefully to the patient that the other woman wasn't likely to get much out of him since he had been impotent since the patient was eight. The patient's reaction to this was to feel warmer toward her parents because it made them seem more human.

As the reader will see, the story fails to make much sense. By now I have learned to view such stories with considerable distrust, but I had less experience then. We felt we saw in the story at least considerable disturbance in her feelings about men, including anger, starting with her father and continuing with her husband. We decided to explore the possibility of brief therapy in the first place, assigning her to a male therapist and offering her a trial period of six sessions.

If we go through the four main selection criteria listed in chap. 9, we will see that none of them are fulfilled:

1. A *focus* could perhaps be found, but it certainly failed to include any detailed understanding of the events of her history.

2. The patient had not really *responded to any interpretation* based on this focus.

3. As far as *motivation* was concerned, the interviewer wrote that her attitude to treatment was that she left the decisions to other agencies and felt it had little to do with her.

4. As far as *specific dangers* were concerned, we can only say that we hardly knew, and that we did not attempt to get further evidence through projection tests.

Despite what I have implied in connection with motivation and focality in chaps. 5 and 9, that sometimes the only way of testing whether brief therapy is appropriate is to try it, experience has taught me also to distrust trial periods of half a dozen sessions with a potential therapist. Too often this reflects an uncertainty about the patient that really should have led to rejection. If something of the kind is to be carried out, it is far better to have more than one interview with the original interviewer, and/or with the psychologist who gives the projection tests, and to watch further developments in terms of focality, motivation, and response to interpretation. There is then no implied offer of treatment, and if the patient begins to appear to be unsuitable, further investigation can be stopped at any point. One pattern that I have twice recently observed with the trial period is that the patient is in resistance for the first five sessions, and then, under the influence of threatened rejection, suddenly makes important communications in the sixth. The therapist has by now become committed to the patient and finds it difficult to stop, and the two settle for further therapy because they can't face the alternative, and of course the patient then immediately goes into resistance again. In the present case the special significance of the sixth session produced exactly this situation, and something more.

The first five sessions were uneventful but quite encouraging in the sense that the patient considered her problems seriously; and the (male) therapist, though inexperienced, handled her sensitively. Nevertheless, no information emerged that made much more sense of the story, and thus the focus became no clearer. Then three days after the fifth session, the therapist received a letter from which the following is an extract:

> Firstly, when young I found that saying my eyes hurt brought a different response from my parents than, say, stomachache. I even discovered that dwelling on imaginary symptoms gave me a strange lurching sensation in my stomach (looking back, an orgasm?). When I first married I found I could only reach a climax in intercourse if my husband was aware of my rather dim sight. To this end I called upon an old habit of unfocusing my eyes. This was completely in cold blood. I acquired a pair of glasses and became "shortsighted." My husband is not a confirmed Christian and I managed easily to forget my lie. Then I told myself that it would be too dramatic to change back and that it would be just as sinful in reverse. Knowing I mustn't use "eyes" as a comforter, I became more remote, depressed. The sin came home to me when I realized that the

damage was for real. I am still not sure that I am not using the "cure," yourself, eye drops, poor sight, etc., etc., to the same ends although I am giving my visits to you as a sign of my good intentions.

This was both a sign of greatly increased motivation, a crucial communication, and a very disturbed and rather bizarre one. Despite the danger of disturbing the patient further, we felt we had to get more information about her and in the next session the therapist asked her to come for a Rorschach. Parts of the report of the (woman) psychologist read as follows:

> The patient's behavior in the interview was extremely bizarre. She made curious repetitive movements while sitting curled up in her chair, and her statements were accompanied by florid expressions of inappropriate affect. . . Her performance on the test revealed severe disturbance of her thought processes, and on several occasions she appeared to go off into a fantasy world of associations to the blots, seemingly impervious to any intervention from me. The quality of intense anger which came through in her voice in the interview was carried over into her percepts on the test, nearly all of which are of violent, destructive forces, or of damaged objects. Her fear seems to be of engulfment by primitive forces. There were two severe breakdowns in her perceptions on the Rorschach, though she was able to make a reasonable recovery after the first. . . Both interview and test clearly indicate the presence of psychotic processes, and though there are some ego resources, her defenses are at best of a rather tenuous nature.

We were now faced with a patient apparently in an incipient psychotic breakdown, with one session left in which to take a decision, who seemed totally unsuitable for our form of treatment, and who had been lulled into a sufficient sense of security to entrust us with her seemingly psychotic world. The consequences of rejecting her at this point might well have been disastrous for her. Here I remembered a previous published case (Malan and Phillipson, 1957): a patient who under the threat of rejection had given a chaotic and psychotic Rorschach, and who was offered treatment nevertheless, and who had then given a second Rorschach that was much less disturbed and revealed far more of his strengths. We therefore took the decision to offer her a further thirteen sessions, making twenty in all, counting the consultation, and to try to keep therapy on the level of sharing her inner world and studiously avoiding anxiety-provoking interpretations.

This the therapist succeeded in doing. I shall not give an account of the rest of therapy because it is not at all clear to me what really happened in it or what significance it had for the patient. On a number of occasions her communications were somewhat bizarre, but she no longer gave the impression of incipient breakdown.

Before the last session she sent a desperate-sounding letter, writing of panicking at the thought of being abandoned, and giving more rather confused details of the sexual significance of her eye symptoms. In this last session the therapist made a transference interpretation about termination: that talking of her eyes to him must have given her sexual excitement, and that she was depressed at having to give this up. She said she had thought the same. Parting was on a note of great sadness. The therapist said she could get in touch with him if she felt the need.

In fact she did not do so. We now have a three-and-a-half-year follow-up through the G.P., an extremely understanding woman who has given her very considerable support. The patient has never broken down, though she has been depressed and has been treated with tofranil. Her eye symptoms have continued but her life appears to be little affected by them. They continue to need treatment by (milder) eye drops. She has had one child and is now pregnant again. She suffered from severe vomiting during the first pregnancy but seems to have coped with being a mother surprisingly well. She has continued to express artistic creativeness in a very successful way. The marriage continues as before.

Thus, the final result of our clinical mistake was at least not to have caused her harm; and possibly, by accepting her and sharing her secret, we may have given her considerable help.

The fourth example was a calculated risk that ended in disaster.

The patient was a single girl of twenty-nine complaining of depression for eighteen months. This was clearly precipitated by the death of her boyfriend, who had attacked her after a jealous quarrel, had gone into an alcoholic breakdown, and had then died suddenly from a coronary thrombosis.

Her family history was appalling. Her father went bankrupt and became progressively demented, her mother became alcoholic, one brother sounded as if he was schizophrenic, and another brother was withdrawn and schizoid.

She was preoccupied with suicidal thoughts, and indeed originally sought help under pressure from her sister who thought she might actually commit suicide, but when asked she said that she wouldn't do it because of her strong religious feelings.

She was given extended projective testing (four interviews). This seemed to suggest that despite her severe disturbance she had a good deal of strength. She was also able to respond to interpretations about her anger. There was a clear lifelong pattern of self-sacrifice resulting in the neglect of her own needs.

We hoped to be able to start with bringing out her guilt about her fiancé's death, and to go on to link it with the anger underlying her pattern of self-sacrifice.

Therapy did not go according to plan. The recent trauma got left out, and the patient and (male) therapist quickly became involved in her need to regress and be looked after and the impossibility of his meeting this. One of her communications in session 7 was that she "imagined herself deep in a grave," the ominous significance of which was missed by me in supervision. The day after the next session she took an overdose of sleeping tablets and died two days later.

Here the risk of suicide, though obviously considered, was underplayed in our assessment, and we took at face value her own statement (and the opinion of the referring psychiatrist) that she would not actually do it. The important warning sign was, of course, the family history. It should also be noted that the patient lived alone in a bed-sitting room and had little support in her environment.

Therapy itself went wrong. I think the therapist was too strictly analytical in his approach. It might have been possible to be more supportive, to develop a therapeutic alliance, and within that framework for therapist and patient together to look at the feelings behind the recent trauma, thus avoiding the patient's need to regress, with its inevitable dangers.

These four clinical stories thus serve both to underline the importance of our selection criteria and to warn us against any ideas of omnipotence.

PART VI

Conclusion

CHAPTER 17

The Present Position

It remains to consider the overall position of brief psychotherapy and to put the present work into perspective.

This work was originally undertaken at a time of complete chaos in the theory and practice of brief psychotherapy, when all possible opinions could be found, from the most conservative to the most radical, on selection criteria, technique, and outcome. As now becomes clear, this illustrates most pointedly how fallacies arise from clinical impression unsupported by systematic evidence:

Anyone who practices long-term psychotherapy occasionally meets a type of patient who may be described as a "ripe plum," ready for picking, a phrase introduced by Henry Dicks in the early discussions in Balint's workshop. This is often a basically healthy patient suffering from symptoms due to an acute conflict, whose unconscious is very close to the surface, and who responds dramatically to a simple piece of insight that, to an experienced psychotherapist, is utterly obvious. Robert Knight (1937) quotes a typical example: a farmer suffering from weakness of his right arm, which was very clearly a conversion symptom designed to prevent him from being able to express his wish to hit people; and which was relieved almost immediately by what amounted to a single interpretation. In this type of situation, what the therapist sees is the dramatic relief of symptoms. He does not, of course, conduct any systematic follow-up; and if he is a well-trained analyst he assumes that since the deep anxieties have not been worked through, the therapeutic effects can go no further. He then reaches a generalization, expressed quite explicitly in this paper by Knight:

> Short psychotherapy of this kind, based on analytical understanding, is valuable in relatively acute but not too severely sick cases in which quick help is needed and in which more prolonged, orthodox psychoanalysis is inexpedient. It should be understood that such treatment is more or less symptomatic and palliative, tends merely to relieve the distressing symptoms and does not alter to any great extent the underlying personality. It may be, however, that the insight gained by the patient from such psychotherapy may enable him to understand himself better and thus strengthen him against breaking down under the stress of similar situations in the future.

Thus is born the conservative generalization about *selection criteria* and *outcome*; and since this type of therapy usually involves neither the transference nor the roots of neurosis in childhood, there are also born conservative generalizations about *technique*.

This kind of generalization is strengthened by various other situations. The first occurs when a patient breaks off treatment in the early stages with apparently little achieved. Here he may later find that he cannot manage and he then returns and undergoes long-term treatment. These are the patients that we know about and who therefore lead to biased observations. We know nothing about the ones who do not return, and we do not take them into account in drawing conclusions.

Similar considerations apply to another situation, when a patient shows dramatic improvement after a short period of treatment and suggests termination. Long, and quite valid, experience has taught us that this is often (always?) a "flight into health," and it is our duty to convince the patient that he is not well at all and to bring him back into treatment. Here there are three alternatives: (1) We fail in this endeavor and he later relapses and returns; (2) we succeed, and he goes on to long-term treatment; or (3) we fail, and he is never seen again. Once more, our observation is biased because it is patients in the first two circumstances whom we know about, and both of these circumstances involve relapse. Thus is born the generalization that no patient can really get better unless he receives long-term treatment and his deep anxieties are resolved.

A third type of situation arises when the therapist is concerned with short-term therapy in a busy psychotherapeutic clinic. Here a large part of the population of patients may well be those in crisis, and the therapist aims to give the patient as much insight into the crisis as possible and to return him quickly to normal life. The observation is often made that the patient may use this as a point of growth, and thus the quite valid generalization is made that the outcome of such therapy may be permanent personality change; but the *in*valid generalization is then made that these patients in crisis are the only types for whom brief therapy is possible.

A fourth type of situation results from the observation of the use of the orthodox psychoanalytic technique in long-term therapy. Here we employ the standard techniques of interpretation of resistance and transference, and after a time we observe the development of the transference neurosis, and we go on to use this therapeutically in a process that is, of course, uniformly time consuming. We do not observe exceptions to this, and reach the generalization that this is the inevitable consequence of techniques based on psychoanalysis, and a necessary condition to the patient's recovery.

There is in all these situations a single common type of fallacy: The circumstances of our work cause us to observe certain phenomena repeatedly, and we come to believe that these are the only phenomena to occur, without asking ourselves whether there may be hidden unobserved exceptions.

In fact, these exceptions *have* been observed from time to time ever since brief psychoanalytic therapy began; and the more often, the more systematic the investigation has been. Among the more recent authors we need to mention Pumpian-Mindlin (1953), Sifneos, and Wolberg; but really priority must be given to Alexander and French. Anyone who reads their case histories can see the clinical (not, of course, the statistical) evidence for the great majority of what has been written in the present work; to generalize, the use of all the basic psychoanalytic principles, especially interpretation of the transference and transference/parent link, in a radical technique of brief therapy leading to radical outcome.

Why then were their conclusions not immediately accepted? It seems to me that their unconscious must have been involved in the way they presented their findings, because they cannot have consciously intended to convey the impression that they were advocating a universal modification of psychoanalytic technique, rather than simply the flexible application of basic psychoanalytic principles to brief psychotherapy. If anyone wishes to be reminded of the effect of their book on orthodox psychoanalytic opinion, he should read the vituperative review by Ernest Jones in the *International Journal of Psychoanalysis* (1946), where, after an attempt to soften what has gone before, the "return of the repressed" occurs with shattering impact in the last paragraph:

> So far this review may appear to be mainly adverse. Nevertheless we consider the book to be a valuable and useful one. To practitioners having little or no knowledge of psychoanalysis, and perhaps holding a position at a clinic attended by a large variety of patients, it should prove not only valuable but illuminating. Such penetration, skill, and tactfulness in the handling of patients as are here demonstrated will show other workers the advantages of an inspired and highly trained team. Our only criticism is that such a reader would be left in ignorance of the important fact that besides the various methods here described there is such a thing as real psychoanalysis.
>
> The word "unconscious" is not mentioned in the index, nor have we been able to find it in the text itself. Perhaps indeed it is not germane to the content of the book.

(After quoting this passage I was relieved to find that the word "unconscious" does occur in the present book, and I will take care to ensure that it is included in the index.)

Jones's last paragraph is, of course, absurd, because the case histories deal with nothing but the patients' unconscious in an entirely psychoanalytic way.

This passage illustrates very clearly how, although a reader might have taken note of the case histories themselves, he was left with the overall impression of an attack on orthodox psychoanalytic technique. As a result the empirical evidence contained in the case histories was totally overlooked.

The trouble was, of course, that quite apart from Alexander and French's presentation, these radical observations stood in complete contradiction to general clinical experience. The effect on opinion has been—to use correctly, I think, a psychoanalytical term for a defense mechanism—a "splitting" between conservative views and radical evidence that has persisted to the present day.

It needs to be said again and again that the successful use of psychoanalytic methods in brief psychotherapy is a tribute to psychoanalysis, not an attack upon it; especially when, as here, it is shown that the more psychoanalytic the technique, the more successful the therapy. The only unpalatable fact to emerge is that patients may sometimes appear to recover without going through the deepest psychoanalytic processes; but this is an empirical observation as surprising to us as to everyone else, and it has to be faced.

In fact, we were started on the road to these discoveries by chance: We stumbled upon the fearless use of psychoanalytic technique, and the treatment of relatively disturbed patients, the first because of our training, and the second because of the relative rarity of "suitable" cases; and the combination of the two generated a momentum of its own. This in turn generated the desire to find out what really happened to patients under a variety of conditions. We have thus filled in some of the gaps left by relying on clinical impression alone, and—as always when any scientific problem is investigated—some of the results have been quite unexpected.

These results may now be summarized in the form of five major generalizations, from each of which important clinical consequences follow:

The first generalization is that *the capacity for genuine recovery in certain neurotic patients is far greater than has hitherto been believed.*

This has the following important clinical consequence:

Brief interventions of all kinds, from the most conservative to the most radical, can be therapeutically effective, and one of the tasks of the clinician is to determine how radical an intervention is needed in any given case.

The second generalization is that *there exists a type of patient who can benefit radically within the limits of brief psychotherapy from partially working through his nuclear conflict in the transference.*

It is important to note that this type of patient is very different from the "ripe plum" as described by Knight. With the type considered here, the therapist needs to do far more than just give a simple piece of insight in one or two sessions. On the contrary, he needs to use the full range of psychoanalytic technique to face the patient with his conflicts, and then a number of sessions to work them through. This is hard psychoanalytic work, involving such basic principles as the interpretation of resistance, watching for the development of the transference, and perceiving and interpreting the link to childhood.

The third generalization is that *such patients can be recognized in advance through a process of dynamic interaction, which must be allied with clinical experience of the dangers of dynamic psychotherapy.*

The principles of selection embodied in this generalization are the most difficult to convey; but it can be said that such patients are responsive, well motivated, appear to have the strength to face their disturbing feelings and to carry on their own lives independent of therapy; that a circumscribed focus can be formulated; and the many possible dangers of dynamic psychotherapy appear to be avoidable.

The fourth generalization is that, with such patients, within limits, *the more radical the technique in terms of transference, depth of interpretation, and the link to childhood, the more radical are the therapeutic effects.*

The fifth generalization is that *there exist certain more disturbed or more complex patients with whom a carefully chosen partial focus can be therapeutically effective.*

This is the area above all that needs further investigation.

Some of these generalizations are new, some are not, but even those that are not have never been generally accepted. They all amount to an extension of the limits of brief psychotherapy toward the more radical end of the spectrum. Perhaps, therefore, one of our major contributions will have been to support this extension with overwhelming evidence.

When these kinds of intensive brief therapy are added to the full range of methods—including crisis intervention, as enumerated by Sifneos; and to these are added all kinds of marital, family, behavioral, and newer techniques—perhaps brief therapeutic methods may make an important contribution, if not to the overwhelming problem of human mental health, at least to the efficiency of psychotherapeutic clinics.

Finally, at a time when psychoanalytic methods are under attack, and when much research evidence is tending toward the conclusion that therapeutic factors in many different kinds of psychotherapy are common and nonspecific, we appear to have shown on the contrary that the application of specific psychoanalytic techniques leads to radical therapeutic outcomes. This is an observation with far more than purely practical implications, which needs to be taken into account in all theories of the human personality that may be written in years to come.

References

ALEXANDER, F., AND FRENCH, T. M. (1946). *Psychoanalytic therapy*. New York: Ronald Press Co.

AVNET, H. H. (1965). How effective is short-term psychotherapy? In: *Short-term psychotherapy* (Ed., L. R. Wolberg). New York: Grune and Stratton. P. 7.

BALINT, M., ORNSTEIN, P. H., AND BALINT, E. (1972). *Focal psychotherapy*. London: Tavistock. Philadelphia: Lippincott.

BARTEN, H. H. (1971). *Brief therapies*. New York: Behavioral Publications.

BECK, D., AND LAMBELET, L. (1972). Resultate der psychoanalytisch orientierten Kurztherapie bei 30 psychosomatisch Kranken. *Psyche* **26,** 266.

BELLAK, L., AND SMALL, L. (1965). *Emergency therapy and brief psychotherapy*. New York: Grune and Stratton.

BERGIN, A. E., AND STRUPP, H. H. (1972). *Changing frontiers in the science of psychotherapy*. Chicago: Aldine.

BINSTOCK, W. A., SEMRAD, E. V., AND BLOOM, J. D. (1967). The role of brief psychotherapy. In: *Proceedings of the 4th World Congress of Psychiatry, Madrid, 1966, Part I* (ed., J. J. Lopez Ibor). Amsterdam: Excerpta Medica Foundation. P. 424.

CAMPBELL, R. J. (1968). Discussion in STRAKER, M., Brief psychotherapy in an outpatient clinic: Evolution and evaluation. *Amer. J. Psychiat.* **124,** 1225.

CAPLAN, G. (1961). *An approach to community mental health*. New York: Grune and Stratton.

CAPLAN, G. (1964). *Principles of preventive psychiatry*. New York: Basic Books.

COLEMAN, M. D., AND ZWERLING, I. (1959). The psychiatric emergency clinic: a flexible way of meeting community mental health needs. *Amer. J. Psychiat.* **115,** 980.

DEUTSCH, F. (1949). *Applied psychoanalysis*. New York: Grune and Stratton.

EZRIEL, H. (1952). Notes on psychoanalytic group therapy: II Interpretation and research. *Psychiat.* **15,** 119.

FINESINGER, J. E. (1948). Psychiatric interviewing. I. Some principles and procedures in insight therapy. *Amer. J. Psychiat.* **105,** 87.

FOX, R. P. (1972). Post-combat adaptational problems. *Compr. Psychiat.* **13,** 435.

FRENCH, T. M. (1958). *The integration of behavior Vol. III*. The reintegrative process in a psychoanalytic treatment. Chicago: University of Chicago Press.

GILLMAN, R. D. (1965). Brief psychotherapy: a psychoanalytic view. *Amer. J. Psychiat.* **122,** 601.

GOTTSCHALK, L. A., MAYERSON, P., AND GOTTLIEB, A. A. (1967). Prediction and evaluation of outcome in an emergency brief psychotherapy clinic. *J. Nerv. Ment. Dis.* **144**, 77.

GUTHEIL, E. (1945). Psychoanalysis and brief psychotherapy. *J. Clin. Psychopath.* **6**, 207.

HARRIS, M. R., KALIS, B. L., AND FREEMAN, E. H. (1963). Precipitating stress, an approach to brief therapy. *Amer. J. Psychiat.* **17**, 465.

HOCH, P. H. (1965). Short-term versus long-term therapy. In: *Short-term psychotherapy* (ed., L. R. Wolberg). New York: Grune and Stratton. P. 51.

HOLLENDER, M. H. (1964). Selection of patients for definitive forms of psychotherapy. *Arch. Gen. Psychiat.* **10**, 361.

JACOBSON, G. F. (1965). Crisis theory and treatment strategy: some sociocultural and psychodynamic considerations. *J. Nerv. Ment. Dis.* **141**, 209.

JACOBSON, G. F., WILNER, D. M., MORLEY, W. E., SCHNEIDER, S., STRICKLER, M., AND SOMMER, G. J. (1965). The scope and practice of an early-access brief treatment psychiatric center. *Amer. J. Psychiat.* **121**, 1176.

JONES, E. (1946). Review of Alexander, F., and French, T. M., *Psychoanalytic therapy. Int. J. Psychoanal.* **27**, 162.

KALIS, L., HARRIS, M. R., CRESTWOOD, A. R., AND FREEMAN, E. H. (1961). Precipitating stress as a focus in psychotherapy. *Arch. Gen. Psychiat.* **5**, 219.

KAUFMAN, M. R. (1967). Discussant on brief psychotherapy. In: Proceedings of the 4th World Congress of Psychiatry, Madrid, 1966, Part I (ed., J. J. Lopez Ibor). Amsterdam: Excerpta Medica Foundation. P. 461.

KERNBERG, O. F., BURSTEIN, E. D., COYNE, L., APPELBAUM, A., HORWITZ, L., AND VOTH, H. (1972). Psychotherapy and psychoanalysis. Final report of the Menninger Foundation's Psychotherapy Research Project. *Bull. Menninger Clinic* **36**, 3.

KESSELMAN, H. (1970). *Psicoterapia breve.* Buenos Aires: Ediciones Kargieman.

KLUWER, R. (1970). Uber die Orientierungsfunktion eines Fokus bei der psychoanalytischen Kurztherapie. *Psyche* **24**, 739.

KLÜWER, R. (1971). Erfahrungen mit der psychoanalytischen Fokaltherapie. *Psyche* **25**, 932.

KNIGHT, R. P. (1937). Application of psychoanalytic concepts in psychotherapy. Bull. Menninger Clinic **1**, 99.

LEVENE, H., BREGER, L., AND PATTERSON, V. (1972). A training and research program in brief psychotherapy. *Amer. J. Psychother.* **26**, 90.

LINDEMANN, E. (1944). Symptomatology and management of acute grief. *Amer. J. Psychiat.* **101**, 141.

LUBORSKY, L. (1962). Clinicians' judgments of mental health. *Arch. Gen. Psychiat.* **7**, 407.

MALAN, D. H. (1959). On assessing the results of psychotherapy. *Brit. J. Med. Psychol.* **32**, 86.

MALAN, D. H. (1963). *A study of brief psychotherapy.* New York: Plenum Press.

MALAN, D. H. (1975). Psycho-analytic brief psychotherapy and scientific method. In: *Issues and approaches in the psychological therapies* (ed., D. Bannister). London: Wiley. P. 201.

MALAN, D. H. (1976). Toward the Validation of Dynamic Psychotherapy. New York: Plenum Press.

MALAN, D. H., BACAL, H. A., HEATH, E. S., AND BALFOUR, F. H. G. (1968). A study of psychodynamic changes in untreated neurotic patients. I. Improvements that are questionable on dynamic criteria. *Brit. J. Psychiat.* **114**, 525.

MALAN, D. H., BALFOUR, F. H. G., HOOD, V. G., AND SHOOTER, A. M. N. (1976). A long-term follow-up study of group psychotherapy. *Arch. Gen. Psychiat.* (in press).

MALAN, D. H., HEATH, E. S., BACAL, H. A., AND BALFOUR, F. H. G. (1975). Psychodynamic changes in untreated neurotic patients. II. Apparently genuine improvements. *Arch. Gen. Psychiat.* **32,** 110.

MALAN, D. H., AND PHILLIPSON, H. (1957). The psychodynamics of diagnostic procedures. *Brit. J. Med. Psychol.* **30,** 92.

MANN, J. (1969). The specific limitation of time in psychotherapy. *Seminars in Psychiatry* **1,** 375.

MANN, J. (1973). *Time-limited psychotherapy.* Cambridge, Mass.: Harvard University Press.

McGUIRE, M. T. (1965). The process of short-term insight psychotherapy. *J. Nerv. Ment. Dis.* **141,** 83.

McGUIRE, M. T. (1968). The instruction nature of short-term insight psychotherapy. *Amer. J. Psychother.* **22,** 218.

MENNINGER, K. (1958). *Theory of psychoanalytic technique.* New York: Basic Books.

MORLEY, W. E. (1965). Treatment of the patient in crisis. *Western Medicine* **3,** 77.

MURPHY, W. F. (1958). A comparison of psychoanalysis with dynamic psychotherapies. *J. Nerv. Ment. Dis.* **126,** 441.

ORNSTEIN, P. H., AND ORNSTEIN, A. O. (1972). Focal psychotherapy: its potential impact on psychotherapeutic practice in medicine. *Psychiatry in Medicine* **3,** 311.

PARAD H. J. (1965). *Crisis intervention: selected readings.* New York: Family Service Association of America.

PHILLIPSON, H. (1955). The object relations technique. London: Tavistock Publications. Glencoe, Illinois: The Free Press.

PUMPIAN-MINDLIN, E. (1953). Considerations in the selection of patients for short-term therapy. *Amer. J. Psychother.* **7,** 641.

SCHOENBERG, B., AND CARR, A. C. (1963). An investigation of criteria for brief psychotherapy of neurodermatitis. *Psychosom. Med.* **25,** 253.

SEITZ, P. F. D. (1953). Dynamically oriented brief psychotherapy in psycho-cutaneous excoriation syndromes. *Psychosom. Med.* **15,** 200.

SEMRAD, E. V., BINSTOCK, W. A., AND WHITE, B. (1966). Brief psychotherapy. *Amer. J. Psychother.* **20,** 576.

SIFNEOS, P. E. (1958). Phobic patient with dyspnea: short-term psychotherapy. *American Practitioner and Digest of Treatment* **9,** 947.

SIFNEOS, P. E. (1965). Seven years' experience with short-term dynamic psychotherapy. In: *Selected Lectures,* 6th International Congress of Psychotherapy, London, 1964. New York: S. Karger.

SIFNEOS, P. E. (1966). Psychoanalytically oriented short-term dynamic or anxiety-provoking psychotherapy for mild obsessional neuroses. *Psychiat. Quart.* **40,** 271.

SIFNEOS, P. E. (1967). Two different kinds of psychotherapy of short duration. *Amer. J. Psychiat.* **123,** 1069.

SIFNEOS, P. E. (1968a). The motivational process: A selection and prognostic criterion for psychotherapy of short duration. *Psychiat. Quart.* **42,** 271.

SIFNEOS, P. E. (1968b). Learning to solve emotional problems: a controlled study of short-term anxiety-provoking psychotherapy. In: *The role of learning in psychotherapy: a Ciba Foundation Symposium* (ed., R. Porter). London: Churchill. P. 87.

SIFNEOS, P. E. (1972). *Short-term psychotherapy and emotional crisis.* Cambridge, Mass.: Harvard University Press.

SIFNEOS, P. E. (1973). An overview of a psychiatric clinic population. Amer. J. Psychiat. **130,** 1033.

SPEERS, R. W. (1962). Brief psychotherapy with college women. *Amer. J. Orthopsychiat.* **32,** 434.

STEWART, H. (1972). Six-months, fixed-term, once-weekly psychotherapy: A report on 20 cases with follow-ups. *Brit. J. Psychiat.* **121,** 425.

STRAKER, M. (1968). Brief psychotherapy in an outpatient clinic: evolution and evaluation. *Amer. J. Psychiat.* **124,** 1219.

STRUPP, H. H. (1975). Psychoanalysis, "focal psychotherapy" and the nature of the psychotherapeutic influence. *Arch. Gen. Psychiat.* **32,** 127.

SWARTZ, J. (1971). Time-limited brief psychotherapy. In: Barten, H. H., *Brief Therapies.* New York: Behavioral Publications. P. 108. Also in *Seminars in Psychiatry* **1,** 380 (1969).

TOMPKINS, H. J. (1966). Short-term therapy of the neuroses. In: *Psychoneurosis and schizophrenia,* (ed., G. L. Usdin). Philadelphia: Lippincott.

USDIN, G. L., ed. (1966). *Psychoneurosis and schizophrenia.* Philadelphia: Lippincott.

WHITTINGTON, H. G. (1962). Experience in a college psychiatric clinic. *Psychiat. Quart.* **36,** 503.

WOLBERG, L. R., ed. (1965a). *Short-term psychotherapy.* New York: Grune and Stratton.

WOLBERG, L. R. (1965b). Methodology in short-term psychotherapy. *Amer. J. Psychiat.* **122,** 135.

WRIGHT, K., GABRIEL, E., AND HAIMOWITZ, N. (1961). Time-limited psychotherapy: advantages, problems, outcomes. *Psychol. Rep.* **9,** 187.

Index